HYPNOTHERAPEUTIC
TECHNIQUES 2E

HYPNOTHERAPEUTIC
TECHNIQUES 2E

ARREED BARABASZ AND JOHN G. WATKINS

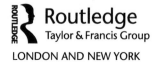

Routledge
Taylor & Francis Group

LONDON AND NEW YORK

First published 2005 by
Brunner-Routledge

Published 2014 by
Routledge
711 Third Avenue,
New York, NY 10017

Published in Great Britain by
Routledge
2 Park Square, Milton Park,
Abingdon, Oxfordshire
OX14 4RN

First issued in paperback 2014

Routledge is an imprint of the Taylor and Francis Group, an informa business

Copyright © 2005 by Taylor & Francis Books, Inc.

Transferred to Digital Printing 2006

Library of Congress Cataloging-in-Publication Data

Barabasz, Arreed F.

Hypnotherapeutic techniques / Arreed Barabasz, John G. Watkins.-- 2nd ed.

p. cm.

Includes bibliographical references and index.

ISBN 978-0-415-93581-4 (hbk)
ISBN 978-1-138-87274-5 (pbk)

1. Hypnotism--Therapeutic use--Handbooks, manuals, etc. I. Watkins, John G. (John Goodrich), 1913- II. Title.

RC495.B337 2004

615.8'512--dc22

2004019944

To Helen Hunt Watkins

Who, like a concert artist, knew how to wield the science
of clinical practice for the betterment of human beings.
And to her colleagues, students, and patients, who will
completely understand the message she wrote:
"All that we have been in life
will live on in the quality of other lives
that we have touched significantly,
and in that way, we are reborn
again, and again, and again."

Preface

Unlike the majority of other treatment modalities and adjuncts to therapy, hypnosis has been around for a very long time. Now, more than half a century of science has demonstrated that hypnosis is one of the most versatile and useful of health care tools for physical and mental health. Clinical hypnosis is securely grounded in an enormous foundation of careful empirical work that substantiates its efficacy under a variety of circumstances (for a recent review, see Lynn, Kirsch, Barabasz, Cardena, & Patterson, 2000; Patterson & Jensen, 2003). Franklin and Lavoisier described science as "disciplined wonderment" in their royal commission report to the king of France on mesmerism (Franklin et al., 1784). This notion is as relevant now as it was 220 years ago. The efficacy of hypnosis is recognized by the National Institutes of Health (*Journal of the American Medical Association*, 1996). The American Medical Association officially approved the clinical use of hypnosis in 1958, and the American Psychological Association approved it in 1960. The two major hypnosis societies, the Society for Clinical and Experimental Hypnosis and the American Society of Clinical Hypnosis, hold memberships in both the American Association for the Advancement of Science and the World Federation for Mental Health.

An increasing number of rigorously controlled studies are showing hypnosis is not just effective but also superior to a number of standard treatment procedures. For example, Lang and her colleagues (Lang et al., 2000; see also A. Barabasz & M. Barabasz, 2000) found hypnosis to have significantly more pronounced effects on pain and anxiety reduction for invasive medical procedures in contrast to structured attention or even intravenous analgesia. The effects are not limited to adult populations. In a comparison of hypnosis and distraction in severely ill children undergoing painful medical procedures, J. Smith, Barabasz, and Barabasz (1996) studied an ethnically diverse sample of children suffering from cancer or blood disorders. Measures of pain and anxiety were obtained from the children and their parents, as well as independent raters. Hypnotizable children (the majority) showed significantly lowered pain, anxiety, and distress scores in response to hypnosis in contrast to low hypnotizable children, and hypnosis was superior to standard pain amelioration interventions. Perhaps of greater interest to the majority of practicing psychologists is the effectiveness of hypnosis as an adjunct to psychotherapy. J. Watkins and Watkins (1997, pp. 162–194) summarized the effectiveness of ego-state therapy and hypnoanalysis. Both procedures were found to be superior to psychodynamic therapies in general. Those using cognitive-behavioral therapies will no doubt be impressed by the comprehensive meta-analysis of hypnosis as an adjunct (Kirsch, Montgomery, & Sapirstein, 1995). The analysis was performed on 18 studies in which cognitive-behavioral therapy was compared with the same therapy supplemented by hypnosis. The results indicated that the addition of hypnosis substantially enhanced treatment outcome, so the average client receiving cognitive-behavioral hypnotherapy showed greater improvement than at least 70% of the clients receiving nonhypnotic treatment. They are particularly striking because of the few procedural differences between the hypnotic and nonhypnotic treatments.

Hypnosis is cost effective. As medical costs continue to soar, new opportunities for those trained in hypnosis are on the horizon. Until recently, the authors of numerous reports have merely alluded to the cost-effectiveness of hypnotic interventions. Recently, a major Harvard Medical School study (Lang & Rosen, 2002) showed findings that are astonishing to those untrained in hypnosis. The average cost associated with standard sedation for a range of outpatient procedures was $638, compared with $300 for sedation with adjunctive hypnosis. The addition of hypnosis resulted in a savings of $338 per case. Hypnosis was shown to reduce outpatient room time, but hypnosis remained more cost effective even if it added as much as an additional 58 minutes to room time. One can only speculate about the cost-effectiveness produced by the greater improvement, an average of 70%, shown with hypnosis by the Kirsch et al. (1995) meta-analysis based on cognitive-behavioral therapies but, similar to the Lang and Rosen (2002) findings, A. Barabasz and Barabasz (2000) demonstrated significantly increased clinical effectiveness and a reduction in treatment time by nearly 50% when hypnosis was added to specific biofeedback treatment interventions.

Therapists who practice approaches (such as psychoanalysis) that require several sessions per week over many months or even years are faced with a severe economic crisis (Goldberg, 1996). Insurance companies, and other third-party payers, will simply not fund such lengthy treatments. Hypnoanalysis, based on psychodynamic theories (Brown & Fromm, 1987; Lavoie, 1990; J. Watkins, 1992, substantially reduces treatment time to as little as 60 to 150 hours. Similar magnitudes of efficiency are achieved with hypnosis in structural and developmental hypnoanalytic treatment of severely disturbed patients (Baker, 1990; Brown & Fromm, 1987; Copeland, 1986). More recently, J. Watkins and Watkins (1997, pp. 162–194) demonstrated that intensive ego-state therapy (an extension of hypnoanalysis) might offer an effective and even briefer approach. On the basis of 15 years of case data, they concluded that therapy of as little as 12 hours often achieves permanent, structural personality changes, including resolution of lifelong disorders.

Although treatment efficacy and cost-efficiency are primary considerations, there is yet another important overlay that makes the study of hypnosis all the more critical at this time. The United States is currently undergoing demographic changes that are entirely without precedent in its history. In 1960, only 16 million Americans did not trace their ancestors to Europe. Today, the number is in excess of 80 million. No nation has ever undergone as rapid and radical a transformation. Immigration to the United States is the largest population transfer in history. People are coming from Asia, Africa, and Latin America. Embracement of cultural diversity in the United States has put an end to the "melting pot," a concept made famous by Israel Zangwill, the Russian-Jewish playwright, in his famous 1908 play of the same name. Diversity in the United States now is a salad rather than an acculturating melting pot. Virtually all psychotherapeutic modalities currently practiced today in the United States, Canada, Europe, Australia, and New Zealand are Western-culture bound. In contrast, hypnosis is multicultural in nature, with experimental and clinical research published in more than a dozen scientific journals worldwide. Hypnosis is the only therapeutic modality that is yet scientifically supported on the basis of Western science that makes it possible, for example, for a psychologist skilled in hypnosis to be accepted simultaneously by Native American healers and those from Eastern cultures. As employment opportunities for both clinical and counseling psychologists continue to shift toward hospital or outpatient medical settings, multicultural adaptability is already becoming increasingly important. The time has come to look seriously at the integration of hypnosis in Ph.D. training. In recognition of this need, the APA Committee on Divisions of APA Relations has provided a grant specifically for "the integration of hypnosis training in Ph.D. programs" led by APA's Division 30 (Society for Psychological Hypnosis), Division 45 (Multi-Cultural), and Division 17 (Counseling Psychology, 2002–2003).

The present book, developed from J. Watkins's (1987) classic text, updates and expands the earlier work. It is specifically intended to meet the current and emerging needs of a university graduate program to train psychologists and medical practitioners in the use of hypnosis. Unlike many other therapeutic modalities, it is still often difficult to get training in hypnotherapy. The majority of top medical schools offer training in hypnosis, but lagging behind are graduate schools of psychology and counseling psychology, where just a minority regularly offers courses in hypnosis. The major scientific societies in the field, the Society for Clinical and Experimental Hypnosis, the American Society of Clinical Hypnosis, and the Society of Psychological Hypnosis (Division 30 of the APA), do offer workshops, up to about three days in length, at their annual meetings and during the year at various centers about the country. These are usually "cram courses" where the beginner is immersed for a very short time in a strange and baffling field that is frequently foreign to his or her previous experience. Fascinating to be sure, but with demands upon his or her own personality and its defenses, that immersion may provoke anxiety. The skilled surgeon, calm and collected in the face of observable physical pathology, may practice his or her skills with high concentration and equanimity. Yet the same person confronted with apparently magical happenings for which he or she has no apparently tangible objective rationale, quails and avoids as if asked to stay in a haunted house. On the other hand, the objective scientific researcher who has dealt with concrete, observable behaviors as variables, and who can trace intricacies of behaviors with the aid of complex designs and mathematical analyses, often wishes to avoid a modality that lends itself to objective formulations only with the greatest of difficulty and complexity.

Of the cognitive, sociocognitive, or behavioral theories available today, none can adequately account for the esoteric phenomena induced by hypnotic trance. There are few competent instructors in this field. Many university graduate schools, as well as many medical schools, still do not have even a single faculty member who is properly prepared to offer regular courses in this discipline. Furthermore, there is a tremendous ignorance on the part of many physicians and psychologists concerning hypnotic phenomena, which is manifested by suspicion and distrust of workers in the field. Despite substantial scientific evidence to the contrary, a number of psychologists confuse the effects of hypnosis with those that can be wrought with suggestion and misconstrue its effects on pain relief as nothing more than the effects of relaxation-suggestion. Some psychoanalysts

continue to parrot objections to hypnotherapy based on unverified theoretical positions voiced by Freud and his associates nearly a century ago.
Accordingly, it is no wonder that so few professionals are skilled in the use
of hypnosis as a treatment modality. The bottleneck seems to be that skill
in hypnotherapy is limited to a few psychotherapists as compared with
many practitioners who have mastered other approaches for dealing with
mental and physical disorders.

In light of the previously mentioned information, and the recognition
of hypnosis as a legitimate scientific and treatment modality by the American Association for the Advancement of Science and the World Federation
of Mental Health, as well as the American Medical Association and APA, it
is clear that hypnosis should be taught along with other accepted methods
of treatment in medical schools and graduate programs in psychology.
Even for those psychology graduate programs that limit their emphasis to
only cognitive-behavioral treatments, dramatic enhancement of outcomes
by the addition of hypnosis (Kirsch et al., 1995) clearly indicates that training in hypnosis should be included routinely as part of these emphases.

Despite the plethora of articles and reference works on hypnosis currently available today, not one of these seems to have been specifically
designed as a teaching textbook. The topics, although often well discussed,
are not arranged in the same systematic way that one would expect a general textbook in physiology or zoology would be arranged. Units of
instruction should be outlined with consideration of the typical three- to
five-credit-hour course for an academic semester or quarter. Lecture and
discussion need be interspersed with practicum experiences that gradually
initiate the new student into the various hypnotic phenomena and the
techniques for eliciting them. Presentations must range hierarchically
from simple to more complex. Theories of hypnosis, often thrown at the
reader in great profusion, should be simplified and directly related to hypnotic experiences. The history of hypnosis needs to be presented in a way
that allows the newcomer to identify with the struggles and difficulties
pioneers had when investigating these phenomena, developing their treatment techniques, and dealing with hostile opposition from colleagues. For
indeed the history of hypnosis is one of repetition. One worker after
another has gone through the same sequence of skepticism, observation,
conviction, overzealousness, effort to maintain scientific respectability,
and problems of explaining his or her approaches to associates and the
public. The history of any field, and especially of hypnosis, ought to be
presented in such a way that the newcomer can identify with the stream of
its development, its heroes, and its innovators. In such training, the newcomer can experience the same changes of perception and understanding

that characterize the professional careers of our predecessors. Students will pass through the initial amazement the same way their instructor did. Whether this turns them on to the field or scares them off will depend on whether the initiation is systematic and stepwise, permitting them to cognitively master new experiences, integrate them into their previous professional background, and develop confidence in the skills of hypnotic induction and therapy. Such skills are essential yet are too frequently superficially learned by those involved only in university-based research in hypnosis.

For decades, we have taught hypnosis to hundreds of psychologists, physicians, dentists, and psychiatrists, as well as to other psychotherapists. Several of them became quite proficient in the modality. Dozens are now distinguished clinical and experimental contributors to the field. But sadly, many left the courses, the workshops, or the institutes in which the instruction was given, interested and fascinated, promising themselves they would really learn to use these techniques but finding themselves many years later using only nonhypnotic procedures. Somehow, their early anxieties, personal blocks, and difficulty in obtaining supervision and mentorship in the field were never overcome.

Many of us who have served as teachers of hypnosis have met former students who report that they enjoyed the course, gained a great deal in understanding their client's personalities, improved their doctor-patient relationships, and developed a greater comprehension of the role of psychogenic factors in causing mental and physical dysfunction. But they then state, "I always intended to practice hypnosis, but I never felt entirely at ease with it." If a student has not started using hypnosis within a month or two after completing a course, he or she often never employs it. Much is lost in the teaching of this modality, because only a minority of those who take workshops have become active users of hypnosis in therapy or researchers of the phenomenon.

Here at Washington State University at Pullman, a four-credit-hour course in clinical and experimental hypnosis has been a regular yearly part of graduate training for counseling psychologists for the past 20 years. In the year 2000, an advanced course in hypnosis and psychotherapy was added and is offered biannually. Students enrolled in the Washington State University APA-accredited PhD program in counseling psychology may begin their use of hypnosis at the university counseling center in practicum experiences in their second practicum year, where nearly all of supervising faculty are experienced and trained in hypnosis. At the University of Montana at Missoula, a course in hypnotherapy has been a regular part of doctoral training in the APA-accredited clinical psychology program for more than 30 years. Teaching in both programs involves demonstrations in class that are continually integrated with lectures and discussion. Audiovisual media also are used. In spite of all this, we found that only about a third of our students were actively using hypnosis in their practices 2 or 3 years later. Students begged for additional supervised training with actual patients, and accordingly an advanced hypnotherapy team was established in the Clinical Psychology Center at the University of Montana for those who had completed the course. At the Washington State University counseling center, a workshop is offered every few years for licensed psychologists. Findings show that initial courses, however well organized, can whet the professional appetite of practitioners and generate research interests for many students. But if these students are to profit from advanced seminars, they need much more actual experience in using hypnosis. In our training, students serve as subjects and as therapists. They work with screened volunteer subjects of known hypnotizability, and they study the literature and relate it first to their experiences in hypnotizing subjects and later to their understanding of clinical cases. Only in this way do they seem to acquire the confidence that permits them to employ hypnosis regularly as a continuous technique in their therapeutic armamentarium.

It is from considering this background that we determined that a teaching text in hypnotherapy was needed that would address specifically the problems of teaching and learning and the personal needs of students wrestling with this as a new modality. This book is, accordingly, designed with a focus on the professor and his or her students. It aims to include that which can be learned, and no more, within a typical academic semester. Given reasonable mastery of this text, a broader background, familiarization with a wider variety of techniques, acquaintance with the many nuances of theoretical controversy, and polished finesse in the practice of hypnotic skills will come later with greater ease.

After having acquired certain basic procedures, having thoroughly convinced themselves of the potential effectiveness that hypnosis can demonstrate in the treatment situation, knowing at least a number of clinical problems within their practices that are amenable to hypnotic approaches, and having mastered the initial awe to the point where they feel some confidence in their hypnotic abilities, clinicians can then develop further through individualized reading of the literature plus attendance at scientific meetings and legitimate workshops. This book, therefore, is dedicated to getting students over the initial hurdles and furnishing the starting impetus necessary to make them into functioning practitioners in the field of hypnosis. One must subsequently develop skills if one is to be an artist, a master of the discipline, and more than a journeyman practitioner.

Many of the books written in this field are written from the standpoint of the writer's attempt to pour his or her experience, and wisdom, into the student—the "big jug and little mugs" theory of education. We also have written earlier books, book chapters, and articles in this field that were presented from that point of view—that of the instructor.

In this book, we are attempting to handle the task before us a bit differently. A theory of the therapeutic relationship presented in an earlier work (J. Watkins, 1978) posited two viewpoints from which we may view another person: the objective and the resonant. When we are objective we observe the actions of a patient from an outside vantage point, much as one might look at a specimen under a microscope. The other is an "it," not ourselves, and our responsibility for "its" actions are minimal. But if we temporarily identify with the other, perceive the world as if through his or her eyes—even view our own self as he or she might—then we are resonating.

This might be viewed as a large step beyond, but certainly in the same direction as, empathy. Resonance is that process by which the individual (therapist) attempts to replicate within himself or herself a close facsimile of another's experiential world. It is approaching a problem from the inner perspective of the other rather than from that of our own. The practice of resonance can be as valuable in the field of education as in therapy. The teacher whose presentations are developed from the viewpoint of the student struggling to master the material should be more effective than the professor who simply "doles it out" and places on the student the burden of mastery. Insofar as it is possible, we shall try to incorporate the resonant point of view in writing this book. This means that when designing each unit we shall try to think not "What is it we wish to tell the students? What should they learn?"; rather, we will endeavor to continually ask ourselves the question, "If I were a new student what would I want to know, what help would I need to master both my own insecurities in this new modality and the techniques necessary to use it skillfully?" Whenever possible, we will assume the student's frame of reference and write the material accordingly. To help ensure a student's perspective, Ciara Clear Christensen, a student naive with respect to hypnosis at the beginning of the preparation of this volume, read and discussed each chapter with the first author as the text was written. Questions such as "Sounds great but what does this mean?" or "Why say it that way?" were addressed. We also owe her a great debt of gratitude for her dedication and weekends of work in typing endless hours of dictation, proofreading, and serving as the subject for photographs in this volume.

The chapter on Hypnosis and Sport Performance was contributed by Erik Dunlap, a Ph.D. student of Arreed Barabasz, who brings his background as a former offensive lineman on the Duke University football team to the subject.

The second author's theories of psychotherapy (J. Watkins, 1963, 1967, 1978; J. Watkins & Watkins, 1982, 1997) emphasize a balance between objectivity and resonance. Therapy is only a kind of education or reeducation, often at unconscious levels. But a good therapist is a good teacher. Here we are not trying to treat problems of a student but trying to inculcate techniques, manners, and approaches effective in the treatment situation.

If this approach can be effectively used in teaching hypnotherapy, then perhaps a beneficial spin-off will also occur. We learn by modeling. Those of us who are psychotherapists often copied manners and skills from the master, the professor or the analyst with whom we studied. In the same way the clinical instructor relates to his or her students, the students will relate to their students—their patients. Manners are contagious, so perhaps the manner of presenting our material may prove of benefit, first, objectively, as the student learns, practices, and masters the necessary skills, and, second, through resonance, as he or she incorporates some of the indirect manners of bringing about the phenomena of hypnosis both with and without a formal induction, use of hypnotic suggestions, and interpretation that might be transmitted by the written and the spoken word. We believe that although the use of hypnosis in therapy may be learned as a science, it is practiced as an art.

Every science-based discipline has its own unique language. Psychoanalysts talk in "psychoanalese." Behavior modifiers write in "behaviorese" terms, and cognitive therapists are forever reframing. Without wishing to offend the psychologist, the psychiatrist, or other professionals, the terminology in the present book is intended to be as clear and simple as possible. When we use technical or professional terms, we do not assume that the student understands them. Because the physician, psychiatrist, psychologist, psychoanalyst, and dentist each have a unique vocabulary, we try to couch the language here in terms that are easily understandable to the broadest range of graduate students. We explain and illustrate specialized terms. Repetition will not harm the sophisticated reader; failure to explain may leave the professional from another discipline confused.

Explanations should be concrete, illustrations and case examples frequent, and specific wordings presented. For example, how often have you read a good psychoanalytic case presentation where the following statement was made: "At this point I interpreted his negative transference"? And how often have you wondered, "Yes, you did. But just what did you say? Exactly what were the words you used, and why did you choose those specifically? Why did you decide to interpret the negative transference at this time? What specific reactions did your patient show to your interpretation—in his or her next remark, his or her behavior during the rest of the session, in the hours and days that followed?" The statement "At this point I interpreted his or her negative transference" may have satisfied the writer. It was objective, but it was not resonant because it did not meet the needs of the student to understand. It did not answer the questions that were on the reader's mind, and it did not develop learning so that the reader would know just how to interpret the negative transference of a patient when required. This is why the present book is made as concrete and specific as possible. We use pictures and diagrams, and we note audio-visual examples that have been made available, because these may be a further aid in the learning process. Study questions and practicum exercises are designed to develop the stages of learning and to maximize retention of factual knowledge and acquisition of technical skill. As much as possible, we present verbatim induction techniques and case materials, together with explanatory notes.

Hypnotherapy must be learned and practiced as a meaningful discipline, not as a collection of scientific facts or as a cookbook of recipes for handling various clinical problems. Elements must not be learned in isolation from one another but be integrated as the whole of understanding that should emerge within the student. As in other professional treatment disciplines, the hypnotherapist should become a clinician, not a technician.

The study of hypnosis usually makes a clinician a better psychologist or physician (or other) and makes him or her a more understanding student of human nature. Perhaps nowhere in the behavioral sciences does the interplay of psychological cause and effect show more clearly than in the psychodynamic movements revealed by hypnosis. Whatever has been one's skepticism about the reality of unconscious processes, no other experience, unless it is that of intensive psychoanalysis, is so convincing as to the reality of covert interactions within the human psyche.

The orientation is psychodynamic and eclectic in this treatise. That is, it is psychoanalytic to the extent that it accepts the existence of unconscious behavior, considers that it is mediated within psychodynamic mechanisms (such as projection, identification, displacement, rationalization, etc.), and takes the point of view that these interactions play significant roles in the etiology of pathological symptoms and maladaptive behavior. However, because many contributions to the treatment of clinical problems have stemmed from the recent investigations of the cognitive behaviorists and have been incorporated in the technology of cognitive-behavior therapy, this work also is eclectic. It is our opinion that some clinical problems are most adequately and efficiently approached from a psychoanalytic point of view whereas others are best approached from the perspective of either behavioral or cognitive-behavioral therapy. Furthermore, the significant, broad and long-range goals targeted by the humanistic-existential therapists, such as the development of meaningfulness, authenticity, and spontaneity in the self, often are required if other than temporary relief is to be granted to many of our patients.

Obviously, this book is not meant to be "purist." Instead, it draws from several alternative theoretical conceptualizations and skills that, practiced within the hypnotic modality, promise maximal therapeutic effectiveness. We include information relating to the major scientific societies and how to affiliate with them. They are key to an individual's continued growth as a clinician who uses hypnosis in his or her practice or research. They furnish continuing education for the initiate and for the expert in the field. There are legitimate national and international societies concerned with research and practice in hypnosis and with ethical codes governing its use. Unfortunately, certain other organizations with lowered professional and ethical standards attract those whose power and exhibitionistic needs exceed their professional sense of responsibility for the amelioration of mankind's ills.

The content of this volume is sufficient for a semester course in graduate school or medical school, or for an intensive introductory workshop. It provides a background history of hypnosis, the phenomena of hypnosis, theories of hypnosis, hypnotizability testing, and, most important, details of hypnotic inductions and deepening techniques. Throughout, the intention of our emphases is to make it possible for students to learn how to induce actual hypnosis in the subjects that they work with to make possible responses that can go well beyond the comparatively weak effects that can be obtained by role playing, expectancy, context, or suggestion without inducing a true state of hypnosis. Students will learn powerful techniques that make it possible to use hypnosis to go beyond the effects that might be wrought by social influence. Recent and rigorously controlled experimental studies show us that hypnosis is clearly much more than social influence or a simple response to suggestion. However, this text recognizes that the use of hypnosis in the treatment of our patients will probably always involve a complex interplay of actual trance induced states and sociocognitive factors. We draw on both domains to maximize the participants' ability to achieve a true hypnotic state that can be substantiated by neural substrates.

Worldwide, the number of clinical and experimental studies being currently published on hypnosis has become exponential. Accordingly, the bibliography of references included can in no way be exhaustive. It is not intended to be. Many excellent books and articles must, of necessity, be excluded. However, we have tried to refer to many of the most significant works, and the serious student will wish to read further in this vast literature.

For those readers who are just starting their acquaintance with clinical hypnosis, welcome aboard and bon voyage. We guarantee an exciting and challenging experience. For those of you who are already working in the field, you know what we mean by the fascination of probing deeper into the mysteries of human psychological and physical experience.

We, the authors of this treatise, are a generation apart. However, it came as no surprise to either of us that as little boys we were both thrilled by tales of exploration. In our very early teens we were both contributing to science. The first author's observations of the aurora borealis were accepted as part of the extension of the International Geophysical Year Studies, while the second author's observations of variable stars were accepted by the Society for the Study of Variable Stars. Alas, we have both mused with sadness that we will probably not be privileged to walk on the surface of the moon or gaze through a porthole window as the terrain of an unknown planet unfolds beneath us. But as this book teaches you how to use hypnosis, perhaps you too, like many of us who began its study earlier, will experience the same intriguing sense of wonder as you see the amazing phenomena that it continually reveals within "inner space," the universe of behavior and experience that constitutes the "self" of every person. Enjoy the adventure and resources that true hypnosis, like no other modality, affords your patients and research participants.

—A.F.B. and J.G.W.

Table of Contents

Chapter 1
The History of Hypnosis and Its Relevance to Present-Day Psychotherapy

Perhaps the earliest recorded description of hypnoanesthesia comes from Genesis 2:21–22: "And the Lord caused a deep sleep to fall upon Adam, and he slept; and He took one of his ribs, and closed up the flesh instead thereof. And the rib, which the Lord God had taken from man, made He a woman."

Now, just imagine that you, as a doctor who has devoted your life to the study of human illness, have discovered a totally awesome new healing principle. You have happened, by good luck, on a new approach that seems to have miraculous results in relieving pain and curing many conditions that have defied the best efforts of your country's most distinguished practitioners. You have watched hundreds of sufferers lose their pains, throw away their crutches, and resume normal living after being invalids for years. As to the effects of your new technique, there can be no doubt.

Furthermore, to account for this therapeutic power, you have developed a theory that is related to what is known scientifically about the operations of natural law. Your waiting room is besieged by patients from near and far. Your reputation as a great healer is established throughout the land. Only one cloud shadows your satisfaction: Your colleagues refuse to listen to you, learn your procedures, and verify them on their own patients. How would you feel? What would you do?

Perhaps in your eagerness to share this great discovery with the rest of the world and to be scientifically recognized for your contribution, you would welcome an official hearing. Let some highly respected members of the medical and scientific societies investigate your practice and see your therapeutic achievements firsthand. Their skepticism will be erased. They can announce to your colleagues and to the rest of the world the truth about your great discovery. Suppose that finally the government appoints such a commission, consisting of several of the most respected names in science. This group visits your treatment office. They study your charts, observe your therapeutic procedures, and interview your patients. Now you surely will be vindicated. Their long-awaited report is finally published. You are devastated. They ignored the concrete examples of your healing. They paid little attention to the reports of your many patients who attest to their cures. They only criticized the theory by which you attempted to explain your therapeutic achievements, and then said that any reported results must be due to "imagination." How would you feel now? Could you carry on being scorned by colleagues and patients alike? Or would you, like Franz Anton Mesmer, leave the country in disgrace, filled with shame and bitterness?

The Discoveries of Mesmer

Mesmer, born in 1734, secured a degree in medicine in 1766. In tune with the times, his doctoral thesis, *De Planetarum Influsu*, attempted to relate changes in human functioning to gravitational and other forces in the surrounding universe. After all, if the position of the moon could so move the oceans of the world, would not such powerful forces also have significant impact on the operations of living organisms, especially humans?

Mesmer was a brilliant man of great imagination. His interests were indeed broad. A musician himself, he was a friend of Mozart, Gluck, and Haydn. Vienna of that day was a city in which the arts blossomed as much as the sciences. But Mesmer was equally a scientist and physician, and as such had been made a member of the Bavarian Academy of Science.

The mid-eighteenth century was a time of great ferment. The impetus for new advances, which two centuries before in the Renaissance had broken the frozen grip of medievalism and stimulated a new flowering in all the arts, especially in Italy, that now swept on into the realms of natural science. Newton, Galileo, Copernicus, Kepler, and others had made significant breakthroughs in understanding the universe and its laws. Gravity, chemical reactions, electricity, and magnetism were being discovered as great natural forces, energies that were soon to be harnessed and enormously increase man's standard of living. The Western world was on the verge of an industrial revolution. And speaking of revolutions, explosive social forces were at work that would soon sweep through the United States and Europe. Monarchies tottered before the increasing clamor of the many common people demanding their rights for liberty, equality, and fraternity.

It was in such a world that Mesmer learned from the Royal Astronomer in Vienna, a priest named Maxmilian Hell, the principle of the magnet. If one would hold a bit of magnetized metal before the eyes of an individual, he or she would become transfixed. Moving and acting as if in another realm, the subject was especially susceptible to healing suggestions that could be administered at that time. His or her pains could be made to leave. Many other complaints could also be banished under the spell of the magnet.

However, Mesmer soon made a most puzzling discovery. A priest named Gassner had been practicing a form of healing much like magnetism, which involved passes of the hands without the use of metal magnets. Mesmer observed Father Gassner's work and found that he himself could also accomplish the same results merely by placing his hand near his patients even without holding a piece of magnetized metal. How could this be? It had been established that a magnet has about it a field that influences other pieces of metal, and when held close to patients it obviously influenced them too, because pain and other symptoms were relinquished. There must be something of the same energy in the hand of the doctor. Therefore, this great healing power apparently was not limited to metals; it could also be found in bodily tissues. So Mesmer coined the term "animal magnetism" to represent a universal force that might account for the healing achieved by "the laying on of hands."

How normal, how natural it was that a brilliant thinker with the searching mind of Mesmer could arrive at such an explanation. Yet here we see an example of what has often occurred in science where, through faulty reasoning, an invalid theory is formulated even though based on apparently sound observational data. Accordingly, Mesmer established his clinical practice on a concept that several years later was invalidated by scientists who were more careful and rigorous in their experimental controls.

Mesmer was not the last to advocate the theory of a fluid, magnetic energy to account for healing effects. A century and a half later, a brilliant, creative psychoanalyst, Wilhelm Reich (1945), formulated theories about the concept of the "orgone," a life energy that could be concentrated in a box and focused back on the human body with healing results. He also treated patients according to his theory and was jailed for refusing to obey a desist ruling of the Federal Food and Drug Administration in the United

States. He died in jail, but perhaps his idea, even now, has not been put finally to rest. Recent "Kirlian" photographs (Krippner & Rubin, 1973) have shown that there is an "aura" of radiation about plant and animal tissue and alterations in it are correlated with healing effects. Maybe, just maybe, Mesmer and Reich were not entirely wrong.

Mesmer's Controversial Case of "Restored" Sight

Maria Theresa Paradis, a young singer and pianist, had been blind since the age of 3 years. The best physicians had not been able to restore her sight. She was brought to Mesmer, who developed a strong interest in her case. With her parents' consent, he took her into his home and treated her. Although a number of prominent physicians had diagnosed her condition as due to destruction of the optic nerve, there was considerable evidence that the blindness might be hysterical.

Maria had performed before Empress Maria Theresa who, being favorably impressed with the girl, had provided for her education and granted her parents a pension. At first, the treatment seemed to be successful, and the girl apparently was able to see again. However, the case created consternation within the conservative medical profession of Vienna. If Mesmer really had such powers, the other doctors might lose their patients to him.

Several influential physicians were able to convince Marie's parents that her cure was not genuine, and they suggested that if she was no longer thought to be blind, the parents might lose the pension. As a result, she was removed by her parents from Mesmer's care and returned to her home, after which her blindness returned.

Here we see an experience from history that is so frequently repeated today, one that society prefers to ignore but that complicates enormously the task of the healing arts practitioner; namely, attempting to treat a patient who has more to gain by remaining ill. Huge malpractice suits are won; workman's compensation, disability payments, and the pensions of neurotically ill veterans are awarded to those who can successfully establish and retain symptoms in the face of treatment, psychological or physiological. To his great chagrin, Mesmer learned about secondary gains and reinforcements in the maintenance of illness long before the investigations of such factors by scientist-practitioner psychologists. This case example also serves to warn us that the first therapeutic question is not how we should treat the patient but whether the patient should be treated at all.

Mesmer's Fascinating Theory of Disease

Mesmer held that because the human body was composed of the same elements as those that made up the universe, it should be subject to the same laws that govern other bits of matter, including the planets. The body, too, should be influenced by light, heat, electricity, and changes in gravitation and even by influences from celestial space. He believed that the two halves of the human body acted in relation to each other like two poles of a magnet and that physiological processes were disrupted when there was a lack of harmony because of the improper distribution of magnetism.

Animal magnetism was viewed as a kind of fluid that could penetrate all matter, that could be concentrated and reflected, and that could be invested by the human will into various parts of the body. Mesmer believed that he could direct this magnetic fluid through his presence, the passes of his hands, the waving of a metallic rod, and contact with the baquet.

The baquet was a large wooden tub about a foot high, which he had constructed within his clinic. It was filled with bits of metal, bottles systematically arranged in concentric rings, broken pieces of glass, and water. It was large enough to allow a number of patients to sit around it. From its upper lid there projected several iron rods. This baquet was supposed to concentrate the magnetism (like a kind of eighteenth-century cyclotron) that could then be transferred by patients to their afflicted members through rubbing against the rods. Being a musician (and undoubtedly somewhat of a showman) Mesmer felt that the experience would be enhanced if the clinic room was darkened and music was playing while he, in a long flowing purple robe, passed among his patients, rubbing their bodies from time to time with his metal rod.

Because patients were expected to go into crises (hysterical seizures) when the concentration of "magnetism" became sufficiently great, it is not surprising that every so often one would writhe and fall into a "fit," thus further impressing the others as to the potency of the treatment. When the number of patients seeking Mesmer's help exceeded the capacity of his clinic, he would magnetize a tree in a nearby park by stroking it. People could then stand around it, basking in its "magnetism" and occasionally going into crises.

Despite all of this apparent foolishness, Gravitz (2004), as a remarkable historian of hypnosis, brought to our attention that Mesmer also recognized that his own belief in animal magnetism was a crucial element and that it "must in the first place be transmitted through feeling" (Mesmer, 1781, p. 25). At some level then, Mesmer understood the criticality of what we speak of when we emphasize the importance of resonance as a key element in helping to bring about the state of hypnosis as an instrument of therapeutic change. Indeed, it would seem that Mesmer had an awareness of key aspects of transference. Although he had no concept of issues of libidinal regression, he was a century ahead of Freud's recognition that the hypnotic state was created from transferential phenomena: "the key to an understanding of hypnotic suggestion" (S. Freud, 1910, p. 51). A complete discussion is cogently presented by Gravitz (2004).

Mesmer's Reception by Colleagues

The same suspicion and criticism by medical colleagues that plagued him in Vienna continued in Paris, and the greater his successes, the greater became the hostility of the other doctors. In 1784, because of the conflicting claims, King Louis XVI appointed a distinguished commission, whose members were suggested by the French Academy of Science, to investigate Mesmer's practice. It is most interesting to note who was included among its members. There was doughty old Benjamin Franklin, who had discovered the relation of lightning to electricity with his kite. At that time, he was the American ambassador to France. There was Lavoisier, the first to isolate the element of oxygen. There was Jussieu, an eminent botanist, and finally (not without symbolic significance for the future of Mesmer's practice) there was the inventor of that device for amputating the head — Dr. Antoine Guillotine (we might also blame him for starting the whole mind–body separation notion that persisted until just a decade ago).

Mesmer's therapeutic zeal was exceeded only by his tendency for exaggeration, his lack of caution in theoretical generalization, and his arrogance, a trait not uncommon in many good therapists today. The commission was soon able, through simple but well controlled experiments, to conclude that the changes in the symptoms of Mesmer's patients could not have occurred through the action of a hypothesized magnetic field. Their report stated flatly that there was no such thing as animal magnetism and that, because it did not exist, reported cures could be only the result of fraud or imagination. Rejected by colleagues and patients alike, Mesmer left Paris, and, after some wandering, settled in Switzerland near Lake Constance, on whose shores he had been born 50 years before. There he spent the rest of his days, unnoticed and unheralded.

How often do individuals who are beaten by the forces of life return to the scenes of their childhood? How often do they simplify their existence, relinquish challenges to competitors, and cease efforts to make further advances? We see it every day in many of our patients. We call it regression. Mesmer's star burst forth like a brilliant nova in the development of psychological treatment, but within a few short years it had returned almost to oblivion. Although personally discredited, broken, and embittered, he left a legacy of findings and questions that have ever since fruitfully stimulated humans' quest for more knowledge about themselves. Mesmer reached to become God; he ended up very much human. Such strivings for power have often been the nemesis of practitioners of hypnosis, who, dazzled by the apparently unbelievable effects they achieve through the hypnotic modality, reactivate their own infantile yearnings for omnipotence. They sometimes lose their raison d'être as practitioners of the healing arts, as servants to men, and seek to use their newfound skills to become masters of humankind. The history of hypnosis has many lessons to teach the would-be hypnotist, and history tends to repeat itself.

The development of modern hypnosis is considered to have started with Mesmer. However, the use of hypnosis in treating human ills is probably as old as the history of medicine. There is evidence that most hypnotic phenomena were known to ancient man. Eighteen hundred years before Christ, hypnosis was apparently practiced in China. The Old Testament Hebrews employed the trance state in the making of prophecies. And the Druids would put suspects into a "sleep" to induce them to tell the truth. In the fourth-century B.C., temple cults developed in Greece (during which an induced sleep was combined with other forms of suggestion for the treatment of illness). Through the dances of whirling dervishes, the ancient Egyptians induced states of trance and ecstasy, during which hypnotic analgesia could be achieved. It would appear that many of these early inductions were successful in establishing true hypnotic trance effects, well beyond what is labeled "hypnosis" by some today. As we reveal in the theories and techniques foci of this text, a number of practitioners and even researchers today seem content to settle for nothing more than the social influence or suggestion and relaxation effects that accompany some insufficient hypnotic inductions. Although these effects can be used to the benefit of our patients, far more can be accomplished with true hypnotic trance, which can now be identified by reliable and rather robust physiological markers of hypnosis (see chapter 3, "Theorizing About Hypnosis").

Mass hypnosis may largely account for the rage of tarantella dancing that swept through Europe during the late Middle Ages. Hundreds of people were seized by the fury, and they gyrated in wild abandon until they collapsed in a state of exhaustion. In India and Tibet, more passive forms of hypnotic meditation were developed that have continued today in the exercises of the Yogis and various forms of Buddhism. Many Indian tribes in the United States used the trance for purposes of medical treatment, making it possible today for psychologists and medical practitioners who are skilled in hypnosis to be accepted by tribal healers. G. Williams (1968) presented a more detailed and documented account of the various hypnotic practices among early peoples. It is sufficient here to note that hypnosis (although called many different names) has been known for many centuries by both primitive and civilized humankind and was employed to treat ills in every part of the world long before it became a serious object of scientific inquiry.

The Development of Hypnosis After Mesmer

Let us now return to trace the history of this interesting phenomenon during more recent years. One of Mesmer's students, the Count Maxime de Puysegur, is credited with being the first to discover the phenomenon of somnambulism, wherein the hypnotized individual can walk, talk, and engage in many activities, yet still remain in a trance state. After Mesmer, a number of people continued to practice in the field, calling themselves magnetists or mesmerists. Some of these, such as de Puysegur, while employing Mesmer's therapeutic techniques, were not convinced that the phenomena were due to an invisible magnetic fluid. They approached close to the more psychological etiologies that are now held. (In 1821, in France, Récamier reported a painless surgery accomplished on a "magnetized" patient.)

Although practice of animal magnetism became almost extinct in France following the discrediting of Mesmer, workers in Germany, especially during the 1840s, continued to employ it. Their efforts were apparently aimed at gaining respectable medical and scientific acceptance, and, in fact, in 1818 the Berlin Academy of Science offered a prize for the best thesis on the phenomena. However, little more was done to bring new discoveries to the field, and none of these men left enduring marks on its development. Sporadic attempts were also made by disciples of Mesmer in France to reactivate interest. They were able to induce the French Academy of Medicine on several occasions during the early 1800s to appoint a commission to examine the therapeutic claims of magnetism. The results were usually inconclusive, and it was not until many years after Mesmer's death in 1815 that renewed study of the phenomenon awakened attention.

Perhaps this illustrates the repetitive nature of the history of hypnosis that has occurred again and again up until the present. Each episode started as a reputable physician or scientist observed hypnotic demonstrations by another worker. The physician's incredulity changed to belief and enthusiasm. These techniques were adopted in their practice and valiant efforts were made to convince professional colleagues. Students and disciples flocked around, and his or her center became a beehive of practice and investigation. The physician would frequently become overly arrogant and pretentious in his or her therapeutic claims, thus antagonizing more conservative scientific colleagues who then tried to discredit the findings. Overenthusiastic followers attempted to treat all conditions, both organic and functional, with hypnotic techniques. Similar to a borderline patient, they made their leader a god. Inevitably they became disillusioned, and interest in the field died down, only to be revived again similarly by a new messiah.

A critical psychiatrist once remarked, "Hypnosis has been tried and abandoned by the human race many times. Why should we study it now?" To which the only appropriate reply is, "No matter how many times hypnosis has been abandoned, people keep coming back to it." Apparently, its efficacy kept rising to the surface well before present-day research and the National Institutes of Health found hypnosis to be officially efficacious.

Not only has the cycle of skepticism, discovery, application, and overenthusiasm leading to abandonment characterized different times and the physicians of different countries; it is a typical experience today by the newcomer who is taking his or her first course or workshop in the field. In fact, you who are now reading this may go through these same stages. You undertake a course in hypnosis because of curiosity or the recommendation of a colleague. Initially you have many doubts and reservations about its reality or potency. You observe the induction of a number of individuals taken into a trance state and learn how to do it yourself. You watch demonstrations of deep trance phenomena, such as pain control, regression, perceptual distortions, and hallucinations. You are astounded. Why had you not been taught these marvelous powers before? Here you have the "magic bullet" that medicine has always sought to cure human ills. You enthusiastically apply the procedures to your own practice with varying degrees of success. If you now seek perfection and omnipotence, sooner or later you will be disappointed. Many of you will forsake the field, as did most of Mesmer's followers. First stage is skepticism. Second stage is overenthusiasm. But if you can persevere through to the third stage, you may reach the point where you recognize that hypnosis is not the magic wand, that it cannot cure all conditions, that it has limits, and that it does not always work. You will then perceive it as simply another useful technique in your therapeutic armamentarium that can often help in the successful treatment of many sufferers. You will find that with this tool you can at times do some things you could not otherwise accomplish, or at least not without a much greater expenditure of time and effort. You are then no longer merely a hypnotist. You are a mature member, along with many others, of the healing arts professions who knows how to use this modality as an adjunct to other aspects of your training for the benefit of your patients. These are a few of the lessons that the study of scientific hypnosis teaches us.

It is 1837 in England, and history is about to be repeated. John Elliotson (1843), a very attractive and brilliant physician, has just observed demonstrations by Monsieur Depotet, a visiting French mesmerist. Elliotson was known for his tremendous energy, his willingness to experiment with new concepts, and his unorthodoxy. He had been the first physician in England to use a stethoscope (curiously, the motivation for the invention of the stethoscope came from the physicians' restraint in placing their ears on the chest of a more than frequently filthy patient). He had translated Blumenbach's *Physiology*, a major text of the day. He had many other original contributions to his credit. He had discovered the value of such drugs as potassium iodide and prussic acid in the treatment of various conditions. Moreover, he was first professor of the Practice of Medicine in London University and president of the Royal Medical and Chirurigical Society.

Obviously, such an inventive and innovative man would be fascinated with the phenomenon of hypnosis. He began practicing and writing about it. He and his students published a journal, the *Zoist*, devoted to the reporting of cases treated by mesmerism. He immediately incurred the anger and scorn of his medical colleagues and was singled out especially for attack by the editor of *Lancet*, the medical journal. Elliotson believed in the magnetic theories of Mesmer and was inveigled into an experiment where he intended to demonstrate that a silver coin (because it contained magnetism) would induce the trance state, whereas a lead coin would fail. Unfortunately, one of his opponents switched coins. The subject was hypnotized by the lead coin, hence responding to Elliotson's words and not to the "magnetized" coin.

Elliotson was bitterly attacked. He continued his work against all opposition, but he was denied the pages of the medical journals and forced to resign his post on the staff of the University Hospital. He was especially noted for his treatment of children, with whose sufferings he could so well identify. Ridiculed, despised, and abused, he died in 1868, vainly attempting to interest his medical colleagues in the practice of mesmerism and to regain his scientific respectability.

Times are better now for clinicians and researchers interested in hypnosis. Courses in the modality are offered in many medical schools and in graduate departments of psychology and counseling psychology. One can specialize in this area and retain professional acceptance. But even yet, the shades of reactionary ignorance linger on. If you return to your hospital or clinic and practice what is taught in this book, do not expect to be automatically received by your more conservative colleagues with open arms. And if you are an academic professor of psychology, your department might indicate it would prefer that you study such respectable areas as learning theory, motivation, or perception. Yet my (A.F.B.) own appointment at Harvard Medical School and early promotion to associate professor was made possible only because of my work in hypnosis. The similar acceptance and career rewards have come to many of my former PhD students who rapidly became chiefs of their psychological services units or repeated winners of major National Institutes of Health grants for research. The second author's (J.G.W.) stellar lifelong career features appearances on national TV (*60 Minutes*, etc.), and his international reputation of fame as the "Father of Ego-State Therapy" is unquestionably due to his work in hypnosis.

Now, the time is 1845 and the place is Calcutta, India. A skilled surgeon by the name of James Esdaile (1957) has been conducting dozens of operations using mesmerism as his anesthesia. He induces profound trance states in his patients and during a period of 7 years has performed more than 2,000 painless operations. Some 300 of these would be classed as major surgery. They involved amputations, removal of scrotal tumors, cataracts, and so on.

At first, Esdaile attracted favorable attention, especially from the deputy governor of the State of Bengal. Through his auspices, Esdaile was given a hospital devoted to mesmeric practice. He even succeeded in convincing a number of prominent physicians of the validity of his work. However, when he returned to Scotland in 1852, he too was the recipient of the rejection that had been hurled at Elliotson. In Calcutta, hypnoanesthesia was for the first time practiced on a grand scale. True, scattered operations had been reported earlier in the United States, England, France, and Germany, but no one had before employed mesmerism for the wholesale relief of pain in hundreds of surgical cases, and no one has employed it so extensively since that time. Ether and chloroform were discovered. The more general applicability of chemoanesthesias, coupled with the unreliability of the mesmeric trance and the greater skill required for its use, soon settled the matter. However, at least one finding of Esdaile's has not been challenged to this day and is deserving of much further research. Although a high proportion of surgical cases died in surgery (or shortly afterward) of shock, almost none of those whose operations were conducted under mesmerism did so. This favorable ratio held even when compared with the ratio of successful surgeries conducted under chemical anesthesias.

One other great contributor of the day came from the English-speaking world. James Braid (1843) was a Scottish ophthalmologist. In November 1841, he visited the demonstration of La Fontaine, a French magnetist. Initially skeptical, he denounced the first séance. But he stayed, continued his observations, and changed his mind. Within a year, he presented a paper, which was rejected, to the Medical Section of the British Association in Manchester.

Braid received attacks, not only from the medical profession but also from the clergy with whom he got into a controversy as to whether the effects of mesmerism were due to the influence of "Satanic agency." Braid could not accept the magnetic theories of Mesmer. He was the first to insist that the phenomenon was psychological in nature and due to suggestion administered while the patient was in a unique state. Extrapolating on the work of Faria (1819) who coined the term *sommeil lucide* (lucid sleep) as an alternative to the animal magnetism explanation of the behaviors elicited by Mesmer, Braid saw a neurological basis and termed it "neuro-hypnotism," or nervous sleep. Soon he referred to it as simply "hypnotism" and the one who practiced it as a "hypnotist." Braid derived the word from the Greek term that means sleep. However, hypnosis is not sleep at all. As Herbert Spiegel (1998) pointed out, both sleep and hypnosis involve a contraction of outside awareness. But it goes in opposite directions: in sleep it dissolves, in hypnosis it intensifies.

Braid did not suffer as much from the darts of jealous colleagues as did Mesmer and Elliotson. But then he was not a man who was driven to seek prestige as much as the others were, nor was he as argumentative in his claims. His career leaves us with a constructive thought. He who returns from his first acquaintance with hypnosis to trumpet enthusiastic claims for its superiority as a therapeutic modality can expect the mobilized opposition of his colleagues. Resistance is not engendered nearly as much when assertions of its value are tempered.

Interest in magnetism reached the United States during the 1830s and 1840s and a number of operations under trance were reported, facilitating an active society of mesmerists in New Orleans in 1845. Phineas Quimby practiced hypnosis in the United States, but he is not as well known as his most celebrated pupil, Mary Baker Eddy, who founded Christian Science. Although the latter method of healing greatly resembles hypnotic interventions, its founder and followers, contrary to controlled research showing that hypnotic phenomena are present in eye movement desensitization and reprocessing therapy (R. Alexander, 1997), insist that it has nothing to do with hypnosis (see Janet, 1919/1925).

Almost a half-century after the death of Mesmer, the focus of hypnotic practice returned to France. In 1864, Ambroise-August Liebeault, a poor man's doctor, settled in Nancy after finishing his medical degree in 1850 at the University of Strasbourg. After reading a book on mesmerism during his medical studies, he had been successful in hypnotizing several subjects. However, it was not until 1860 that he began to practice the modality seriously.

Liebeault was a simple and modest man. To induce his French peasant patients to submit to hypnotic treatment (because they were accustomed to drugs and physical manipulations), he offered to treat them free with hypnosis while charging for the more traditional therapies. By offering such free treatment he, unknowingly, was testing the effects of hypnosis versus those of expectancy. During the late 1900s, expectancy was thought by those of the sociocognitive perspective (Kirsch, 1990; Kirsch & Council, 1989) to account for much if not all of what could be wrought by hypnosis. Such notions, originally refuted by the therapeutic results produced by Liebeault more than 100 years ago, are only now being brought to requestioning (A. Barabasz, 2001b; Russell & Barabasz, 2001). Liebeault acquired much respect among the poor people of the area and is pictured as a great humanitarian, interested in the welfare of others regardless of recompense to himself. Bramwell (1956, p. 57) described a typical incident that he observed in Liebeault's clinic:

> Two little girls, about six or seven years of age, no doubt brought in the first instance by friends, walked in and sat down on a sofa behind the doctor. He, stopping for a moment in his work, made a pass in the direction of one of them, and said; "Sleep, my little kitten," repeated the same for the other, and in an instant they were both asleep. He rapidly gave them their dose of hypnotic suggestions and then evidently forgot all about them. In about twenty minutes one awoke and, wishing to go, essayed by shaking and pulling to awaken her companion, her amused expression of face when she failed to do so being very comic. In about five minutes more the second one awoke, and, hand in hand, they trotted laughingly away.

Liebeault believed that the phenomena were psychological in nature, and he completely discarded the magnetic theories. After 2 years of hard work he published a book titled *Du Sommeil et des Etats Analogues, Considères Surtout au Point du Veu de l'Action de la Morale sur le Physique* (On Sleep and Related States, Considered Especially from the Point of View of the Action of the Mind on the Body). Perhaps initially the most unsuccessful book ever published, only one copy of the book (Liebeault, 1866) was sold then. He continued treating as the poor man's doctor, unknown, for some 20 more years, when great recognition belatedly came his way.

Liebeault practiced actually and figuratively on "the wrong side of the tracks." On the other side lay the great University of Nancy, and at its medical school resided an eminent doctor, Hippolyte Bernheim, professor of neurology. Liebeault was successful in treating a patient who for many years had resisted Bernheim's therapeutic efforts, and the eminent professor decided to pay a visit to Liebeault. Highly skeptical at first, Bernheim might have felt that he was carrying out this investigation for the purpose of exposing a quack.

However, if he came to jeer, he stayed to cheer. Liebeault's work interested him greatly, and he became one of the country doctor's best friends. In 1886, he published his own textbook, *Suggestive Therapeutics* (see Bernheim, 1964), describing the techniques and giving due credit to Liebeault. After that, visitors from far and near flocked to Nancy to observe and study with Liebeault and Bernheim. Even though now famous and although many purchased his book, Liebeault preferred to treat the poor for little or no fees, and he apparently never profited financially from his newfound status. He and Bernheim developed what came to be known as the Nancy School, a center for hypnotic practice and instruction that emphasized the concept of suggestion and taught that hypnosis was a psychological phenomenon, not a magnetic one.

Another school developed to the north in Paris under the leadership of the distinguished neurologist Jean Martin Charcot (1889). Charcot, who practiced at the Salpetrière Hospital, opposed the views of the Nancy group. He mistakenly believed that hypnotic phenomena were pathological and found only in hysterical people. Although he was aware of the factor of hypnotic suggestion and of psychological influence, he still tried to revive interest in the old magnetic theories (see Figure 1.1).

Liebeault and Bernheim were soon drawn into a controversy with Charcot and a number of joint experiments were set up to test the relative claims of each. The views of the Nancy group prevailed, and magnetic theories of hypnotism were no longer seriously voiced after that time.

Pierre Janet (1919/1925) studied with both Bernheim and Charcot and was a prolific practitioner of the hypnotic art. He considered it a form of dissociation and likened hypnosis to hysteria. He reported an interesting case of a young woman who suffered from anorexia and a glove anesthesia (see p. 246 of this volume) over most of her body. She would eat only while under a state of hypnosis. Once, while Janet was absent from the clinic, he left her under hypnosis so she could be fed. In the hypnotic state, she appeared so normal that when her family came to visit that day they concluded she was cured and took her home. After a week or two, the hypnosis wore off, and her symptoms returned. She was hypnotized by Janet again and sent home once more. During the next 8 years, she was placed back in hypnosis and sent home every few weeks. She died of tuberculosis, apparently having spent 8 years without any further problems caused by anorexia. Janet was aware of unconscious processes and wrote about them.

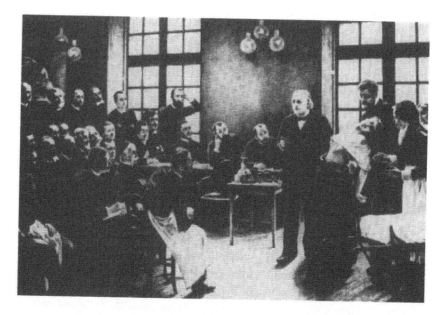

Fig. 1.1 A demonstration of hypnosis by Jean Martin Charcot. *A Clinical Lecture at the Salpetrière.* A. Brouillet's painting shows Charcot at the height of his fame, demonstrating a case of *grande hysterie* to an elite audience of physicians and writers; behind him is his favorite disciple, Babinski. The painter has involuntarily shown Charcot's fatal error: his verbal explanations and the picture on the wall suggest to the patient the crisis that she is beginning to enact; two nurses are ready to sustain her when she falls on the stretcher, where she will display her full-fledged crisis. (Le Salon de 1887, Paris, facing page 62).

However, because it was Freud who described these processes in more detail, Janet was not given the credit for discovering them.

Up to this time, hypnosis had been used as a general therapeutic method for attacking all types of symptoms, whether organic or psychogenic in nature. Hypnoanesthesia and the relief of pain were its most common uses. Also, until this time, most practitioners considered psychiatric illness to be, if not simply malingering, organically caused. Even Charcot subscribed largely to this point of view. But now the time was ripe for the discovery that many disorders were psychologically, not physiologically, caused, and hypnosis was to play an important role in the vanguard of these advances.

Josef Breuer was a general-practice physician in Vienna, highly respected and also a teacher of medicine, although not a professor. He was conservative in nature and given to much equivocation and doubt in pursuing a remarkable discovery he had made. Hypnosis had been used primarily to suppress or eliminate symptoms. Thus, Bernheim and Liebeault would hypnotize their patients and instruct them to relinquish their illnesses. Often this was effective; often it was not. Breuer used "suggestive hypnosis" to treat a young woman known as Anna O., who suffered from a hysterical disorder. He was not successful in relieving her symptoms at first. However, when he induced her to "abreact" or relive early traumatic situations in her life in which she remembered (reconstructed memory may or may not be accurate; see A. Barabasz, 2001a) and expressed feelings, the symptoms left. Breuer and Freud were close friends. In fact, Breuer helped Freud financially during his early medical studies, which enabled Freud to get married. Both men had studied with Dr. Ernst Bruecke, a psychiatrist who espoused a strong physical–chemical approach to the understanding of mental disorders. Freud was most intrigued with Breuer's abreactive method, but he received no encouragement from Charcot when he described it to this teacher, and Bruecke was most violently opposed to hypnosis, which he regarded as rank charlatanism. Accordingly, although Freud had observed Breuer's work as early as 1882, he did not take up the practice of hypnotism until 1887.

Freud's experience with hypnosis brought him to the discovery of unconscious processes and provided the great breakthrough in psychiatric thinking that was to dominate this discipline for the next half century (Breuer & Freud, 1957). However, for a number of reasons he relinquished his use of this technique. In the first place, he was not a very good hypnotist. He was unable to induce a deep state in many of his cases. This might have been due to the fact that Freud, a brilliant, impatient young genius, was not sensitive in interpersonal relationships. Not unlike some noted hypnosis researchers today, he was not sufficiently patient to involve himself in the induction process long enough to secure a profound hypnotic state. Furthermore, Breuer, the modest old conservative, was quite embarrassed when Anna O. developed strong love feelings for him because of the treatment. This caused him to break off his therapeutic relationship with her. Freud was similarly embarrassed when a female patient threw her arms about him. He had not at that time discovered the meaning of transference and did not know how to deal with such manifestations. Also, many patients who relinquished their symptoms under hypnotic abreaction would reinstate them again, and Freud despaired of achieving permanent results by this modality (see J. Watkins, 2001, and J. Watkins & H. Watkins, 1997, for new hypnotic abreactive techniques that minimize this problem).

At any rate, Freud developed a much slower and less effective method of cathartic release by pressing his hand on the patient's forehead and asking the patient to freely associate, that is, tell everything that came to mind. As we see later, this might have actually constituted the induction of a light hypnotic state, but the material that emerged was less emotionally laden. As Freud was better able to handle and understand this, he was able to study the process more logically and with less emotional distraction. Perhaps this was best for the development of psychoanalysis because it brought to therapy a slower and more rational approach.

Unfortunately, Freud masked his own inadequacies at working within the hypnotic relationship by maintaining that psychoanalysis began only with his discarding the hypnotic method and introducing that of free association. The daughter (psychoanalysis) rejected its mother (hypnosis), and it was the parent that was regarded as illegitimate during the next few decades. Most of the objections that Freud raised about hypnosis, such as that its results were temporary and that it "bypassed the ego," have since been disproved by investigators in the field.

It should be noted also (see Kline, 1958) that when Freud practiced psychoanalysis, he was content to listen passively to the associations of his patients, but when he used hypnosis, his own manner of treatment changed. He became the authoritarian and commanded the symptoms to disappear. In fact, he said that he became bored with the monotonous arbitrary prohibitions used in treatment by hypnosis. Whether Freud's different therapeutic manner when he used hypnosis compared with when he was psychoanalyzing was because of his having been taught that hypnosis was an authoritative approach involving command and entreaty or whether something within his own counter-transference needs was stimulated by the hypnotic relationship, we will probably never know. Hypnosis gives the hypnotist the illusion of great power, and many a modest man has been seduced by power into becoming a tyrant. At least it does teach us that therapeutic hypnosis is much more than an altered state of consciousness achieved by manipulations of the operator. In the treatment situation, it is a sensitive mode of communication, and its effective use is subject to the quality of the interpersonal relationship between hypnotherapist and patient. There is little doubt now that Freud's failure with hypnosis was largely due to his personality rather than to an inherent weakness in the modality. It is a pity that this point seems unknown by the majority of analytic psychotherapists. But the aura of Freud, the great master of psychoanalysis, remains and still keeps many of his disciples from learning to recognize that his prejudices withheld from the psychoanalytic field a most fruitful technique that can uncover repressed material, assist in its ego integration, and frequently produce permanent results in a much shorter time than can free association.

In spite of his rejection of hypnosis, Freud could never quite abandon it completely. Time and again, he would toy with the idea, although he personally could not bring himself to reexamine his position and use it again on his patients. In 1919, he wrote, "Hypnotic influence might find a place in it [psychoanalysis] again." He also stated that practical psychoanalysis might constitute an alloy of "the pure gold of analysis" with the "copper of direct suggestion" meaning hypnosis (S. Freud, 1900–1953, p. 402).

The days of the 1890s were a boom time for hypnotic practitioners. Everybody hypnotized everybody for every known disorder. Carcinomas, brain tumors, viral diseases, and so forth were subjected to hypnotic suggestion, of course with a high number of failures. Doctors who wished for omnipotence and thought that they had arrived there became disillusioned. Then, with the rising interest in psychoanalysis among physicians, hypnosis fell once more into disuse. Only a few isolated practitioners and lay entertainers continued to employ the modality.

A Harvard psychiatrist, Morton Prince (1906), investigated multiple or dissociated personalities by hypnosis and, in World War I, Simmel in Germany and Hadfield in England employed it to treat war neuroses. Simmel (1944) developed a modified abreactive technique in which his German soldier-patients were induced to release their angers by tearing to pieces under hypnosis a dummy wearing a French uniform. Hadfield integrated hypnosis with psychoanalytic techniques and was probably the first to coin the term *hypnoanalysis.*

Modern Hypnosis

In 1933, Clark Hull, a distinguished experimental psychologist, published the first book that presented controlled research investigations on hypnotic phenomena. He and his associates looked into such matters as the relation of postural sway to hypnotizability, age differences in hypnotizability, the relation of hypnotizability to general intelligence, the ability of individuals under hypnosis to transcend normal motor and sensory abilities, and so forth. These were the first carefully controlled investigations. Up to that time, nearly all data about hypnosis had been secured from clinical observations on patients. Such reports had inherent in them the subjectivity and biases that are characteristic of case studies. Hull was the first to map out hypnosis as a legitimate field of study by modern experimental science.

The world of academia proved to be just as conservative as the province of medicine, and Hull was the recipient of much criticism by other psychologists, who regarded hypnosis as within the field of magic and not science. Hull's pioneering studies did much to break down academic prejudice against investigators in this area, because his own scientific credentials were impeccable. He was widely renowned as a researcher and theorist in the field of learning, and in 1936 served as president of the American Psychological Association (APA). Hull and his students were a powerful influence in making hypnosis respectable among experimental scientists, just as Bernheim and Charcot had been in relation to the medical profession.

During the 1930s, another boost to physicians and psychotherapists came in the form of a flood of innovative papers emerging from the pen of Milton H. Erickson (see Haley, 1967). This psychiatrist experimented with a wide variety of ingenious techniques for inducing hypnosis and eliminating symptoms. He became a master in the art of using language to communicate with his patients at unconscious levels. Erickson did not subscribe to the psychoanalytic goals of achieving insight into the causes of neurotic disorders. Rather, he would bypass resistances and make his patient's defenses untenable, thereby forcing a relinquishment of symptoms. As first president of the American Society for Clinical Hypnosis, and as the first editor of the *American Journal of Clinical Hypnosis,* he achieved worldwide recognition. He was also a controversial figure during the societal quarrels that broke out among hypnotic specialists during the late 1950s and early 1960s. That is another story, which we describe later.

During World War II, the second author of the present text (J. Watkins, 1949), while at the Welch Convalescent Hospital in Daytona Beach, Florida, was given the unusual opportunity of developing a hypnotherapy program for returning soldiers. The abreacting of war experiences had been found valuable by Grinker and Spiegel (1945), but in their work they, as well as most other military psychiatrists, relied on the use of such drugs as sodium amytal and sodium pentothal to induce the altered state of consciousness that would permit emotional release. At that time, only a few military practitioners were employing hypnotic techniques in the treatment of war neuroses. In 1945, the Welch Hospital included some 2,500 soldiers who were psychiatric casualties, and an entire company of patients was allocated to treatment either by hypnotherapy or by "narcosynthesis," the term Grinker and Spiegel (1945) applied to their approach. Much latitude was given in this "Special Treatment Company" to develop and experiment with a wide variety of hypnoanalytic procedures.

During the years immediately after the war, there was a great upsurge of interest in the applications of hypnosis to dental practice. The anxieties and dental phobias shown by many patients have always been a source of difficulty to these practitioners. Hypnosis offered an approach for dealing with them. In addition, hypnotic anesthesia might prove of value in either replacing or supplementing chemoanesthesias for the relief of dental pain. Burgess (1952) and Heron (1953), two psychologists in Minnesota, taught hypnotic techniques to many dental practitioners. "Hypnodontia" societies were organized, and there were more than 300 dentists within that state using hypnotic procedures almost before dentists in other parts of the country had heard of such procedures.

A pioneering group of some 25 psychologists and psychiatrists organized the Society for Clinical and Experimental Hypnosis (SCEH) in 1949. The leaders in this group were Jerome M. Schneck, a psychiatrist and psychoanalyst, who served as its first president, and Milton H. Kline, who became the editor of the *Journal for Clinical and Experimental Hypnosis,* published by the society. To counter the criticism focused on hypnosis by psychoanalysts, conservative physicians, and academic psychologists, membership in this organization was purposely restricted by the extremely high membership requirements. To become a member one was required to have had many years of experience and have published significant contributions. Accordingly, the organization grew very slowly, and during the following 8 years, it did not number more than 100.

In 1955, a report by a lay hypnotist was published that described a participant who, under hypnotic regression, purported to be the reincarnation of a young Irish woman called Bridey Murphy. Bridey gave many details of her supposed "life" of 150 years earlier. Although reputable scientific study could find no realistic basis for this claim, the case attracted much public attention. *Time, Life, Look,* and many other magazines devoted space to it. Both lay people and professionals were intrigued. The publicity given to Bridey Murphy tended to emphasize the unscientific and spectacular claims that had so often in the past brought repudiation of hypnosis by reputable physicians and scientists. It smacked of Mesmer's showmanship. Interest in hypnotic "reincarnation" died down, but a number of scientists and mental health practitioners were induced to commence serious study of the therapeutic potentialities in hypnosis.

Milton Erickson organized a teaching team that gave 3-day seminars throughout the United States to physicians, psychologists, and dentists. Many new recruits to the field received their initial training at these courses. However, these newcomers found that they did not have the extremely high requirements for membership in the SCEH. They were considerably dissatisfied at their inability to affiliate with the only hypnosis society existing at that time.

After a battle over efforts to lower the entrance requirements for the SCEH, Erickson and his associates organized, overnight, a new society called the American Society of Clinical Hypnosis (ASCH). Filled from the ranks of the students in seminars, this organization grew rapidly and became much larger in size than the SCEH. A bitter conflict ensued between the parent group, centered in New York, which insisted on the extremely high standards of membership, and the new vigorous young ASCH, centered in Chicago, which argued that hypnosis was too valuable a modality to be so restricted. This split occurred in 1957 and was followed by more than 5 years of bitterness, name-calling, and raiding of each other's memberships. Competition for new members, especially of those who had achieved status in the field, was keen. The SCEH prided itself on its quality and had at that time, as it does today, the better-established journal. The ASCH, with its large and increasing membership, was much stronger financially, had a built-in recruitment system for new members in the seminars, and held out its shingle as "the most representative" organization in the field.

The SCEH, threatened by the large membership and financial solvency enjoyed by the ASCH, countered in 1958 by developing two new organizations that were to make significant impact. Specialty boards existed in the field of medicine, dentistry, and psychology that certified practitioners who could demonstrate certain high-level qualifications. Thus, medicine had the American Board of Obstetrics and Gynecology, the American Board of Psychiatry and Neurology, the American Board of Surgery, and so forth. Specialty certification existed in such dental fields as periodontia and orthodontia, and in psychology the American Board of Examiners in Professional Psychology certified highly qualified practitioners in the fields of clinical, industrial, and counseling psychology. These usually involved 5 years of specialized experience plus examinations.

Accordingly, the SCEH undertook to organize and launch the American Board of Clinical Hypnosis with three subboards: the American Board of Medical Hypnosis, the American Board of Hypnosis in Dentistry, and the American Board of Examiners in Psychological Hypnosis; the latter issued separate certificates in clinical and in experimental hypnosis.

Reception of these boards was mixed. The psychology board was approved by the APA, and its "diplomats" were officially listed in the association's directory. The medical board did not receive official recognition by the American Medical Association (AMA), although the association had approved hypnosis as a legitimate medical discipline. The dental board did not receive the approval of the American Dental Association, nor would the association even recognize hypnosis as a legitimate study for dentists at the time.

To complicate the picture of conflict further, the AMA, stimulated by its psychiatric members, tried to restrict the use of hypnosis only to medical practitioners and to exclude psychologists from the field, especially clinical psychologists who were employing it psychotherapeutically. In general, this effort was not successful, except for a few states where medical practice laws were amended to limit the use of hypnosis to physicians. Within the two societies, the SCEH and ASCH, physicians, psychiatrists, psychologists, and dentists enjoyed a close congenial relationship, and quarrels between disciplines were largely avoided.

The second move by the SCEH at that time was in organizing the International Society for Clinical and Experimental Hypnosis (ISCEH). The ASCH had been more successful in developing the field within the United States, but its very name limited its member-getting ability in other countries. Accordingly, the ISCEH, with the SCEH as its U.S. division, soon initiated divisions in some 30 different countries. Bernard B. Raginsky, a Canadian psychiatrist who was president of the SCEH at the time, requested John G. Watkins to form and chair the International Organizing Committee. The committee contacted leading workers all over the world to become the international directors of the new society and to organize the various national divisions. Raginsky (1963), who was also a president of the Academy for Psychosomatic Medicine, was a distinguished contributor to the field and had published numerous papers, especially on the applications of clinical hypnosis to the treatment of psychosomatic disorders. Widely known and respected, his leadership as the first president of the ISCEH was strongly instrumental in getting it accepted on a worldwide basis. The second author (J.G.W.) served as its executive secretary during the first 4 years, and later served as its president.

The ASCH initially perceived the boards and the ISCEH as inimical to its interests, and it boycotted both organizations. However, as time passed and as the bitterness of competition between the SCEH and ASCH declined, it became rather inevitable that these two groups were complementary to each other and that each had something constructive to offer the field. The ASCH had many more members and a continuous educational program. The SCEH had the boards, the ISCEH, and a widely accepted journal, the *International Journal of Clinical and Experimental Hypnosis*. Many people who were members of both societies pressed for unification. As of 2005, such a uniting had not taken place, but the old quarrels, the bitterness, and the competition have disappeared. The two societies now cooperate in many matters, and joint national conference meetings are planned. Reports of each other's conventions and papers are published in both the *American Journal of Clinical Hypnosis* and the *International Journal of Clinical and Experimental Hypnosis*.

The ISCEH held meetings about every 2 to 3 years (Chicago, 1958; São Paulo, 1960; Portland, Oregon, 1962; Kyoto, 1967; Mainz, West Germany, 1970; Uppsala, Sweden, 1973; Philadelphia, 1976; Melbourne, Australia, 1980; Glasgow, Scotland, 1982; Toronto, Canada, 1985; The Hague, 1988; Jerusalem, 1992; Melbourne, Australia, 1994; San Diego, 1997; Munich, 2000; Singapore, 2004). In 1973, it was reorganized and its name changed to the International Society of Hypnosis. Both the ASCH and SCEH are now affiliated with it.

The Institute for Research in Hypnosis was also originally organized by the SCEH as a training and research unit. It was chartered by the Board of Regents of the State University of New York as a nonprofit educational foundation and served as the medium through which a number of courses, workshops, and international congresses were presented. The institute developed a treatment facility in New York City called the Morton Prince Center for Hypnotherapy. In the APA, Division 30 (formerly known as "Psychological Hypnosis" and recently renamed "Society of Psychological Hypnosis" [SPH]) also was organized to promote research and practice in the field of hypnosis. The SCEH, the ASCH, and to a much lesser extent the Society of Psychological Hypnosis sponsor workshops in hypnosis, as do various local hypnosis societies. APA's Division 17 (Counseling Psychology) started a Special Interest Group in Hypnosis in 1997. An increasing number of medical schools and graduate departments of psychology and counseling psychology from the larger universities now offer training in hypnosis. The year 2002 is another milestone. APA's Committee on APA Divisions Relations awarded a grant to the first author of this text (as president of the Society of Psychological Hypnosis 2002-2003) to develop a basis for the Integration of Hypnosis Training in PhD Programs (in clinical psychology and counseling psychology). The grant was developed in cooperation with APA's Multicultural and Counseling Psychology Divisions.

At long last, hypnosis has largely overcome the prejudices in the medical profession and academia. Hypnosis is accepted as a legitimate scientific and treatment modality. The substantive National Institute of Mental Health supported research from the 1960s to 1980s at laboratories, such as those headed by Ernest Hilgard at Stanford, Martin Orne at the University of Pennsylvania, and Theodore X. Barber at the Medfield Foundation. More research and clinical application is focused in medical settings led by Harvard University Medical School, where hypnosis is the standard non-pharmacologic analgesia for interventional radiological procedures (see

Lang et al., 2000; Lang & Rosen, 2002), and by Stanford University Medical School, where hypnosis is routinely used to prolong life and provide cancer pain relief (see Spiegel, 1997.) At the University of California (Davis) Medical Center, hypnosis is in regular use to reduce blood loss and speed healing in spinal surgery patients (see Bennett, 1993). The APA Division — Society of Psychological Hypnosis program at the APA National Conventions has been overflowing with attendees. The national conventions of the SCEH and ASCH are attended by hundreds of members where the latest research papers, clinical studies, symposia, and training workshops on hypnosis are presented. Awards are annually made to outstanding contributors. Hypnosis appears to have outgrown its boom-or-bust cycles and is here to stay, intriguing legitimate scientists into investigating its strange phenomena and converting reputable clinical practitioners within the medical, psychological, and dental professions into using it to help their patients.

As a final note, we should remember that this current stage of growth and acceptance was achieved only at the cost of much conflict. The pioneers in this field fought hard to secure its recognition and to maintain their own professional status. Mesmer, Elliotson, Braid, and Esdaile battled constantly with the establishment of traditional medicine. Liebeault treated for 20 years in obscurity. Charcot engaged in bitter controversy with the Nancy practitioners. Freud drew from hypnosis his first understanding of unconscious processes and then abandoned it. His followers rejected it. Professional quarrels raged over the question of training. Hypnosis societies battled over standards of membership and fought for respective status. Practitioners or investigators in this field survived and flourished only if they could demonstrate outstanding abilities and could maintain their professional integrity in the face of attacks and pressures from many directions.

Perhaps this resulted in a selecting process that was all to the good, because the field today is peopled by many able clinicians and scientists. The major North American societies, the European Society, the Australian Society, plus the international organization, and numerous societies by individual country now number among their members many outstanding contributors who are continually adding to our knowledge of this fascinating modality and developing an even more effective therapeutic technology. If humanity is to survive, the understanding of man's inner space may be of greater importance than the conquest of outer space, and in this realm, hypnosis can play a significant role.

A Chronological Outline of the History of Hypnosis

Prehistoric period   Hypnosis is probably used by primitive man as almost his only "medical" treatment.

Ancient historical   Hypnosis is used in India by yogis and in Greek temples as "sleep therapy."

Medieval period   Trance states involve dancing frenzies and cures by the "laying on of hands."

1775–1784   Mesmer develops and practices his theories of animal magnetism.

1784   The French Commission evaluates and rejects Mesmer's theories.

1784   De Puysegur discovers the state of somnambulism.

1821   A painless surgery reported in France by Récamier on a "magnetized" patient.

1837–1868   Elliotson fights for scientific and medical acceptance.

1841   Braid develops the term *hypnotism* as a psychological phenomenon.

1845–1853   In Calcutta, India, Esdaile performs more than 2,000 operations with patients under hypnoanesthesia.

1864   Liebeault begins his practice of clinical hypnosis in Nancy.

1864   Phineas Quimby practices hypnosis and teaches it to Mary Baker Eddy, founder of Christian Science.

1882   Bernheim visits Liebeault and is converted to the value of hypnosis.

1882   Freud observes Breuer's abreactive method.

1885   Bernheim publishes his book *de la Suggestion.*

1886   The Nancy School of Liebeault and Bernheim prevails over the Paris School of Charcot, and hypnosis is established as a psychological, not magnetic, phenomenon.

1887   Freud takes up the practice of hypnotism.

1894   Freud abandons hypnosis and begins the development of psychoanalysis.

1906   Morton Prince treats a case of dissociated personality with hypnosis.

1933   Hull publishes the first book on experimental hypnosis, *Hypnosis and Suggestibility.*

1933   Milton Erickson begins publication of a series of papers reporting unique and innovative approaches in hypnotherapy.

1945–1946	Watkins develops hypnoanalytic techniques in the treatment of war neuroses.
1947	Dental hypnosis begins in the state of Minnesota.
1949	The SCEH is founded.
1953	The *Journal for Clinical and Experimental Hypnosis* begins publication.
1957	The ASCH is formed.
1957	The American Board of Clinical Hypnosis with three subboards, the American Board of Medical Hypnosis, the American Board of Hypnosis in Dentistry, and the American Board of Examiners in Psychological Hypnosis is formed.
1957	The ISCEH is founded.
1957–1962	Much strife exists between the two hypnosis societies, the SCEH and ASCH.
1958	The therapeutic use of hypnosis by physicians is approved by the AMA.
1960	The American Board of Examiners in Psychological Hypnosis receives the official approval of the APA.
1973	The ISCEH is reorganized, broadened in membership, and renamed the International Society of Hypnosis.
1983–2000	A series of experimentally controlled studies apply advanced EEG and brain scan technologies to reveal the neural substrates of the hypnotic state.
1996	National Institutes of Health technology assessment panel recognizes hypnosis in the treatment of chronic pain, insomnia, and other disorders and recommends its integration into medical interventions.
2002	The APA Committee on APA Divisions Relations provides a grant to the APA Division 30 — Society for Psychological Hypnosis (in collaboration with the APA divisions of Counseling Psychology and Multicultural Psychology) to study the integration of hypnosis in Ph.D. training.

Chapter 2
Hypnotic Phenomena

"Even the best hypnotic subjects pass through life without anyone suspecting them to possess such remarkable ability until by deliberate experiment it is made manifest." Then they are hypnotized and "no ordinary suggestions of waking life ever took such control of their mind." (James, 1890, p. 600)

Most of us in the general population respond to hypnosis. We are not usually gullible; neither are we more responsive to placebos, social pressure, or authority figures than those unfortunate nonresponders. Furthermore, research shows that responses to hypnosis do not correlate with most types of suggestibility (Killeen & Nash, 2003). Hypnosis predates the study of psychology and has outlasted just about any other medical or psychotherapeutic modality known to modern science quite simply because it makes it possible for people to use their own natural talents to achieve goals without the negative side effects wrought by other means (A. Barabasz, 2003a).

Despite historical controversy about what hypnosis really is, many are in agreement as to its phenomena. Whether it is instituted as a formal hypnotic induction, self-induced, or spontaneous, there is general agreement as to the behavioral and perceptual changes possible once one is experiencing a state of hypnosis. The ability of hypnotized individuals to exhibit unusual behaviors and to transcend normal limits of function has never ceased to amaze the average person who observes it for the first time. Even

27

experienced workers, who have become accustomed to observing certain responses to hypnosis and view reactions not normally obtainable in unhypnotized individuals, frequently reexperience a sense of awe. It is truly astounding to see the remarkable possibilities in human functioning, which become amenable to initiation and new self-control, simply obtained by the hypnotic modality.

When a class of scientifically trained professionals, such as physicians or psychologists, first sees a demonstration of deep trance phenomena, including posthypnotic hallucinations, amnesia, or regression, the common reaction is one of shock and disbelief. With seeming ease the therapist accomplishes miracles. Participants appear to recall and relive emotionally encoded details of their lives long ago forgotten. They can evince disturbances of perception that are usually seen only in psychotic patients. They can compulsively carry out actions that they might not perform if they were in complete control of themselves. It is no wonder that objective observers, who have been educated not to believe in miracles, immediately find their rational processes challenged to account for such apparently weird happenings. The strange behavior flies in the face of common sense.

In an attempt to explain the happenings, some say simply that it is not really occurring, it is a trick, or the participant is acting only to please the therapist and fool the viewers.

Professionals might find it easier to retreat into explanations of dissociative reactions. Hypnosis cannot be science; it belongs to the realm of fairies and goblins. Hypnosis also challenges the ideas held by those with religious background, and often times these natural talents are mistaken as works of the devil. This being said, one can clearly understand why therapists during the Middle Ages were often burned at the stake for practicing witchcraft.

Here we have observable human behavior, which is contrary to normal expectations, and we have no completely adequate theory or rationale to account for it. Reasonableness promotes reasonableness. Likewise, irrational behavior stimulates irrational reactions. It is not uncommon for beginners in the field to experience strange feelings of awe, perplexity, disbelief, anxiety, or laughter. Primitive transference reactions stemming from early fantasies of power and omnipotence are frequently mobilized. Clinical teachers of hypnotherapy often view with concern the early experiments of some of their students who are suddenly imbued with the idea that they have acquired godlike powers, which they can use to control others and build up their own prestige.

John Watkins was once dismayed to hear about how one of his workshop students, a physician, used his new knowledge to hypnotize patients, anesthetize their arms, and then stick needles through them before colleagues to impress them with his newly acquired powers. It is with difficulty that the serious instructor in hypnosis guides students safely between the early Scylla of skepticism on one hand and the Charybdis of overinvolvement on the other.

Hypnosis is a phenomenon that can initiate strange behaviors in the therapist and in the participant. Those of you who are reading this book, or perhaps are studying it as part of a course, should be ever mindful of this factor and strive to keep an even emotional keel, even though you remain highly curious and motivated. The hypnotherapists who learn to use this modality for helping others are those who also have learned to react to it constructively within their own selves. A "therapeutic self" (J. Watkins, 1978) finds in hypnosis a powerful adjunct to one's healing abilities, but a pathologic self can employ this modality for the release of one's destructive tendencies.

Regardless of whatever little remains of the argument as to whether an altered state is necessary to elicit hypnotic behaviors, let us take the position held by the majority of therapists using hypnosis (A. Barabasz, 2000; E. Hilgard, 1992; Kirsch, 1993; H. Spiegel and D. Spiegel, 2004). We recognize, as the EEG and brain imaging studies discussed in the next chapter show, that such a state can be made manifest. Now let us assume that hypnosis has been induced and deepened (by one of the techniques to be described in later chapters) and that the therapist is now administering suggestions aimed at influencing the participant's reactions. We shall also assume that a moderately deep degree of such trance has been secured. What hypnotic responses are now possible?

Motor Behavior

One of the characteristics of hypnosis is a loss in criticality. Hence, if the therapist were to say, "You will sit on the floor and cross your legs," participants will act as if under a compulsion, that is, as if they were no longer "critical" or able to resist carrying out such strange behavior, as they would be in the nonhypnotic state (see Figure 2.1). Almost any motor behavior can be suggested and, if it is within their physical capabilities, the participants will probably carry it out as if they were a dutiful automaton. Sometimes they can even be induced to behave in ways that transcend normal functioning. Watkins and Showalter reported the case of a 19-year-old participant who was told that she was 29 years old, a genius, and a doctoral graduate of a famous university. She could then read with amazing speed and facility, and she increased her reading speed 63% with no loss in comprehension (see LeCron, 1968, p. 159). This response was sub-

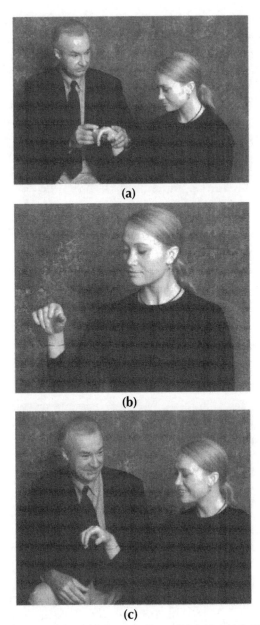

(a)

(b)

(c)

Fig. 2.1 Hand wagging compulsion. (a) In hypnosis, the participant is told that her right hand will wag up and down and that it will be unable to stop after emerging from hypnosis until the therapist touches the hand. Therapist also gives the hypnotic suggestion nonverbally as the waging is initiated by moving the hand up and down. (b) The participant is brought out of hypnosis and is surprised to see her hand wagging automatically. (c) The participant is quite amused to see that she cannot stop her hand from wagging up and down.

jected to experimentally controlled investigation with a group of participants and was fully supported (A. Barabasz & Barabasz, 1994b). However, the increases were maintained for only a short period of time.

The participant who has been given a suggestion of an action to be carried out, such as walking across the room and examining a certain book, usually carries this through as if there were no other possibility. Such participants might be unable to remember, after having been removed from hypnosis, that they ever performed the action. Sometimes, when the hypnotic state is very light or for certain inner dynamic reasons that may not be known to the therapist, the participant will sit motionless and refuse to carry through the action. The person is actually in a state of hypnosis but does not respond, and it appears that the suggestion has been recorded and processed, the inhibition of the suggested action might have been achieved at the cost of anxiety and inner conflict. This sort of reaction on the part of the participant can be used to further enhance rapport or, we hope, resonance between the participant and the therapist by interpreting that the occurrence demonstrates how hypnosis remains ultimately in the control of the participant. Indeed, as pointed out by H. Spiegel and Spiegel (2004), all hypnosis is essentially self-hypnosis. The skilled and considerate therapist will either remove the suggestion, which has not been executed, or simply instruct the participant during or after hypnosis to carry it through. An unresolved suggestion may leave the individual burdened with inner turmoil after the session is finished. In my (A.F.B.) initial training in hypnosis, my instructor suggested, after inducing and deepening hypnosis, that a member of the class had a coin in the palm of his hand. The student said he could not feel any coin there. Unfortunately, my instructor forgot to remove the suggestion. Later that night the student phoned him to ask about "feeling something warm" in the palm of his hand. The hypnotically suggested coin was getting a bit warm in his hand! Relief came only when my mentor removed the suggestion. In another interesting case, one of John Watkins's participants did not carry through a suggestion to pick up a teacup and put it down. He seemed pleased to mention that he had successfully resisted the suggestion. However, he reported the next day that he had been unable to sleep that night.

Accordingly, failure to carry through a hypnotic suggestion may mean simply it was not heard. However, it might mean that the trance state was not deep enough to induce the lowered criticality or that some need to resist has been mobilized in the participant. We believe this is a far too common problem in a large number of university studies of hypnotic phenomena that use inexperienced graduate students to induce hypnosis and collect data. In any event, be sure to remove all uncompleted suggestions.

Compulsive behaviors are not the only suggestions that can be made; compulsive inhibitions can also be suggested. Hypnotized participants who are told that they cannot rise from the seat can be quite unable to do so no matter how hard they try. Individuals who are told that they cannot speak their names can find themselves unable to respond. Hypnotic suggestions of inhibiting behavior have been used as part of the treatments aimed at stopping smoking, overeating, drinking, or other bad habits and addictions. There are complications that can occur when hypnotic suggestion is used to counter normal reactions or habitual responses, which is why therapists should be psychologically trained and sophisticated. Those who use hypnosis in their practices act first, according to their training as a psychologist, medical practitioner, or dentist. Any suggestion is an intervention in a human system of equilibrium. Previous responses, even though unconstructive, can have been established for specific reasons. Intervening in them with hypnotic suggestions for compulsions or inhibitions can change that equilibrium and release a train of subsequent reactions that might be worse than the ones that the suggestions are aimed to supplant.

Sometimes the therapist tries to facilitate or improve behavior suggestively. During World War II, John Watkins, as an army psychologist, suggested to a soldier that he would be exceptionally clear-sighted and steady while firing on the rifle range. On that particular day the soldier made an almost perfect score and qualified as "Expert," a level of behavior substantially above what he had previously achieved. That temporary improvement in behavior achieved through hypnosis has been so frequently demonstrated that it no longer requires proof. However, much research needs to be done on the conditions that preceded or accompanied the administration of the successful suggestions and their potential duration. There is great variability. One report was made of a suggestion given a hypnotized individual, which was carried out 30 years later.

It should be noted that sometimes suggestions are aimed directly at changing a specific behavior: "You will rise out of your seat and yawn." At other times a situation is suggested that results in a desired behavior as a consequence; for example, "Your muscles will feel tired and stiff," causing individuals to rise from their seats, stretch, and yawn.

Influencing Attitudes

Hypnotic suggestions are sometimes intended to modify attitudes that underlie behavior rather than the behavior itself. Thus, a suggestion directed toward improving morale — "You will begin to feel hopeful about getting well and will view your doctors as genuinely concerned in helping you" — can have the effect of stimulating more cooperative behavior on the part of a hospitalized patient.

Not only is it possible to induce individuals to concentrate more highly when studying or to motivate themselves to a greater degree of interest, individuals also can often be helped by hypnosis to reason selectively. Television news stories indicated that something of this nature was done by the North Koreans in brainwashing prisoners of war so that they perceived information that was made available to them as only anti-American and procommunist. The same strategy was employed in the famous case of Cardinal Mindzenty in Budapest during the 1950s. Through what was termed hypnotic brainwashing he was induced to renounce his normal allegiances and accuse himself at a public trial staged by that communist regime. More recently, the Chinese soldiers that attacked and captured students retreating from Tiananmen Square were exposed to days of monotonous systematic misinformation about the students while being held in a train station. Hypnotic-like pressures can thus be used for malevolent and benevolent purposes.

Alteration of Perceptions

Easy behaviors can be carried out from simple directions without hypnosis, mere suggestion, or the simple consequence of the individual's need to please the therapist by role-playing (Sarbin, 2004). However, hypnosis is required to obtain more difficult suggested disturbances to perception. When such changes are produced by hypnosis, they are surprising and sometimes alarming to the participant. Such alterations in perception are the most convincing of the potency of hypnosis.

The research thus far indicates that hypnosis is used most to influence perceptions directed against pain. It is quite amazing to the lay observer to hear therapists say to their patients, "When I count up to five you will be wide awake, alert, and you will no longer have the headache that has been troubling you." The individuals emerge smiling and report, "It doesn't hurt now." Has the pain really stopped, or are they merely saying this to please the therapist? Does it make any difference that the physiological marker of pain can still be present? As E. Hilgard (1992) pointed out, pain is what hurts and when the hurt is gone the pain is gone.

E. Hilgard and Hilgard (1975) completed several carefully controlled experiments that show rather conclusively that at the overt or conscious level the participant is indeed not experiencing pain. However, at a covert or unconscious level the pain is apparently being recorded. The football player who completes a game suffering from an undiscovered fractured clavicle demonstrates the same phenomenon. Even though a pain is initiated organically in some part of the body, the individual must receive it at a higher level of brain function before one feels the hurt (Hilgard, 1992). If it is dissociated from perceptual centers, one does not sense the pain. Such an ability to block off pain stimuli is routinely done with hypnosis in the interventional radiology clinic at Harvard Medical School (Beth Israel Deaconess Medical Center, Boston) (Lang & Rosen, 2002), and it can be of great help to a suffering patient. Furthermore, anesthesia or analgesia hypnotically induced in one part of the body can be transferred to other parts by rubbing these other parts (or placing them in contact) with the anesthetized area (see Figure 2.2).

The fact that such a manipulation of pain perception is possible by hypnosis does not mean that all patients can achieve it. Nonetheless, the majority of research studies support the finding that all but the least hypnotizable can benefit to some substantial degree. Differences in hypnotizability, the depth of trance that a patient can reach, the skill of the therapist, and many other factors will determine just how much pain relief a given patient receives. There is great variability.

Hallucinations can be induced in good hypnotic participants. For example, they can be told that they will hear voices calling their names, hear a fly buzzing around, or smell the flowers and the good green earth (see Figure 2.3).

In contrast, Milton Erickson (1938a, 1938b) used hypnosis with the suggestion for total deafness so that the participant did not flinch at a loud noise. Long ago Kline, Guze, and Haggarty (1954) showed that this apparent deafness, while similar to that found in hysteria, could not be equated with organic hearing impairment (see also Kramer & Tucker, 1967). For a time, our understanding of this phenomenon became even further clouded when the Erickson report was brought into question by a clever experiment. Scheibe, Gray, and Keim (1968) employed Orne's (1979) real simulator design (see A. Barabasz & Barabasz, 1992) and asked unhypnotizable individuals to fake being in hypnosis. This form of social influence, known as experimental demand characteristics, induced them to approximate the same behavior even though they were not hypnotized. Alas, it seemed that social-influence role-playing rather than a true hypnotic effect could account for the apparent deafness.

It was not until decades later when advances in EEG measurement and analysis made it possible to study the phenomenon to determine how hypnosis can change the way the brain responds to a hallucination for deafness. Role-playing is no longer a viable explanation for those who actually experience hypnosis. We (A. Barabasz et al., 1999; Jensen, Barabasz, A. Barabasz, & Warner, 2001) discovered that when highly hypnotizable indi-

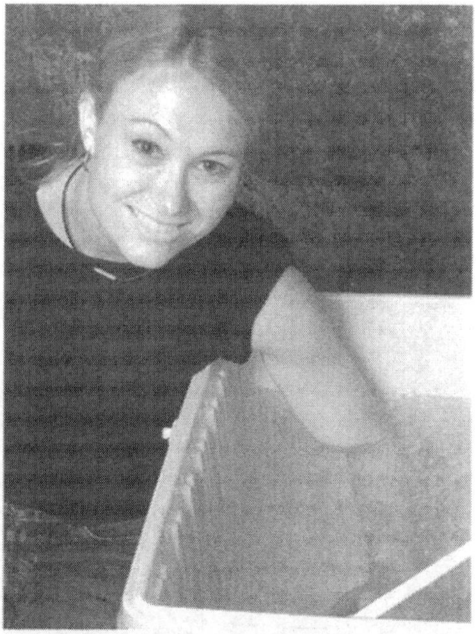

(a)

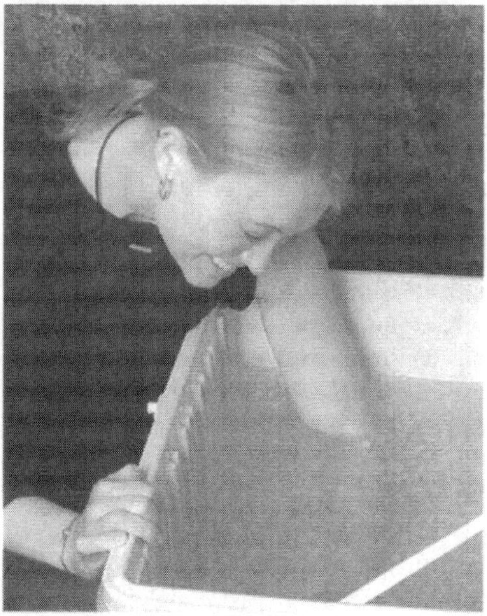

(b)

Fig. 2.2 Hand anesthesia. (a) Without hypnotic anesthesia the participant's left hand hurts painfully in the ice water. (b) Because of posthypnotic anesthesia the participant's hand is rendered painless in the ice water.

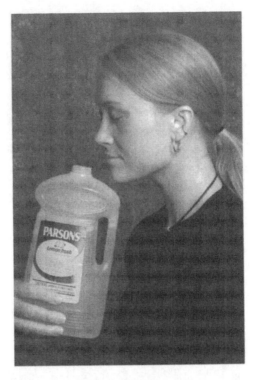

Fig. 2.3 Olfactory hallucination. (a) Hypnotized, the participant is told to take a good sniff of some beautiful perfume. She is now enjoying the perfume, which really is ammonia.

viduals were deeply hypnotized and given a suggestion for total deafness, versus when given a suggestion to imagine placing ear plugs in their ears that would attenuate sounds produced by a computer tone generator, EEG brain activity reacted in opposite ways. Because the hallucination for total deafness was contrary to the way the brain responds to hypnosis (participants have to hear the sound before they can block it out at the executive-control level; see E. Hilgard, 1992; D. Spiegel & Barabasz, 1988), participants were surprised that they heard anything at all. This surprise effect produced an increase in their EEG event-related potentials. When given the ears plugged suggestion, just the opposite happened and the brain reacted with a decreased event-related potentials. The findings were consistent with controlled experiments using olfactory hallucinations and visual hallucinations (A. Barabasz et al., 1999; A. Barabasz & Lonsdale, 1983; D. Spiegel, Cutcomb, Ren, & Pribram, 1985). Those who still insist that hypnosis is nothing more than a product of social influence might consider that the nonhypnotizable control participants in all of these studies were, at best, able to fake overt responses. They were not able to change their EEGs, as were those actually experiencing the hypnotic state. Social influence could not produce the EEG event-related potential changes that could be wrought only by the high hypnotizable participants in the hypnosis condition. The auditory attenuation effect was tested again (A. Barabasz, 2000) in a situation where the individuals were first given the suggestions in a hypnosis free context. Again, the event-related potentials could be altered only in the true hypnotic condition but not in the hypnotic context condition, which used the identical suggestions. This later study showed that the hypnotic induction, given sufficient hypnotic depth, produces effects far beyond those that could be produced by suggestion or social influence alone.

Even more dramatic are the effects produced by hypnosis that appear when inducing visual hallucinations (see Figure 2.4), either negative — "You will be unable to see anybody in this room" — or positive — "You will see a large white dog sitting in the middle of the room." The deeply hypnotized individual responds so realistically that it is quite amazing to watch. However, participants might also experience a form of amnesia when emerging from the hypnotic state, disclaiming any awareness of the hallucination. For example, some individuals coming out of hypnosis will report, "There was an idea of a white dog in my mind, like a dream. I could see it even though I knew it wasn't really there." Another reaction participants might have after coming out of hypnosis might be complete denial of their behavior. Those participants with top scores on the better scales of hypnotizability can even produce complex positive and negative visual hallucinations with clear brain activity indicants (A. Barabasz et al., 1999; D. Spiegel & Barabasz, 1988), which reflect the subjective experiences of individuals rather than a simplistic hypnotized-unhypnotized correlate (see Figure 2.5).

A common demonstration of suggestion distortions in the olfactory sense is to tell hypnotized persons that they will smell a most beautiful perfume. A bottle of ammonia is then held under the noses. If the trance state is deep enough the individuals will smile and describe this "beautiful perfume." Later if told that they will smell some ammonia, and a bottle of water is placed under the nose, reactions can involve grimacing and violent withdrawal just as if the liquid were truly ammonia. Furthermore, the taste sense can also be altered so that if individuals are told they will enjoy a "nice apple" but in actuality are given a piece of lemon, they will eat the lemon with much gusto and report how enjoyable the "apple" was. In addition, the taste hallucination has been used to alter the taste of junk foods and add desired flavors, such as a butter taste

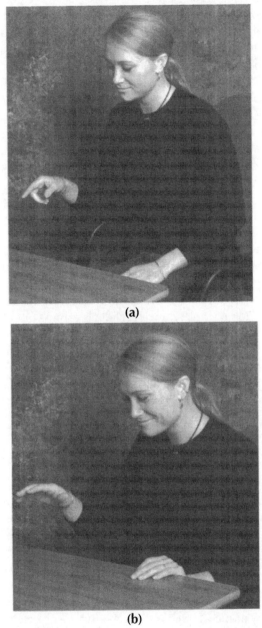

Fig. 2.4 Visual hallucination. (a) Hypnotized, the participant is given the posthypnotic suggestion that there is a rabbit on the table in front of her. (b) Responding posthypnotically, the participant pets the rabbit.

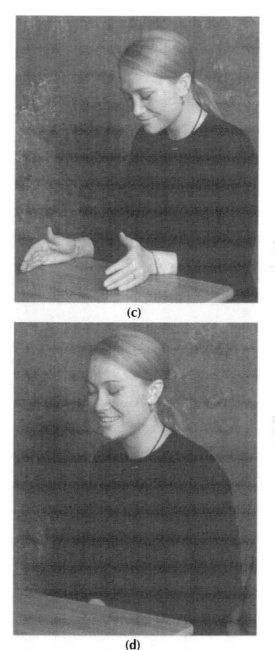

(c)

(d)
Fig. 2.4 *Continued.* (c) The participant demonstrates how long the rabbit is. (d) The arranged signal of the therapist's touching the participant's shoulder removes the posthypnotic suggestion. The participant is amused to discover the rabbit has disappeared.

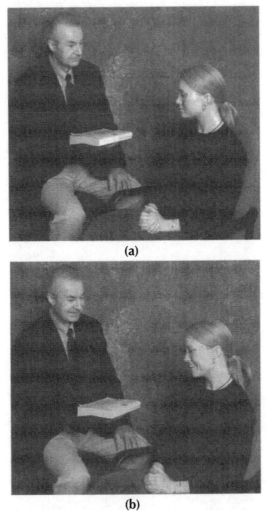

(a)

(b)

Fig. 2.5 Negative posthypnotic hallucination. (a) In hypnosis, the participant is told the therapist is invisible. The book, held by the therapist, appears to be floating in midair. (b) The therapist raises the book up and down, and the participant laughs as she sees the book floating up and down on its own.

without butter, to healthy foods with my (A.F.B.) patients in treatment for weight management.

Every one of the senses is subject to influence under hypnosis. The degree can range from slight alterations to profound hallucinations, which are astonishing to observers and most baffling to the participants. Little work seems to have been done investigating how long such severe distor-

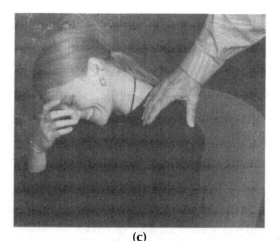

(c)

Fig. 2.5 *Continued.* (c) The hypnotic suggestion is released by the therapist's touching the participant's shoulder, and the participant giggles with surprise as the therapist becomes visible to her.

tions of reality perception can endure. It is obvious that to insist that a dog is present when one is not there or to maintain that there is nobody in a room that is actually filled with people, one must require a great amount of energy in the denial of reality calling heavily on the dissociative and the focused concentration aspects of the hypnotic trance. There are limits in each situation related to the hypnotizability of individuals and the intensity of their relationship with the therapist. If the therapist pits his or her authority against reality, the closeness to the participant must be quite intense, or the participant will relinquish the therapist instead of the reality ("I know you told me to see a dog there, doctor, but I don't see it"). Undoubtedly, this variable has come into play in a number of laboratory studies of hypnosis leading to the misinterpretation that only social influence could be at work once the hypnotic trance, if actually achieved by the researcher in the first place, is relinquished under the ultimate control, always held at some level by the participant.

Not only the perception of hot or cold (temperature sense) but also body temperatures have been influenced hypnotically (A. Barabasz & McGeorge, 1978; Maslach, Marshall, & Zimbardo, 1972). If participants are told that the furnace has been turned on very high, that it is becoming insufferable, and that they feel as if they are in an oven, they will fan themselves, sweat, roll up sleeves, and so on. If the image of being in a wintry blizzard is suggested, they will shiver, huddle for warmth, blow on the hands, and engage in other compatible behavior.

By suggesting to individuals that their hands were being placed in a basin of hot water, we raised the skin temperature of their hands more than 4 degrees as measured instrumentally. At first glance, this seems miraculous, but if one considers that by suggesting a most frightening situation to individuals or showing them a gruesome film, the adrenal glands will increase the release of adrenaline into the blood stream, the phenomenon does not appear to be so unusual. The hypnotic hand-warming technique has been used as an aid in the treatment of migraine headaches (A. Barabasz, 1977), precluding the need for patients to be dependent on elaborate biofeedback devices or medications with dangerous side effects.

Influencing Autonomic Processes

Suggestions can be directly given for behaviors requiring activity of the striated muscles. Organ behavior usually has to be influenced indirectly by picturing to the participant emotional situations that will normally stimulate such activity (Ikemi & Nakagawa, 1962). Thus, suggestions of hunger combined with images of delectable foods will result in an increase in gastric acidity (Hall, 1967).

Pulse rate and blood pressure can be modified using hypnosis, but the effects produced thus far have been transient rather than of treatment value to patients for which such management might be of value. In one extreme case, Bernard Raginsky (1963) reported a complete cessation of heart functioning during the hypnotically regressed reliving of a previous emotional situation. Salivation can be increased by suggesting that participants visualize biting into a rich, juicy orange, or it can be decreased when the participants are told that there are dry crackers in their mouths. This latter manipulation has been of value for some patients during dental treatment.

Influencing Mood and Affect

One of the most frequent symptoms for which patients consult psychiatrists and psychologists is depression. Because depression is commonly based in some underlying guilt or inhibited anger, direct suggestive therapy is seldom successful in achieving a permanent resolution. However, temporary elevations of good mood can serve to provide the necessary lift and revival of hope, which then can be used to therapeutic advantage. Manic individuals can also be temporarily quieted, thus increasing the likelihood of their cooperation in treatment programs. A continuous, but not severe, depression could accordingly be lifted for a day or so to permit, for example, a student to take and pass a crucial examination. Over the past decade considerable progress has been made in the use of hypnosis to enhance the cognitive-behavioral treatment of depression (Yapko, 1992, 1997).

Influencing Cognition

It is quite obvious to everyone that the set, orientation, theory, or political position individuals have adopted materially influences the way they think. A piece of economic news will be evaluated quite differently by a conservative than by a liberal person. Not only perceptions but also cognitions are filtered selectively through pre-established belief systems. It is accordingly not surprising that hypnosis does not easily or quickly reverse those beliefs of which we are convinced. However, skillful suggestions implanted in individuals while in hypnosis will quite often result in a modification of selective cognitions. Specific instructions to concentrate and think about an interpretation given by their therapist can often result in their becoming convinced of a previous error in judgment and a willingness to modify their point of view much more quickly than would be the case if the argument were presented in the conscious, nonhypnotic state. Hypnosis does not provide magical change or instant reversal of previous sets, but it does offer a modality for strongly influencing thought processes. It is this ability, which hypnosis presents to the psychotherapist who is trained to work with it, the opportunity to shorten the time for achieving constructive therapeutic change in many patients. Hypnoanalytic therapy, although not suitable for all patients, tends to progress much more rapidly than traditional psychoanalytic therapy (J. Watkins & H. Watkins, 1997).

Posthypnotic Amnesia, Hyperamnesia, and Regression

A typical characteristic of the deeply hypnotized individual is the appearance, spontaneously upon emerging from trance, of an apparent amnesia for that which had transpired while in the hypnotic state. Most frequently, it will be partial, but it can be total. It can also be selective in that the participant sometimes reports to the therapist an inability to remember but does remember when questioned by others. This brings up the question as to whether the amnesia was real or faked. At other times, the suggestions given by the therapist not to remember can result in amnesia for hypnotic events that otherwise the participant would normally recall (the most thorough science-based coverage of amnesia remains that of Kihlstrom & Evans, 1979).

Although there is controversy over the theoretical rationale for this phenomenon, there seems to be substantial agreement that it is not the same as simple forgetting (E. Hilgard, 1977; Orne, 1966). Thus, researchers have viewed the phenomenon as a product of hypnotic suggestion, direct or implicit, and also as a special form of dissociation. Kline (1966) emphasized the psychodynamic needs of the participant as an initiating cause, whereas Wright (1966) called attention to the unique interpersonal relationship between therapist and participant. J. Watkins (1966) viewed the selectiveness of the amnesia (specifically as related to the therapist versus others) as inhering in intrapersonal gestalts or "ego strategies" that "forget" that which is cognitively inconsistent between the hypnotic and the posthypnotic conditions. Often the participants will remember an item suggested during hypnosis but will manifest "source amnesia"; that is, forget where they first learned it. Source amnesia has been suggested as a criterion to distinguish between genuinely hypnotized individuals and simulators.

Among the phenomena of hypnosis, which are most surprising to the uninitiated, is hypermnesia, or the ability of many individuals to seemingly reconstruct memories of details of their earlier life that they were not normally able to recall. Deeply hypnotized individuals can be quite capable of naming every classmate in their first-grade class and describe clearly all the features of the room. They might be able to recite poetry that they had learned early in school and had not repeated for many years. A 40-year-old school principal was asked (by J.G.W.) if he had ever "spoken a piece" as a child in school. He stated that he had been valedictorian of his eighth-grade class. No amount of conscious effort, however, could enable him to remember even the title of his address. After a deep hypnotic trance was established, he apparently regressed back to the eighth grade and, once "introduced on the graduation platform," he delivered a 15-minute speech quite worthy of an intelligent 14-year-old. There were no hesitations in his delivery, and the nature of the speech was such that it was quite unthinkable that it could have been concocted on the spur of the moment merely to please the therapist. Afterward, he corroborated the title and the content. However, he was still not able to reproduce it as a speech without entering a hypnotic state. In another case, a 30-year-old individual sat down at the piano and performed the number that she had played at her first recital about the age of 13. Prior to being hypnotized and subsequently, she was also completely unable to execute it.

Hypermnesia is much easier to achieve than regression. In the latter, a reexperiencing seems to occur with the emotions and motor movements that are presumed to have accompanied the original incident. The phenomenon of hypermnesia seems to have been well substantiated experimentally (E. Hilgard, 1965). It is widely accepted and used in clinical practice. However, despite the sometimes convincingly high level of emotionality that can accompany hypnotically reconstructed memories, such reconstruction is no more likely to be accurate than nonhypnotic interventions aimed at reconstruction (E. Hilgard & Loftus, 1979; Orne, 1979).

The reality of hypnotic regression also remains controversial. Many hypnotherapists use it in clinical practice (J. Watkins & H. Watkins, 1997). A given participant may demonstrate a true or apparently real regression, another participant may demonstrate a partial regression, and another participant demonstrate only a simulated one. Furthermore, the same individual may manifest various degrees of involvement in regression at different times. (Experimentalists have not always been able to achieve in the controlled laboratory studies the kind of regressed experience reported by clinicians with their patients.) Accordingly, there are some workers who consider it as an artifact, an "acting as if." There is but one experimentally controlled laboratory study available to date to shed light on the issue (A. Barabasz et al., 2003).

Watkins once hypnotized a 19-year-old college sophomore and regressed her to ages 6, 9, 12, and 14. At each of these regressed ages, she was administered standardized reading tests and her eye movements were photographed on an opthalmograph. When hypnotically regressed to 6 years and 10 months (June at the end of the first grade), she demonstrated a reading age of 6-10 in word recognition, 7-3 in sentence reading, and 7-4 in paragraph reading as measured on the *Gates Primary Reading Tests*. When regressed to the age of 8-10 (June at the end of the third grade), she achieved reading levels of 9-6 in vocabulary, 9-10 in level of comprehension, and 7-9 in speed of reading on the *Gates Reading Survey*. This averaged exactly to an age of 8-10 in general reading ability. Reading specialists, masked as to actual age of the participant and the focus of the experimental demonstration, judged her eye movements as being typical for a first grader and third grader, respectively (see Figure 2.6). At the upper ages there seemed to be greater variance between her reading achievement scores and what would have been expected at those ages. A truly definitive study would involve comparing test scores and eye-movement photographs under regressed hypnosis with those that had been made years before when participants were actually at the age to which later they had been hypnotically regressed (LeCron, 1968).

Age regression is closely related to hypermnesia, and an increase in memory detail is usually found in hypnotically regressed participants or patients. However, the fact that the hypnotized individual is highly susceptible to suggestive influence throws doubt as to what extent the reenacting of the early experiences may have been initiated or altered by the therapist's influence. Both researchers and therapists must be extremely careful to avoid suggesting happenings that did not occur. Regressed participants may relive fantasies rather than actual historical occurrences. The experimental reliving by patients of such fantasized events is generally useless in

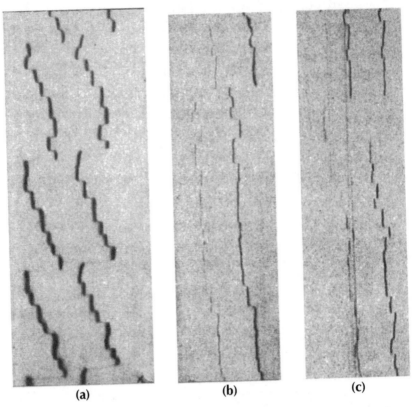

(a) (b) (c)

Fig. 2.6 Photographs of eye movements in experimental participants. (a) Eye movements of a normal college student while reading. (b) Eye movements of the same participant while reading when hypnotically regressed to the third grade. (c) Eye movements of the same participant while reading when hypnotically regressed to the first grade.

establishing accurate memories unless fully corroborated. However, the same reliving techniques can be meaningful and constitute valid therapeutic material because they generally have personal if not historical validity. The reliving of known circumscribed past events is an enormously powerful tool in accelerating progress in ego-state therapy (Emmerson, 2003; J. Watkins & H. Watkins, 1997).

J. Hilgard (1977) proposed three interpretations of hypnotic regression: one is the "ablation" theory, which holds that earlier experiences can be reactivated by hypnotically ablating away later ones. This rationale has been more accepted by clinicians and earlier workers but is supported by rather weak experimental evidence.

A second conception, the "age-consistency" theory, proposes that participants will behave in ways appropriate to their regressed age rather than

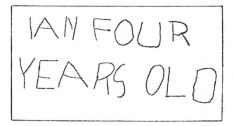

Fig. 2.7 Handwriting samples of a participant hypnotically regressed to various ages.

simply relive actual experiences (see Figure 2.7). Researchers have been divided on these points for decades.

Finally a "role-enactment" theory was first introduced by the studies of Troffer (1965). She found that the most realistic performances of childlike behavior occurred when the experimenter became involved in the role enactment, hence, behaved in a manner appropriate for an adult speaking to a child. This finding held for all three of her groups: the unhypnotizable simulators, the hypnotizable but not hypnotized simulators, and the hypnotically regressed hypnotizable participants. Her study suggests doubt as to the necessity of ensuring that the participant is in a hypnotic state to secure regression worthy of use in psychotherapy. However, because both hypnotizable groups did better than nonhypnotizable simulators, the possibility remains that the hypnotizable simulators were actually hypnotized while enacting the simulating role. This study also supports the concept that hypnosis may be not only an altered state of consciousness, which inheres in the participant, but also an interpersonal transaction between therapist and participant, hence a "state relationship" as proposed by Kline (1958) and J. Watkins (1967). Hypnosis in the individual cannot be divorced from the role, manner, and involvement of the therapist. It is a bipolar phenomenon.

The reality of hypnotic regression rejected by some experimentalists remains controversial among clinicians. Therapists use it widely and consider it a valuable tool, especially in hypnoanalysis and in ego-state therapy. When a highly experienced clinician is involved, it is possible, even highly likely, that the intensive, regressed hypnotic relationship, which inheres in a therapist-patient interaction, cannot be obtained in the more artificial laboratory setting. If so, clinicians and academic researchers may simply not be observing the same phenomena.

Dissociation

E. Hilgard (1977, 1992) recalled that hypnosis has been closely associated with the process of dissociation. Whether or not hypnosis is a form of dissociation, there is little doubt that dissociation can be induced by hypnosis. Thus, participants can be told that they are somebody else, perhaps a well-known celebrity, and they will act accordingly, often most convincingly. In addition, they can be given hypnotic suggestions, which they carry out and then show a complete amnesia about later. They can also be told under hypnosis that they will be unable to remember certain experiences that they have had while hypnotized or that they will forget, for example, the pain that they had endured during a surgical procedure. Hypnosis, accordingly, is a modality in which dissociation can be established or resolved. It is no wonder that some variation of hypnosis becomes the therapy of choice in treating cases of amnesia and dissociative identity disorder (multiple personality). In the book *Sybil* (Schreiber, 1974), the analyst noted that the changes occurred much more rapidly when she was using hypnosis than during the more traditional psychoanalysis.

John and Helen Watkins have been systematically using hypnotic dissociation in the development of a type of therapy that they termed "ego-state
therapy" (J. Watkins & H. Watkins, 1981, 1997). "Normal" individuals are
dissociated into ego states, or "part persons," by hypnosis to evaluate intrapsychic conflicts, and "family therapy" techniques are employed to resolve
them (Emmerson, 2003; J. Watkins & H. Watkins, 1997). This approach
will also be described in more detail in our Volume II, *Hypnoanalytic Techniques* (forthcoming).

Altering Subject-Object Relationships

Closely associated with dissociation is the ability of hypnosis to alter subject–object relationships. Thus it is possible to create the feeling in individuals that a member of their bodies is no longer a part of them, hence, that
they are "object" instead of "subject." This is similar to what occurs spontaneously without hypnosis in a hysterically paralyzed patient. By reversing this subject–object maneuver, a part, which has been experienced by
such individuals as "it" rather than "me," becomes once more incorporated into the self. Ideas, or entire patterns of behavior and thinking, also
can be altered as to subject and object. Through hypnotic manipulation,
individuals can be induced to throw themselves into some "role" or to act
out and live out a facet of their own selves. They are then experiencing this
role as "me." Later the entire role can be hypnotically changed over into an
"object," and they will then experience it as "him" or "her," as if watching
this behavior in another person. These complicated maneuvers require
considerable training and experience to be used effectively in the sophisticated strategies of hypnoanalytic and ego-state therapies.

Time Distortion

Another rather puzzling hypnotic phenomenon is the apparent ability of
hypnotized individuals to experience greater or lesser amounts of experiential time within a given period of clock time. This should really not
seem so unusual, because most of us commonly experience time as passing
rapidly when we are involved in interesting meaningful activities, and we
feel that time is dragging when our immediate environment is providing
little stimulation or when we are assigned to boring tasks. The manipulation of time sense is spontaneous under such conditions.

A typical behavioral demonstration of time alteration using hypnosis
involves setting a musician's metronome at 1 beat to the second. The hypnotized participant is told, "You will hear a tick each second, 60 to the
minute. You will not consciously be aware of this ticking sound, but it will

be recorded in you unconsciously, and you will know that a second passes between each of the ticks. Tick-tick-tick. One second, 2 seconds, 3 seconds," and so on. Suggestions of this type are repeated until the ticking is built into the participants' time sense. The participants are then asked to write their names over and over again, either on paper or at a blackboard. After a norm is established for the number of times, they normally write their names within a 1- or 2-minute interval, and the metronome is increased to 120 beats per minute. The participants respond by increasing their speed of writing, sometimes inscribing their names furiously. The metronome is then slowed to 30 beats to the minute. The participants now decelerate their writing speed, appear depressed, and write their names in slow motion. Experiential and behavioral time seem to be tied to the ticking rate of the metronome. If questioned posthypnotically, the individuals may maintain that they wrote at a constant rate. This apparently hypnotic phenomenon is in need of controlled experimentation in a laboratory setting to determine how much of the response is due to hypnosis versus other factors. A few early attempts provided only partial information, which remains subject to alternative interpretations.

Cooper and Erickson (1959) reported a series of studies involving the manipulation of time experience by hypnosis. They compared "world time" or "clock reading" with experiential time, which they termed "seeming duration." A typical experiment involved suggesting to hypnotized individuals that they would engage in the continuous activity of picking cotton for a "personal time" of 1 hour and 20 minutes. Actually the participants were given only 3 seconds of actual time. They then signaled the number of cotton balls that they had picked, which generally were in the hundreds. Sutcliffe (1965), in his role as a sociocognitivist, criticized this study in that no actual behavioral referents were used. He argued that the participants were only conforming to suggested expectations and that we have no proof that they actually experienced 1 hour and 20 minutes within a 3-second interval, which is true, because one's internal subjective experience is not perceptible to another person. Here again, the debunker and the credulous worker can interpret the data differently.

Zimbardo, Marshall, and Maslach (1971) found that hypnotic participants given suggestions of "expanding the present" behaved differently from simulators, both in subjective reports and in behavior involving playing with clay. They were also able to distinguish between hypnotized participants and simulators on the basis of their ability to translate the verbal suggestion of a synchronicity between clock time and personal time into behavioral reality on a task involving the regulation of lights by pressing a key. Their carefully controlled studies added substantial experimental evidence to an acceptance of the reality of time distortion that can be produced by hypnotic trance.

Therapeutic possibilities for the use of time distortion were demonstrated by Aaronson (1968), who found that when the present was expanded, a state of euphoria ensued and a schizophrenic-like state "followed removal of the present time sense." This entire area shows considerable promise for employment in therapeutic tactics but needs much further exploration.

Hypnosis as an Altered State and Interpersonal Relationship

Except for instances of spontaneous hypnosis in everyday life (see chapter 3), we view hetero-hypnosis and self-hypnosis developed under the guidance of the therapist, as both an altered state of consciousness and an intensive interpersonal relationship. The following question arises then: How much of the participant's behavior is due to the effect of trance and how much inheres in the interaction between therapist and participant? Fortunately, when we practice hypnotherapy we are interested in maximizing all factors that will facilitate the treatment. Throughout this book we, therefore, typically employ techniques of hypnotic induction and deepening, which, at the same time, use all constructive interpersonal relationship aspects possible that exist in any good therapist-patient interaction. As therapists, we are interested in the outcome for the patient, not in the purity of each contributing factor.

Summary

In this chapter, we tried to describe the many different types of phenomena that can be elicited under hypnosis. By this we mean what is possible with some participants or patients, not that every person is capable of exhibiting all of these phenomena. The more complex phenomena seem to require a greater hypnotic depth. Because of the controversies in the field, research findings must be evaluated with the recognition that enthusiastic therapists often over-evaluate their accomplishments, and overly critical experimenters may simply have failed to elicit the phenomena. However, even the most critical and rigorous workers generally agree that, regardless of what hypnosis is, unusual alterations in behavior, perception, affect, and cognition can be achieved by means of it.

Chapter 3
Theorizing About Hypnosis: Recent Breakthroughs Shed New Light

Visiting Ernest (Jack) Hilgard's Stanford Laboratory of Hypnosis Research, Milton Erickson demonstrated classic hypnotic dissociation with a highly hypnotizable student volunteer. The student, already hypnotized [by Professor Hilgard], was asked by Erickson to hold up his right arm, straight from the shoulder. Holding gently the upraised hand, Erickson explained that he was lowering the upraised hand and arm. Upon letting go of the still upraised hand, he touched the student's lap, as if still holding it, to indicate that the hand was now resting there. To validate the subject was hallucinating the hand on his lap, Erickson encouraged him to place his left hand over his right hand on his lap and to hold it there. Once the subject accomplished this, Erickson, using his fingernails, pinched the hand of the upright arm with great intensity. Then, observing no apparent response to the painful pinch, he immediately, yet calmly, inquired as to whether the subject had just felt anything. With no mention of anesthesia, or any mention of expected performance, the subject casually reported he felt nothing. Indeed, how could he feel something in the hand that was, as he knew it, somewhere else. (E. Hilgard, personal communication to Arreed Barabasz, August 16, 1991.)

This fascinating demonstration of hypnotically produced dissociation (ca. 1960) was repeated by Hilgard and his colleagues with dozens of students who tested high on the Stanford Hypnotic Susceptibility Scale. This, in combination with other examples of dissociation dating back to Pierre Janet (1889), served as the basis for E. Hilgard's (1977) neodissociation theory of hypnosis. Numerous experiments, based on Hilgard's theory, were conducted using hypnosis for pain relief at Stanford in the 1960s to 1979. The findings are now in widespread use for the benefit of our patients in treatment for conditions in which pain is prominent, when an alternative to dependence on chemical analgesics is preferred, or when hypnosis is used adjunctively in combination with analgesic medications. (we discuss Hilgard's theory in greater detail later in this chapter).

Theories are, by their nature, oversimplifications. In a sense, the more simplified a theory can be elucidated, the more useful (and perhaps more likely to be used) it becomes as a decision guide to practitioner scientists and research scientists. Both groups can draw on a stated theory to conceptualize their clinical treatment plans or experiments, and then test them for effects. Psychotherapists are better equipped in their work when they recognize that all clinical interventions are, in essence, mini experiments. As a basis for the intervention, a theory, if useful, predicts the outcome with reasonable reliability. A theory is not necessarily true or false. The usefulness of a theory then depends on whether its predictions are borne out and whether treatment outcomes can be controlled when it is applied. The theory that most succinctly provides an explanation of a phenomenon, which can also be applied to real life treatments for our patients, therefore, becomes the best science can offer practice.

Anyone curious about psychopathology, psychotherapy, psychology, or many aspects of medicine will find the study of theories and applications of hypnosis compelling. Behaviors such as analgesia, controlled hallucinations, age regression, amnesia, and trance logic can be elicited by hypnosis in less than an hour. As Kihlstrom (1987, p. 1449) explains, hypnosis can produce "experiences involving alterations in phenomenal awareness, memory, and actions." How many other situations can you think of in which all of these behaviors can be elicited in those that have the abilities to create them? Accordingly, it is not surprising that a number of theories have been proposed to explain hypnosis. Most are merely descriptive; some only deal with a single aspect of the modality. A few try to account for hypnotic phenomena by relating them to other psychological concepts that are already in use. Hypnosis, derived from the Greek word *hypnos* meaning "to sleep," is a misleading metaphor in itself, given that it is long established as a scientific fact that hypnosis is not nocturnal sleep as defined by EEG brain waves (reviewed by Evans, 1979). William Coe (1992), citing the use of the term *hypnosis* by different groups and different theorists to mean different things, went so far to say that hypnosis is indefinable. Perry (1992) pointed out cogently, "Regardless of whether this is true, the existence of competing interest groups does not warrant a wholesale rejection of the term, anymore than the existence of competing religious groups implies that there is no such thing as religion." On August 7, 2003, the executive council of Division 30 of the American Psychological Association voted unanimously in favor of a new official definition of hypnosis (Green, Barabasz, Barrett & Montgomery, in press). It reflects recent research that stimulated new ways of thinking about hypnosis. I (A.F.B.) was honored to chair the definition committee and to serve as president of the division. The executive council at the time of the unanimous vote had prominent members from divergent theoretical positions.

The new definition still lacks of an explanation of a hypnotic trance that is satisfactory to all serious workers in the field, but this shortcoming does not deny existence of the phenomenon. We still lack an adequate definition of *personality* despite decades of wrestling with the concept. Knowledge and research on sleep and dreams was enhanced by the discovery of rapid eye movement sleep and the EEG stages of sleep, but we did not deny the reality of nocturnal sleep or dreams prior to these advances (E. Hilgard, 1992). Until the recent breakthroughs and discoveries of physiological markers of hypnosis (e.g., see A. Barabasz, 2000, 2001b; A. Barabasz et al., 1999; Kosslyn, Thomas, Constantini-Ferrando, Alpert, & Spiegel, 2000; Rainville, Hofbauer, et al., 1999) the study of hypnosis was very much the same as the study of sleep years earlier. So, why should there be such concern about a precise explanation of the trance phenomenon and such a quest for absolute certainty about what we are studying?

The expectation for complete information leaves one immobilized by indecision. In one *Star Trek* episode, Captain Kirk, for whatever reason, had lost his communicator, thus leaving him stranded on a strange planet and unable to return to the starship *Enterprise*. The *Enterprise* then comes under attack from (you guessed it) Klingons. Spock takes command. Spock obtains information on the location of the enemy but is unable to act because the data is incomplete. Time to act has nearly run out. Captain Kirk then returns and, of course, saves the day because he can act without complete information. The episode's writer misunderstood both Spock and rationality. Certainly Spock, as the supremely rational being, would not have been immobilized but would have taken the course of action that would have the highest probability of benefit to the *Enterprise* and crew based on the incomplete information available. If absolute certainty was essential to make a decision (draw a conclusion, develop a treatment plan) few decisions could ever be made by rational beings. As is the case with most decisions, one must select a single theoretical position explaining hypnosis from those theoretical positions available at the time. The decision is based on the incomplete information available without knowing with absolute certainty whether it is correct.

Alternative conceptualizations have led to conflict between those who adopt the generally accepted (for a review, see E. Hilgard, 1992) view of hypnosis and those who adopt an opposing standpoint. The primary view sees hypnosis as a distinct psychological state characterized by focused attention allowing one to dissociate perceptions and sensations, to attend with intensity and precision to thoughts and events, and to rally innate resources in unusual ways (A. Barabasz, 2000, 2001b; A. Barabasz & Barabasz, 2002; A. Barabasz & Lonsdale, 1983; A. Barabasz et al., 1999; Fromm, 1992; E. Hilgard, 1965, 1977; E. Hilgard & Hilgard, 1975; Kihlstrom, 1987, 1997; D. Spiegel, 1991b; D. Spiegel & A. Barabasz, 1987, 1988; H. Spiegel & D. Spiegel, 2004; J. Watkins & Johnson, 1982; J. Watkins & Watkins, 1979-80). Those who accept the state conceptualization of hypnosis may or may not embrace "hypnotic trance," but they recognize that the major hypnotic phenomena have been established well enough by controlled experiments and clinical practice to provide investigatory avenues in psychology and medicine. The state conceptualization explains (perhaps incompletely) the demonstrated utility of hypnosis in a variety of psychological and medical practices. Those with psychodynamic orientations accept hypnosis as an altered state of consciousness. Erika Fromm (personal communication to E. R. Hilgard, January 23, 1991) saw hypnosis as an altered state of consciousness into which people go if they have the talent to do so: They experience heightened ego receptivity and ego activity, attention changes, more primary process thinking, more imagery, dissociative phenomenon, regression in service of ego, and a fading of the generalized reality orientation. Fromm saw hypnosis as an altered state of consciousness in which the repressed returns more easily.

Sigmund Freud (see J. Watkins, 1987) was intrigued with hypnosis with his observation of Breuer's use of hypnotic abreactions in the treatment of hysteria. Freud's period of using the modality occurred before he developed his understanding of the dynamic processes involved in interpersonal relationships. Hypnosis was a medium he did not understand (his induction techniques were inept) and could not master. He was faced with reactions from his patients he was not then able to handle. He abandoned its use. Freud did make efforts to understand the phenomenon. He apparently linked hypnosis with hysteria, as had Jean Martin Charcot and

Janet. Thus, he concluded that evocation of the hypnotic state facilitates the discovery of painful aspects of repressed character underlying hysterical phenomena. This conception about hypnosis, first promulgated by Freud and later emphasized by Anna Freud (1946), has been most instrumental in turning psychoanalysts away from using it. Sigmund Freud (1938, p. 27) reported

> on an experiment, which showed me in the coldest light, what I have long suspected. One of my most acquiescent patients, with whom hypnotism had enabled me to bring about the most marvelous results, and with whom I was engaged in relieving her suffering by tracing back her attacks of pain to their origins, she woke up on one occasion, threw her arms around my neck. The unexpected entrance of a servant relieved us from discussion. From that time onwards there was a tacit understanding between us that hypnotic treatment should be discontinued.

Freud conjectured that hypnosis obliterated the ego and made it impossible for the integration of unconscious material to be uncovered during its use. This progress impeding conception was shown to be an error (Gill & Brenman, 1959) and is no longer held by those analysts who are knowledgeable and experienced with hypnosis. However, the notion was very close to theories that view the hypnotic state, at least in part, as a special relationship or transference. In fact, Sigmund Freud (1922) stated, "From being in love to hypnosis is evidently only a short step."

Hypnosis as an Interpersonal Relationship

Ferenczi (1926) specifically depicted hypnosis as a form of transference, describing it as a parent-child relationship. He went on to delineate two different types of hypnoses, which he called "father hypnosis" and "mother hypnosis." The first hypnosis exemplified that kind of relationship exhibited during authoritarian hypnosis where the therapist dominates his or her participant. This was related to the typical German family of that time, wherein the father exercised a commanding power over his wife and children. The second hypnosis was a typical form used in clinical treatment, where the practitioner maintains a more gentle and persuasive attitude, using a soft voice to lull the participant into a trance state, and where the therapeutic suggestions are couched in a diplomatic manner — the way Victorian mothers were reputed to handle their children. Viewed from this standpoint, hypnosis becomes a special type of state or relationship that facilitates the responsiveness to suggestions in hypnosis. Perhaps the conceptualization of mother hypnosis was the first recognition that hypnotic trance could be brought into treatment without the need for a formalized induction ritual.

J. Watkins (1954) at one time attempted to equate the hypnotic state with transference, but later (1963) modified this stance and maintained, rather, that hypnosis was much more than transference. He explained the phenomenon by elucidating that transference needs in the hypnotic individual and countertransference motivations in the therapist determined whether a hypnotic state could be induced easily, with difficulty, or not at all, and whether that state was light or deep.

Kline (1958) also recognized the interdependence of the hypnotic state on the quality and intensity of the interpersonal relationship between therapist and participant. Thus, he concluded that there is no constancy of itself in the hypnotic relationship, but there is constancy to the hypnotic trance state. The trance state was seen as a very basic and fundamental reorientation in perceptual and object relationships. Kline brought to light the point that hypnosis is not a unitary "something" or "either-or." It exists quantitatively to different degrees and in different depths, and qualitatively in different forms depending on the nature of the unique relationship between the two parties before the induction, during the induction, and during nonhypnotic therapeutic interventions. We can conclude from this that the state of hypnosis induced in Participant A by therapist B is not the same as that induced in the same person by therapist C, that it is not the same in Participants A and D when both are induced by therapist B, and that it is not the same in Participant A when induced by therapist B at one time and at another time. The differences in each of these cases are quantitative and qualitative in nature. The hypnotic state should, therefore, not be regarded simply as a unitary state without considering the relationship in which it occurs.

Adequate rapport, the special kind of relationship, accounts for the fact that many individuals may become more hypnotizable after they are better acquainted with the therapist, whereas at other times they may be responsive to strangers onto whom they can project unrealistic transference feelings. It also explains the observation made by experienced practitioners that many research studies showing negative results with hypnosis are often conducted by insensitive investigators who are more knowledgeable in the intricacies of experimental design than they are experienced in the subtle interpersonal relationships involved in working with hypnosis. As J. Watkins (1987) noted, such experimenters crudely read off standardized instructions, secure perhaps some degree of relaxation, and then conclude that the hypnotic phenomena are not "real" but merely role-playing. It is considerably more likely that these folks never succeeded in activating a genuine hypnotic state. Recent findings support this hypothesis (Barabasz et al., 2003; Barabasz and Christensen, submitted).

A. Barabasz and Barabasz's (2002) invited address at the annual convention of the American Psychological Association cited numerous studies coming from the sociocognitivists where nothing more than a superficial induction was employed, and then no attempts whatsoever were made to ensure any depth of hypnosis had been achieved at all before exposing the participants to demanding test suggestions that, consistent with the expectations of the sociocognitive experimenter, were doomed to failure.

We believe that the recent data demonstrates the hypnotic state can be shown as an essentially pure psychological state with replicable neural correlates. The simple fact is that the sensory alterations experienced by the person in hypnosis are accompanied by task-related brain function changes whether or not a hypnosis-related brain region lights up every time. We also opine that the clinical application of hypnosis is incomplete if we do not endeavor to also recognize that the human interpersonal factor is always the prerequisite essential part.

The Hypnotic State as Regression in the Service of the Ego

The famous Menninger Clinic analysts Gill and Brenman (1959) conceptualized the hypnotic state as a temporary and nonmalignant kind of regression. They characterized it as a "regression in service of ego." This was contrasted with "regression proper." Essentially, the concept is that the ego engages primary process in its service to make use of it for the purposes at hand. Of course, primary processes are primitive both cognitively and behaviorally, characteristic of the experience of a small child. Operating in the realm of primary process, ideas are simply accepted at face value and need not be integrated within a broader matrix of meaning. In classic psychoanalytic theory, primary process characterizes the "id" wherein two opposing concepts can reside yet not contact each other or struggle for resolution. As reconceptualized by Orne (1979) in his concept of hypnosis as "trance logic," primary-process thinking does not follow the principles of Aristotelian logic. The psychopath who groups a sink stopper and a cigarette together in an object assembly test, not because they are both round but because he once saw a man who "was smoking a cigarette while he was fixing a sink," is functioning at the level of primary-process logic. Functioning at the primary-process level will not solve mathematical equations, but it may be an open door to creativity. When regression takes place in the service of the ego, it is possible for the strong ego to relinquish its need for full integration and to simply "enjoy" the childhood play of a regression to primary processes.

The concept of hypnosis as an altered state of consciousness was viewed by Gill and Brenman as a state of altered ego functioning that was elicited by transference; that is, the ability of the hypnotized individual to regress into a more passive and childlike state in which the relationship with the therapist changes the nature of the participant's functioning so that it involves a greater degree of primary-process thinking and behavior. This change, however, unlike that of the psychopath, is temporary and can be reversed at the will of the participant's ego, hence, is voluntary in nature. Michael Nash (1992), editor of the *International Journal of Clinical and Experimental Hypnosis* from 1998 to 2002, shed considerable light on the similarities and differences between hypnosis, psychopathology, and psychological regression. Those wishing to explore this aspect more thoroughly are referred to Nash's 1992 chapter in which he critically examines in what sense there is and in what sense there is not a shared process underlying hypnosis and psychopathology. He explored temporal regression, topographic regression, and hypnosis as a division of consciousness. In 1959, Gill and Brenman characterized regression in the service of the ego as (a) more likely to occur as the ego becomes more adaptive and less likely to occur as the ego grows less adaptive; (b) marked by a definable beginning and end; (c) reversible, with a rapid and full reinstatement of normal organization of the psyche; (d) terminable under urgent conditions by the unaided participant; (e) occurring only when the participant judges the circumstances to be safe; and (f) voluntarily sought by the participant and is in contrast to "regression proper," which is an active rather than passive regression.

Only the notion of reversibility with total reinstatement of normal neuronal organization of the psyche has been subjected to the rigors of controlled scientific experimentation. On the basis of Gill and Brenman's conceptualizations, Reyher (1964) reasoned that hypnosis and sensory restriction are manifestations of the ascendance of lower levels of neuronal integration in the organization of brain functions and behavioral regulation. Conditions that restrict or homogenize sensory input prevent adaptive behavior with adaptive neuronal integration. Regression to primary process involves the replacement of fully adapted neuronal integration by a phylogenetically older and lower level of integration. Removal from restricted environmental stimulation should then reactivate higher neuronal integration.

Men isolated by winter in Antarctica became significantly more hypnotizable (A. Barabasz, 1979, 1980c). Inspired by these findings, obtained under field conditions with a crude measure of hypnotizability, a controlled laboratory experiment was devised (A. Barabasz, 1982) to test Reyher's theory directly. Restricted environmental stimulation (REST) procedures were used with ten subjects. The *Stanford Hypnotic Clinical Scale: Adult* (A. Morgan & J. Hilgard, 1978-1979) was modified to include a posthypnotic suggestion for an analgesic reaction, then ferodic shock was used to determine pain threshold and tolerance levels prior to REST, immediately after REST before removal from the REST environment, and 10 to 14 days later. To mask the hypnotic focus of the study and to obtain physiological data — for example, skin conductance — researchers collected peripheral, core, and chamber temperature data during 6 hours of REST. Researchers used a control group to assess the effects of repeated hypnosis on hypnotizability scores and any potential effects of social influence and context of the experiment.

Multivariate analysis of variance results showed hypnotizability and pain tolerance scores to be significantly enhanced only for participants exposed to REST immediately after REST and 10 to 14 days later. The maintenance of the enhanced hypnotizability and pain tolerance at follow-up failed to support Reyher's (1964) theory of brain function and this single feature of the concept of regression in the service of the ego. The qualitative, independent postexperiment inquiry findings were revealing. Apparently, sensory restriction forced the organism to focus, perhaps as seldom before, on internally generated imaginal activity. This defensive maneuver might better be conceptualized as a dissociative reaction, which serves to maintain neuronal integration in the organization of brain functions.

J. Hilgard (1974, 1979) found imaginative involvement and strict childhood discipline to be positively related to high hypnotizability, which could not be explained by conformity behavior. Apparently, the child learned to mitigate the effectiveness of punishment through the imaginative involvement of practiced dissociation. Perhaps in the A. Barabasz (1982) study, and its replication (M. Barabasz, Barabasz, Darakjy-Jaeger, & Warner, 2001), participants learned to develop imaginative involvements in REST as a mechanism of coping with the reduced external stimulation. Consistent with J. Hilgard's findings, these skills, once acquired, may account for the higher levels of hypnotizability found after REST and the maintenance of this ability over time. The data seemed to be more cogently explained by E. Hilgard's (1977) neo-dissociation theory of hypnosis rather than regression in the service of the ego. However, it seems important to note those experiments disproved only one aspect of Gill and Brenman's conceptualization of hypnosis as regression in the service of the ego. In any event, both theoretical explanations are consistent with the overall state conceptualization of hypnosis in contrast to the social influence and role-playing explanation.

Meares's Concept of Regression in Hypnosis

Meares (1961) also viewed hypnosis as a regression, but he differed from the Gill and Brenman point of view in that he focused not on regressed behavior but rather on regressed mental functioning as included in the concepts of Reyher (1964) and addressed, in part, by our experimentally controlled laboratory experiments (A. Barabasz, 1982; A. Barabasz et al., 2003). Meares saw the hypnotized person, especially the deeply hypnotized one, as one who thinks and functions at a primitive level much like that which must have characterized humans during their phylogenetic development from animal to primitive man. Meares held that in this early stage the process of hypnosis must, in some way, have determined the acceptance of ideas, hence intellectual functioning was at an archaic level. Logical thought in man developed later. Meares explained that it is precisely this logical thought that is set aside during the regression into the hypnotic state. J. Watkins (1987) explained this atavistic regression coincides closely with Kline's (1966) "lowering of criticality" as a central feature of hypnosis.

Hypnosis as Superego Modification or Reparenting

Kubie and Margolin (1944) emphasized the mechanism of identification in their psychoanalytic theory of hypnosis. The state of hypnosis and the hypnotic induction are carefully distinguished. They emphasize that the induction involves a gradual elimination of normal sensorimotor relationships as environmental stimulation is restricted. The hypnotic state is viewed as evolving from the obliteration of all channels of communication with the outer world except one, that with the therapist. Through monotony and immobilization (eye fixation, etc.) the participant withdraws all attention from exteroreceptive stimuli, except those presented by the therapist. Once the hypnotic state is fully established in the participant, the participant's ego once more expands to contact the outer world. This time, however, "his or her own ego" is changed by its incorporation of the therapist within it. The image (voice, behavior, etc.) of the therapist is now fused with the previously incorporated images of parents. This allows the replacement or modification of the superego. The voice of the therapist is like the voice of the parent within and is obeyed as such. Hypnosis, then, is viewed as becoming an experiential reproduction of the natural developmental process that represents the early parent-child relationship. Kubie and Margolin emphasized that hypnosis may be necessary, perhaps essential, in any psychotherapy that aspires to replace the authority of early critical superego figures with a more benevolent reparenting.

As in the work of Brenman and Gill, Kubie and Margolin's work incorporated the concept of regression as predominant. However, unlike Brenman and Gill, who conceived of it as a regression to an early state of thinking and behavior, Kubie and Margolin perceived it as regression to the earliest child-parent relationship. Because Kubie and Margolin incorporated identification with the therapist by the participant, this accounts for the fact that the participant experiences and carries out the therapist's suggestions as if he or she were ego-syntonic; that is, originating within the participant's own self.

Object Cathexes: Hypnosis as a Modality for Ego Manipulation

Paul Federn (1952), a close associate of Freud's, formulated a theory of personality structure that was never well understood by psychoanalysts or other psychologists, perhaps partly because of his difficulty in clearly expressing his views. Although Federn's theories were aimed not specifically at hypnosis but rather at the general structure and functioning of the ego, they appear to be especially relevant. He held that the essence of self was an energy that he called "ego cathexis." Any physiological or mental process invested with this energy was experienced as belonging to "me." Hence, "my" hand is experienced as part of me because it contains ego cathexis. The same would be true of "my" thought. This ego energy is "the self" and is distinguished from "object" cathexis, a kind of nonself energy that can also activate various physiological and psychological processes. If my arm is invested only with object cathexis, I experience it as not part of me, as if it were a board simply attached to my shoulder or as it would be sensed if it had been hypnotically anesthetized and made immobile. It has no feeling and appears to be detached from the body ego. My arm is no longer "me" but has become "it."

According to Federn's theory, "me" or "it" depends on whether an item (either physical or mental) is "cathected" with ego energy or object energy. Thus, an idea that breaks out of repression into the ego without being invested with ego energy is experienced as an object, as "not me." In the schizophrenic such an idea (e.g., the thought of his dead mother) breaks into consciousness without being invested with ego cathexis. Accordingly, it is experienced as a hallucination, as if it had originated in an object outside the self. The schizophrenic experiences this as if he were "seeing" his dead mother, not "thinking" about her.

Federn did not write much about hypnosis per se. However, when through hypnosis we resolve an amnesia, initiate or remove a paralyzed limb, lift a repression, or inculcate within a participant suggestions that are acted on as if they were his or her own ideas, we are definitely manipulating object and ego energies as these have been defined by Federn. From his ego-psychology viewpoint, hypnosis becomes a modality for the manipulation of cathexis, a way of reversing subject and object either in parts of the body or in ideas and perceptions.

Federn further delineated ego structure by hypothesizing that it is normally divided into states. Each ego state represents a body of self behaviors and experiences bound together by a common principle and separated by a boundary from other states that have been integrated about other factors. Thus, Ego-State A may represent those behaviors and experiences that are united by the common factor of having occurred when the participant was in the first grade. Ego-State B may represent a similar set of items that are included within the concept of relationship to parent figures. Ego states may be large or small. Another way to think about ego states might be similar to the setup of the United States, which includes states, counties, cities, school districts, and national forests, each organized around a central concept, including a set of items bound by a common jurisdiction and separated by a boundary from other states.

J. Watkins (1978) modified and extended Federn's concepts to provide the rationale for a manner of psychotherapy, which can be hypnotic or nonhypnotic. He conceived of normal personality structure as being organized into ego states because of the economy of jurisdiction, such as leaving to the federal authority the interaction of the entire nation with other countries, whereas specific responsibilities are left to local jurisdictions. Within the personality at any given time, one state is usually "executive." It constitutes the "self" in the "now." It includes those behaviors and experiences that are currently being activated and that are being felt or acted on. At that time, the executive state is the one most highly energized with ego cathexis. Other states, separated by a boundary from the executive state, are for the moment relatively immobilized. Their impact on the entire individual is "unconscious." For example, when individuals are at a party one state is executive and one set of behaviors and experiences is operative. When they are at work the next day the party state has ceased to be executive and is replaced by another. One behaves and experiences differently. Likewise, a hypnotized person is in a different state, so a different set of behaviors and experiences are activated. Hypnosis, by its ability to manipulate cathexis, can deactivate a present state and make another executive, just as in regression to an early age participants are induced to relive their earlier experiences and repress present awareness.

The boundaries between ego states vary in permeability from person to person and probably within a single individual from time to time. At one end of the continuum there is almost complete communication between elements in different states. The boundaries are permeable, and the federal jurisdiction over all the person makes him or her highly integrated. At the other end are the true multiple personalities (dissociative identity disorders), wherein the boundaries between the respective states are so rigid and impermeable that "Mary" is completely unaware of the existence of "Joan," and when one is executive, it is amnesic to the period during which the other was activated. Most people lie somewhere in between. There is also partial dissociation, and there are many latent multiple personalities. Such an ego state or covert multiple personality might account for Hilgard's "hidden observer." E. Hilgard and Hilgard (1975) wrote, "It does not mean that there is some sort of secondary personality with a life of its own — a kind of homunculus lurking in the shadows of the conscious person." The hidden observer is merely a convenient label for the information source tapped through experiments with automatic writing and automatic talking. They apparently did not attempt to rule out the possibility that this hidden observer might be an ego state or a latent multiple personality.

J. Watkins and H. Watkins (1979–1980) extended Hilgard's inquiry to a number of hidden observers located in a good hypnotic participant by the responses to such questions as "What is your name?" "Where do you come from?" "How long have you been in the person?" "Under what circumstances were you born?" "What is your function within George?" and so on. They found that these entities described themselves as having identity, content, and specific functions within the psychological economy of the entire individual and could often indicate their origins — sometimes related to traumatic events. In other words, they acted like "covert multiple personalities." Further exploration of the hidden observer phenomena would seem to have significant implications for personality theory.

Federn's ego-state theories appear to parallel and to predict the kind of findings reported by Hilgard except that they are couched in a psychoanalytic rather than a behavioral terminology. If this is true, cognitive control systems and ego states are simply two names for the same phenomena, hence, dissociated parts of the ego. If hypnosis is to be considered as a modality for the manipulation of cathexes, then it has the ability to change subject to object and vice versa; that is, it can be used to change part(s) of "me" into an "it" and back again. Psychoanalysts have used the term *introjection* to represent the internalization of an object. However, once it has been internalized they then treat it as if it is now part of the self. Kubie and Margolin do that when they speak of the "incorporation" of the therapist into the participant's ego.

There has been great confusion in many psychoanalytic writings because of failure to distinguish between subject and object. An "introject" can be compared to an internalized objectlike piece of undigested food within the stomach. It is within the person but not a part of him or her. Once food has been metabolized, assimilated, and incorporated into the protoplasmic structure of the individual it is no longer an object but truly part of the physical "me." This is analogous to identification wherein a mental object is incorporated into the self. Federn clearly distinguishes between subject and object in that a mental object is activated only by object cathexis. When this has been replaced by ego or self energy, the previous "object" has now become "subject." Identification has taken place.

The use of the word *identification* represents a process and the entity created by that process is confusing. Because there is no noun term that represents the entity created by the process of identification in the same way that *introject* is the entity created by the process of introjection, J. Watkins and Watkins (1981) proposed the term *identofact*. Through identification (the investment of an internalized object with ego cathexis) the object has been changed into subject and is now termed an identofact. This distinction is important in understanding various hypnotic manipulations. Hypnosis makes it possible for us to change introjects into identofacts and vice versa. Kubie and Margolin spoke of the incorporation of the therapist into the ego of the participant so that the voice of the therapist now becomes the thoughts of the participant and is experienced as such. This means that an initial introjection during the induction process is followed by a change of that introject into an identofact through its investment with ego or self energy. This is accomplished through modified attention, concentration, and the directing of ego energies within the hypnotic relationship.

J. Watkins and H. Watkins (1997) developed a therapeutic approach that they called "ego-state therapy" based on the concept that anxiety is caused by inner conflict between different ego states. Both with and without hypnosis they activate the different component states of the conflict in turn (make executive), ascertain the role each plays in the "family" of ego states, and attempt to resolve the conflict. Ego-state therapy involves the application of group and family therapy techniques to the treatment of conflict within the "family of ego states" that constitutes a single person.

Trance Logic as the Essence of Hypnosis

Orne (1959, 1979) held that the essence of hypnosis, and that which distinguishes truly hypnotized individuals from simulators, is the ability of hypnotized participants to freely mix perceptions derived from reality with those that stem from this imagination. This characteristic of tolerance of logical inconsistencies Orne termed *trance logic*. Trance logic might be manifested as follows. Truly and deeply hypnotized participants ("reals") are given the hallucination that they will see a certain friend sitting in a chair in front of them. The participant is then brought out of trance. The participants see their "friend" and may engage in conversation with the friend. The participants are then asked to look behind where the real friend is seated and are asked, "Well, then, who is this?" The real participants demonstrate logical inconsistency or trance logic by indicating that the real friend and the hallucinated image are seen. Participants who are faking or simulating hypnosis, having already reported seeing the hallucinated image, tend to deny seeing the real friend. They feel the need to demonstrate logical consistency.

Trance logic is closely related to the concrete thinking or primary process that characterizes the reasoning of psychotics, dissociative reactions, primitive peoples, and children (see Kasanin, 1944). Whether or not trance logic represents the essence of hypnosis, there is substantial evidence (Sheehan, 1977) that it is a significant factor in assessing true hypnotic behavior in contrast to behaviors that are merely obtained by suggestion alone or role-playing.

An Ego-Psychological Theory of Hypnosis

Erika Fromm's (1992) theory is based, to a great extent, on concepts developed in classical and neoclassical psychoanalysis. She noted, foremost, that hypnosis is an altered state of consciousness, a state different from the waking state. Until about 1885, psychology acknowledged only two states: the waking state and the state of sleep. The waking state was defined as one in which we operate with consciousness. Sleep was considered to be a non-consciousness state and, therefore, not worth exploring. Then, at the turn of the century, Freud (1900-1953) made his great discovery: the unconscious. He identified three mental states: the conscious (that which at a given moment is in full waking awareness), the preconscious (that which is not in full awareness but can be brought into consciousness by simply turning one's attention to it), and the unconscious (those mental contents, memories, fantasies, thoughts, and affects that resist being brought into consciousness). He conceived of dreams as a special state of consciousness of great significance; namely, as "the royal road to unconscious activities of the mind" (Freud, 1900-1953, p. 608). Fromm contended that dreams are clearly not the only royal road to the unconscious. Hypnosis is another. Consistent with neodissociation conceptualizations of hypnosis, in general, Fromm highlighted William James's (1890, 1935, p. 298) first research on altered states of consciousness where James emphasized that our normal waking consciousness is but one type of consciousness and that parted from it by the flimsiest of screens lie potential forms of consciousness entirely different. James emphasized that we may go through life without suspecting their existence, but in the presence of an appropriate stimulus they are, in all their completeness, definite types of mentality that are discontinuous with ordinary consciousness.

Fromm also recognized that as a cognitive-perceptual state that is different from the waking state, it has its own felt reality. She embraced an involuntaryism or nonconscious involvement as elucidated by Shor (1979). Simplifying the concept further, she noted that the individual might recognize the hypnotically altered state of consciousness as being "different from the waking state." However, subjectively, very vividly altered states do not necessarily translate into overt behavior that is easily measurable or observable by an outside observer (Fromm, 1979; Shor, 1979). Given these antecedents to her ego-psychological theory of hypnosis, Fromm (1992) contended that hypnosis does not circumvent the ego. Rather quite the contrary; the hypnotic individual can hear, see, and smell and can produce imagery, thoughts, and even defenses. All of these are, of course, ego functions.

Fromm viewed E. Hilgard's (1977) model of hypnotic consciousness as a horizontal one in which all subsystems are on the same level. Rather than conceptualizing hypnosis as a neodissociation process, she (Fromm, 1965, 1976) interpreted the dissociation process that takes place with such great ease in the hypnotic state as a dissociation of the experiencing ego from the observing ego. Her psychoanalytic model of consciousness, preconscious, and unconscious awareness in trance, then, is a vertical one in which, as in psychoanalytic theory, the unconscious, the preconscious, and the conscious are viewed as mental states arranged in an ascending order (Gill & Brenman, 1959).

Fromm (1977, 1992) viewed hypnosis as an adaptive regression consistent with regression in the service of the ego. She saw the hypnotic state as one that causes an ego-modulated relaxation of defensive barriers, allowing a return to earlier, less realistic, primary-process thinking. She emphasized that this is also temporary and limited to the time of relatively deep hypnotic trance. The major point is that Fromm viewed regression in the service of the ego as healthy. She noted that letting go of one's usual controls and going backward a step on the developmental ladder to be able to take steps forward is indeed the definition of "regression in the service of the ego" or, as Hartmann (1939/1958) called it, "adaptive regression."

Fromm (personal communication, August 11, 2002) explained that this should all be quite obvious that, for example, a person suffering from a cold might well curl up in bed "just like a child," watching hours of senseless lightweight TV programs, letting himself or herself simply be taken care of by others. This regression helps the person to get well, healthy, and independent once again more quickly. She further likened the activity to taking a vacation in which one engages in entertainment, napping, or reading nondemanding materials. Clearly, these regressions in the service of the ego are nonpathological and healthy. Fromm emphasized that secondary-process thinking occurs in words and in sentences rather than in imagery. It is a result of the impact of reality and is, therefore, reality oriented and goal directed thereby operating by logically ordered practical or abstract concepts. It is the dominant everyday cognitive mode of the normal adult. When primary process occurs spontaneously in the healthy adult, it represents an input from the drives or from the unconscious ego, both of which can enrich waking logic and otherwise ordinary modes of thought. Fromm emphasized that primary-process thinking is not given up when secondary-process thinking is in operation. The point is that our thoughts are hardly ever devoid of some minor form of imagery and even in the very deepest stages of trance or perhaps even in nocturnal dreaming there always remain elements of realism and logic. There is simply no sharp line of distinction separating one from the other. Healthy primary processes are particularly characteristic of intuitive thought and creativity,[1] whereas pathological primary processes are schizophrenic hallucinations and psychotic thinking. In the psychotic, primary process overwhelms the secondary-process logic and reality orientation. Neither primary-process nor secondary-process energy can be invested in imagery.

Consistent with E. Hilgard's (1977) neodissociation conceptualization and the plethora of other state-oriented theorists, Fromm's argument convincingly states that the state of hypnosis is anything but the "special process" proposed by Spanos (1982). Individuals in the waking state are mainly reality oriented and at the secondary-process level. The balance shifts toward the primary-process pole of mental functioning when one enters a state of hypnosis. Waking trance, then, is a form of primary-process imagery in which the individual is fascinated and in some depth of hypnosis while apparently wakeful. Fromm also differentiated between concentrated or focused attention in one instance and expansive or free-floating attention in another (Fromm, 1979). She saw that attention, absorption (Tellegen & Atkinson, 1974), and the general reality orientation (Shor, 1959/1969) are also important parts of the hypnotic state. Although originating from cognitive psychology, Fromm saw both attention and absorption as representations of ego functions. As persons' capacities for absorption are realized when they enter the hypnotic state, the general reality orientation fades into the background of awareness. Attention is a cognitive process, and cognition is a function of ego. Absorption is a product of ego receptivity and concentrated attention.

During the 1980s, Fromm and her colleagues at the University of Chicago focused their attention on the identification of structural variables that characterize the state of hypnosis (Fromm, 1981, 1988; Fromm & Kahn, 1990). These variables include absorption (Tellegen, 1981), concentrative and expansive (free floating) attention (Fromm, 1969), ego activity, and receptivity. The general reality orientation (Shor, 1959/1969) fades into the background of awareness, as the individual enters the hypnotic state. The context of the hypnotic state may typically include increased imagery; hypermnesia; a wide variety of thoughts, emotions, hyperactive dreams, and self-suggestions of sensory; and motor phenomena (Fromm, 1988). The extent to which, these characteristics are experienced by individuals is dependent on trance depth.

Unlike the majority of other psychoanalytic authors, Fromm subjected a number of her hypotheses about hypnosis to experimentation. For example, to test whether hypnosis is regression in the service of the ego, a research team administered the Rorschach to 32 participants in waking and hypnotic states. The findings revealed that in hypnosis there was a significant increase in primary-process thinking. However, this increase was not uniformly reflected in increases in defense and coping functions that would be predicted by the psychoanalytic conceptualization.

Furthermore, they found that hypnosis had no effect on Holt's *Adaptive Regression Scale* scores (Holt, 1963). Predominately flexible and far-ranging ego activity and a higher level of coping mechanism activity characterized the hypnotic state. Uniquely, males produced significantly more primary process in the hypnotic state than in the waking state as compared with females (Fromm, Oberlander, & Gruenewald, 1970). The findings were replicated and extended by Levin and Harrison (1976), who used the *Thematic Apperception Test* and the Rorschach to induce dreams. They also found a significant increase in primary-process thinking in hypnosis, but again the participants did not universally demonstrate the increase of controls and defenses under hypnosis that should make it possible to adaptively use regression. Importantly, Levine and Harrison recognized that they may have failed to obtain full confirmation of adaptive regression because of the fact that the participants may have only been lightly hypnotized rather than at a level of adequately deep trance.

Research from our lab (A. Barabasz, 1982; A. Barabasz et al., 2003) disproved one of the six Gill and Brenman characteristics of regression in the service of the ego, whereas research from Fromm's lab and those replicating her work statistically isolated two relatively independent factors and experimentally found support for one but not the other. Fromm et al. (1970) showed that hypnotic trance significantly increased primary-process (childlike) mentation. However, contrary to the investigators expectations, hypnosis had no significant effect on adaptive regression, which was thought to involve going backward developmentally then making forward progress.

Given these data, Fromm did not relinquish the idea that hypnosis is a form of regression in the service of the ego but went on to conclude that the increase in primary process alone simply cannot be all that is needed to demonstrate adaptive regression. She insisted there must be a combination or balance of the two factors to constitute regression in the service of the ego (Fromm, 1992).

Perhaps Fromm's greatest contribution to our understanding is that her work disproves Freud's notion that hypnosis circumvents the ego. Hypnosis is better conceptualized as an altered state of consciousness in which the ego functions in a way that is quite different from the way in which it functions in the waking state. Although hypnotized individuals retain the capacity to observe and reflect, even to think and experience as they wish, these are all clearly ego functions. The deeply hypnotized individual, one in which the trance state has been actually accomplished, may hallucinate objects that cannot be so hallucinated in the reality-oriented secondary-process-based waking state. Hypnosis, to one degree or another, involves a shift toward primary process while retaining some aspects of secondary process. Rather than circumventing the ego, the hypnotized person shows greater ego receptivity than a person in the waking state. The person relaxes his or her vigilance and defenses while allowing internally generated stimuli (A. Barabasz, 1982) to become established at the hypnotic level of awareness.

The receptivity is clearly one of the most essential aspects of hypnosis and is frequently mislabeled *suggestibility*. Receptivity facilitated by hypnosis facilitates the freedom to allow unconscious fantasies, memories, thoughts, and affects to rise into awareness while in the hypnotic trance. The hypnotic state is characterized then by a greater intensity of affect than the waking state and the tendency to experience imagery as reality.

Fromm (personal communication, August 11, 2002) recognized that her theory of hypnosis does not include the all-important aspects of the transference relationship and its role in bringing about hypnotic trance, which is emphasized by the present authors.

The Neodissociation Theory of Hypnosis

During dissociation, certain behaviors and experiences seem to be split off from others. In psychoanalytic terms there is a division in the ego that separates it into two or more different states. If the dissociation is severe enough, we have multiple personalities (dissociative identity disorders) in which each of the entities is oblivious of the existence of the other. These two different personalities may take turns being "executive." Hence, during the period when Personality A is functioning, Personality B is dormant, asleep, or unconscious. When Personality B appears, it is amnesic to the period during which Personality A was active. These alternating multiple personalities had been observed by Janet (1889) and classified as a form of hysteria in his 1907 Harvard lectures. Janet recognized that dissociation need not be complete, as in the case of dissociative identity disorder, and he supported partial dissociation in the sense that dissociated ideas might still affect the emotional life of the patient (James, 1890).

Hilgard's attraction to dissociation first became apparent in the early years of his writing in his first book on hypnosis (Hilgard, 1965). Hilgard found the term *dissociation,* particularly *partial dissociation,* to be more useful than *regression* as an interpretation of hypnotic phenomena (pp. 392–393, 395–396). Well in advance of the upsurge of interest in multiple personality disorders (dissociative identity disorders), Hilgard's Stanford Laboratory of Hypnosis Research was involved in numerous experimental studies that revealed less pervasive types of dissociation, such as those found in routine hypnosis, as illustrated by the profound example given at the beginning of this chapter.

Hilgard's original focus on dissociation was entirely based on his interest in investigating the hypnotic relief of pain. These involved, primarily, the administration of hypnotic suggestions of analgesia in an arm that was placed in cold water. Apparent pain-free responses were elicited in which the participants evidenced no overt pain behaviors and reported that they did not feel pain. Such phenomena, of course, have been well documented since the time of Esdaile. However, when questioned under hypnosis as to whether there was "some part" of the person that experienced the pain, most participants responded affirmatively. Communication was established with this part by the automatic writing method, in which a hand is dissociated from the rest of the body and asked to write independently about the felt experience. Because of the slowness of this procedure the communication was shifted to "automatic talking" in which the voice is dissociated and speaks for this part independently and separately from the rest of the person.

The studies of E. Hilgard and Hilgard (1975) showed that although there was often little evidence of *overt* pain when analgesic suggestions had been hypnotically inculcated, the experience of pain and memories of it were being *covertly* recorded and could be reported by this part as a hidden observer. A typical classroom demonstration by E. Hilgard at Stanford University, and now in our own classes, might involve something like suggested deafness. It is after hypnotic induction has been successfully completed that it is suggested that the individuals may be hearing at some level whereupon when one tells them, even though hypnotically deaf, they might be hearing at some level and, if that was the case, to signal by lifting the index finger. Invariably the finger rises.

A similar experiment can be conducted using anesthetic suggestions after hypnosis has been successfully induced to cold pressor pain instead of hypnotically suggested deafness. This procedure involves hypnotically anesthetizing the hand and then placing it in circulating ice water. Even though participants consciously report no pain, a finger signal can be used to indicate that the pain was being experienced somewhere by some part of the participant. Hilgard's theory holds that this "something" was an underlying "cognitive structural system," which he termed "hidden observer" (E. Hilgard, 1977).

Hilgard regarded the hidden observer as merely a metaphor or convenient label for the information tapped, and not as a secondary personality with a life of its own. In contrast, J. Watkins and Watkins (1997) viewed the hidden observer as the same phenomena as ego states. Accordingly, J. Watkins and H. Watkins replicated parts of these studies for hypnotically induced deafness in hypnotically induced anesthesia to cold pressor pain, using his verbalizations for making the suggestions. For participants they used patients who had once been in ego-state therapy with Hellen Watkins and whose major ego states were already known to her. They then activated hidden observers using Hilgard's verbalization and then inquired about them further. They found different ego states, many of whom they had observed in therapy (J. Watkins & Watkins, 1979-1980).

Hilgard became more explicit and proposed that the human personality was divided into "cognitive control systems" and that the covert pain was, in these experiments of deafness, being recorded by a secondary cognitive control system that did not normally have communication either with the outside world or with other primary systems that had been hypnotized.

Hilgard hypothesized that this was a secondary cognitive control system separated by "barriers" from the primary one and from communication with the outside but that under hypnosis these barriers could be broken by the techniques of automatic writing or automatic talking, thus making it possible to verify the existence of covert pain in the absence of normal overt indicators.

Sutcliffe (1961), coming from the sociopsychological (social influence) explanation of hypnosis, accused Hilgard's participants of deluding themselves. If they achieved pain reduction but did not evidence the physiological indicants identical to those found through the use of local or general anesthetics, Sutcliffe saw them as deluded. Sutcliffe's logic is narrow, for pain is the feeling that something hurts, and less pain means that it hurts less. Physiological changes such as blood pressure, heart rate, or other concomitants of felt pain need not be alike for insensitivities to painful stimulation to be genuine. When the pain is gone, the hurt is gone, and the hidden observer phenomenon clearly explains these issues. J. Hilgard and Hilgard (1975, 1983) discussed physiological and psychoanalytic explanations for this phenomenon, ranging from consideration of the duality of right and left hemisphere action within the brain to "temporary partial structures within the ego" similar to multiple personalities. They suggested that the hypnotic suggestions could apparently "shift controls from one system to another" and propose that if these systems were more intensely investigated they would prove to represent "broader mechanisms than those applicable to only pain and suffering." Hypnotic procedures can then be employed to rearrange "the hierarchies of control over systems other than those involved in pain." Years later, D. Spiegel, Bierre, and Rootenberg (1989) tested the brain's reaction by means of event-related potentials (ERPs) (see A. Barabasz et al., 1999) and showed convincingly that hypnosis served to attenuate the brain's reaction to painful stimuli. Sutcliffe's (1961) assertion that pain reduction achieved by hypnosis was not supported by physiological indicants was disproved.

This line of thinking from E. Hilgard and Spiegel revived the theory of hypnosis as a kind of dissociation. This carries significant implications for a reappraisal of what constitutes normal personality structure and functioning. General Norman Schwarzkopf (1992) provided an interesting example in his post–Gulf War autobiography: "As I walked out the gate, I had the same odd sensation that I'd experienced for much of the afternoon: a dissociation from my actions. It was a kind of out-of-body experience, as though I stood watching at a safe remove while Schwarzkopf went back outside the perimeter at risk of being blown away. But there was nothing eerie or mystical about it. I was kind of on automatic pilot."

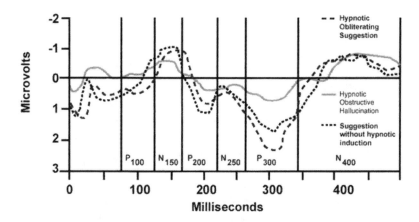

Fig. 3.1
EEG event-related potential (ERP) brain responses to alternate hypnotic suggestions for deafness in hypnosis and nonhypnotic conditions. (Data from Barabasz et al., 1999.) *Note:* Downward deflections indicate greater brain ERPs. In the hypnotic state, the demnd for complete deafness shows a strong retention, while an obstructive suggestion (ear plugs) attentuates the brain's response.

Hypnosis as Intense Focal Concentration

H. Spiegel and D. Spiegel (2004) emphasized, as do most theorists, that there is no absolute dividing line between nonhypnotic and hypnotic alterations in consciousness. Dissociated experiences where one's usual pan awareness of the surrounding world is suspended are naturally occurring. They include (a) daydreaming, (b) intense concentration in a work or play activity, (c) absorption in (a book or audio or video stimuli), (d) natural childbirth when pain is not experienced, (e) spontaneous fugue states involving waking activity without later conscious recall (see A. Barabasz, 1980), and (f) the intensity of two people who are in love with each other where they are so involved with each other that they are unaware of other people or counter cues around them. Spiegel and Spiegel agreed with the sociological notion that placebo effect occurs in response to a situational context (for the most comprehensive review of the complex placebo effect, see Shapiro & Morris, 1978). However, in sharp contrast to the sociopsychological conceptualization, Spiegel and Spiegel explained that placebo effect can be due to spontaneous trance states. Spontaneous hypnosis was first experimentally addressed by E. Hilgard and Tart (1966) and then revealed in a number of other studies (A. Barabasz, 1990a, 1990b, 1990c, 2000).

A quarter of a century ago, H. Spiegel and D. Spiegel (1978, pp. 22–34) conceptualized hypnosis as a psychophysiological state (we discuss numerous recent experimentally controlled studies supporting this position elsewhere in this chapter). The hypnotic state is characterized by the participant's ability to sustain a state of attention, receptive, intense focal concentration with diminished peripheral awareness. Rather than a form of relaxation, the hypnotic state occurs in an alert individual who has the capacity for intense involvement with a single point in space and time. Thus, the hypnotic state involves a contraction of awareness or involvement with other points in space and time. The intense focal attention necessitates the elimination of distracting or irrelevant stimuli, thereby creating a dialectic between focal and peripheral awareness. Individuals with the ability to enter hypnosis attend only to a given task while simultaneously freeing themselves from distractions. This special capacity for absorption has been supported by several research studies (A. Barabasz, 1980c, 1982, 1984a; M. Barabasz, Barabasz, & Mullin, 1983). The trait can be tested using a simple true-false scale developed by Tellegen and Atkinson (1974), who also showed that high hypnotizability was correlated with absorption.

To further elucidate the nature of the hypnotic trance phenomenon, H. Spiegel and Spiegel (2004) liken it to one's central visual field (macular vision capacity) that is but a small arc of 5° to 7°. Humans can see only a very small part of what surrounds us in detail, with the remainder of the visual field hazy and colorless. Our brain makes presumptions and assembles a relatively detailed, stable, and colorful visual environment based on snapshot samples. It is our choice to focus on detail or access the wider visual environment. Analogous to macular vision, the hypnotic state is intense and detailed yet highly focused. Consciousness, then, is the result of the dialectical tension between intense and less intense focal experiences and the integration of experiences focal and peripheral. Spontaneous hypnotic trance, then, is a normal and frequent experience of any individual with hypnotic capacity without the need for any formal hypnotic induction.

Spontaneous hypnosis is elicited either by internal arousal such as imaginary involvement (A. Barabasz, 1982) or by trauma external cues such as an accident resulting in physical injury (Ewin, 1986a). The formal hypnotic induction brings discipline to the elicitation of the trance state and adds the complexity of the interpersonal transference factor. Although formal trance induction does not involve control of one person by another, the relationship factor can substantially influence the willingness of the individual to suspend critical judgment. The individual capable of entering hypnosis will then be more likely to stretch the limits of usual responses.

The *Hypnotic Induction Profile*, a test of hypnotizability developed by H. Spiegel and Spiegel (1978–1987, pp. 35–78), is one method for inducing trance while measuring it simultaneously. The participant learns to identify the special state of attention involved in hypnosis, thereby facilitating his or her ability to use self-hypnosis. The Spiegels view all hypnosis as a form of self-hypnosis.

The Sociopsychological Explanation of Hypnosis

In opposition to those who adopt the major (see E. Hilgard, 1992) view of hypnosis are the critics of hypnosis who adopt an opposing standpoint based on social-psychological theories (T. X. Barber, 1969; Kirsch & Lynn, 1995; Sarbin & Coe, 1972; Spanos & Chaves, 1989; Spanos & Coe, 1992; Wagstaff, 1981).[2] Proponents of the sociocognitive explanation of hypnotic phenomena address their theorizing and experiments to deconstructing most of the ordinary beliefs, research, and clinical observations about hypnosis, such as the genuineness of posthypnotic amnesia or of hypnotic hallucinations. As E. Hilgard (1992) explained, they reflect a distaste for any interpretation that favors distinct identifying characteristics of hypnotic phenomena as compared with more mundane forms of social interaction. They view even the most responsive of hypnotic participants as purposeful agents who are responding to contextual demands and who guide their behavior in terms of their understandings of those demands and in terms of the goals they wish to achieve (Lynn, Rhue, & Weekes, 1990; Spanos, 1986). The sociocognitivists conceptualize hypnosis as mere role enactments, deliberate constructions, or doings of highly motivated individuals. For example, contrary to the numerous experimentally controlled studies discussed later in this and other chapters and the countless numbers of painless surgeries conducted with hypnosis as the sole anesthetic is explained away simply as being the result of the participant's motivation, context of the situation, simple distraction, or mere role-playing to please the therapist.

Sarbin (1950) explicitly rejected the research and clinical observations supporting the hypnotic state. Instead, differences in hypnotic responding were viewed as simply differences to the extent to which individuals become involved or absorbed in hypnotic role-playing. Fifty-two years later, Sarbin (2002) maintained his position that hypnosis is nothing more than contextually supported social action.

Spanos & Coe (1992) summarized the sociopsychological position as one that views that individuals organize sensory information into categories that are then used to guide their actions. The idea is that people use implicit understandings to negotiate social situations. This provides for smooth social interaction, because the interacting parties share similar understandings of a common situation and of the reciprocal roles that they are to play within the confines of their shared definition of the situation at hand. Hypnosis, defined as role enactment, is an interaction with the therapist that proceeds in terms of some sort of mutually negotiated self-presentations and reciprocal role validation. All of this involves tacit understandings of the "actors" concerning the definition of the situation (hypnotic context) and the behaviors that they must play to be considered appropriate to that definition. The sociopsychological conceptualization emphasizes the notion that hypnotic responding may involve faking and lying on the part of the participants, such as acting deaf when they actually hear or raising an arm even if it does not feel right. Sociocognitivists also believe that participants may be deluding themselves into thinking they do not feel pain or that their arm is rising involuntarily. The position acknowledges disinterest in isolating the essence of hypnosis in favor of attempting to account for all that can be wrought by it into some general theory of social activity. Spanos (1991) placed the word *hypnosis* in quotation marks to emphasize the sociocognitive position that he believed does not in any way refer to a state or condition of the person but rather refers to the matter in which historically rooted conceptions of hypnosis are held by the participant in a context labeled "hypnosis." Spontaneous hypnosis and the evocation of hypnotic responses outside of such labeled contexts are ignored.

Spanos & Coe (1992) dismissed the eight experimentally controlled investigations of hypnosis versus waking suggestion on EEG ERPs with a footnote. Differences in the wording of suggestions in hypnosis leading to increased or decreased ERP amplitudes between the A. Barabasz and Lonsdale (1983) and the D. Spiegel, Cutcomb, Ren, and Pribram (1985) studies are dismissed despite the existence of two explanatory articles (D. Spiegel & Barabasz, 1988) that appeared before the Sarbin paper. Later, the Spiegel and Barabasz hypotheses were subjected to tests in a series of fully controlled experiments (A. Barabasz, 2000; A. Barabasz et al., 1999; Jasiukaitis, Nouriani, & Spiegel, 1996; Jensen, Barabasz, Barabasz, & Warner, 2001) and were fully confirmed. As in the *Star Trek* example at the beginning of this chapter, Sarbin also apparently wanted absolute certainty about the psychological functioning that can be drawn from the late component ERP amplitude changes before he is willing to recognize that the issue is not whether a "hypnosis" part of the brain lights up but that the state of hypnosis can be demonstrated with distinct physiological correlates that reflect alterations in consciousness that correspond to participants' experiences of perceptual alteration. Contrary to numerous studies that consistently show such changes due to hypnosis but not suggestion alone there is no evidence to support the idea that such EEG changes can be produced by social-influence role-playing without the presence of hypnotic responding.

Theory Convergence, State Theory Breakthroughs, and a New Focus

Taking on the difficult task begun by Spanos and Barber (1974, p. 508), Irving Kirsch and Steven Jay Lynn, once again, engaged in an attempt to converge current theories of hypnosis. Their article "The Altered State of Hypnosis," which appeared in the *American Psychologist* (Kirsch & Lynn, 1995), became widely cited. They accomplished much in the interest of helping to guide the writers of introductory psychology texts away from the traditional oversimplified tack of portraying the field as dominated by two diametrically opposed warring camps most frequently referred to as state and nonstate conceptualizations of hypnosis. The article argued that "virtually all substantive differences between [among] theorists cut across this apparent distinction" and a more accurate description is to view the trance state versus the sociopsychological phenomenon position "as points on a continuum" (p. 846). Many of us in the field might find much to agree with in the Kirsch and Lynn article, especially concerning what Hilgard (1992) termed the "domain of hypnosis"; that is, what happens when an attempt is made to induce hypnosis in a consenting individual. However, many of us would recognize that the article, written by two of the best-known sociocognitive theorists, might assume a bit too much commonality, in the attempt to accommodate state conceptualizations within sociocognitive theory. Since the article was published, new data has shed additional light on the issues (A. Barabasz, 2000, 2004; A. Barabasz & Barabasz, 2002; A. Barabasz et al., 1999; Barnier & McConkey, 2003; Killeen & Nash, 2003; Koch et al., 2003; Ray & Tucker, 2003; Vermetten, 2004; Woody & McConkey, 2003). This new work shows that the complexity of hypnosis involves more than response to suggestion, social influence, and expectations. Barnier and McConkey (2003) concluded that now there is almost as much divergence as there is convergence at the theoretical level. Commendably, Kirsch and Lynn did draw attention to unresolved issues and questions. The concept of convergence of theories was short lived because it served to obscure features of the phenomenon that allows us to seriously study the problems of interactions between conscious and unconscious mental life. To shed further light on the matter we shall focus on three salient issues while attempting to dispel one of the remaining myths or misconceptions that unnecessarily continue to divide the field.

Although research by Kinnunen, Zamansky, and Nordstrom (2001) cast new doubts about notions regarding compliance and expectation and new evidence showing the criticality of assessing subjective experience has emerged (Milling, Kirsch, & Burgess, 1999), our guess is that many were drawn back toward trance-state conceptualization because of the striking findings from what has now become a wide range of recent experiments.

Recent research has dealt directly with the limitations that plagued the earlier experiments on markers of hypnotic trance. Critical control conditions have been added and researchers are benefiting from the exponential advances in measurement and computer technology that was unavailable less than a decade ago. Once thought "unlikely to be found" while holding out the "possibility that subtle indicators will eventually be found" (Hilgard, 1973, p. 978), measurable, repeatable, and parsimoniously logical markers of hypnosis were, at last, available to test the reality of trance — a subtle, yet, clearly identifiable altered state of consciousness. Consistently controlled experiments with replication after replication involving more than a dozen different researchers in labs as far apart as England, Italy, New Zealand, and the United States have revealed robust physiological markers of hypnosis.

The first substantive response to the Kirsch and Lynn article came from John Kihlstrom (1997). Kihlstrom elucidated the rationale for persistence of the controversy between the state and nonstate views. Let us recognize that even without physiological markers, the trance state of altered consciousness denied by Kirsch and Lynn back in 1995 does exist. Cogently, Kihlstrom (1997) reminded us there is a state of altered consciousness in hypnosis and that "it matters not one wit whether it can also occur without a formal induction"; "Amnestic subjects cannot remember things they should be able to remember; analgesic subjects do not feel pain that they should feel; subjects asked to be 'blind' or 'deaf' do not see or hear things that they should see and hear." Even simple motor responses involve alterations in consciousness: "We feel heavy objects in our hands that are not there, forcing our outstretched arms down to our sides; we feel magnetic forces, forces that do not exist, pulling our extended hands and arms together" (Kihlstrom, 1997, p. 326). The behavioral markers of alterations in consciousness are simply blinding flashes of the obvious to many clinicians and researchers. Behavioral indicants have been there for our experimental pleasures and our patients' wellness for a very long time. Now, in addition to the long list of behavioral markers, neoteric science has made it possible to identify some rather subtle, yet robust, physiological markers of hypnotic responding that cannot be produced by those lacking hypnotic talent, by relaxation alone, or by suggestion alone.

Kirsch and Lynn (1995) acknowledged, "If physiological markers of hypnosis could be identified, it would support the idea that hypnosis is a unique altered state of consciousness" (p. 855). But in that same article they persevered in their sociocognitive position and claimed that hypnosis is nothing more than social influence, that suggestions can be responded to with or without hypnosis, and that the function of a hypnotic induction is merely to increase suggestibility to a minor degree. In scholarly support of their skepticism about the existence of physiological markers of hypnosis, they cited Dixon and Laurence (1992, p. 50), who believed that conclusions about the "physiological distinctiveness of an alleged hypnotic state" could not be supported because of an "unfortunate but customary lack of replication." The recent findings regarding physiological markers of hypnosis were reflected earlier in Kirsch's (2003) revised theoretical perspective that now recognizes "states" of hypnosis. Still currently relevant were Dixon and Laurence's criticisms about psychophysiological studies of hypnosis that failed to examine nonhypnotic relaxation. This maybe a potential trap for the unwary researcher unaware of the work of Hilgard and Tart (1966), who used the now all but forgotten experimental control of "state reports" in their series of experiments, affirming the phenomenon of spontaneous hypnosis as discussed earlier in this chapter (see also H. Spiegel, 1998; H. Spiegel & Spiegel, 2004). Spontaneous hypnosis can and does occur for those who are hypnotizable, in a variety of contexts without a formal induction, such as in response to relaxation instructions. Yet another related element brought to us by Dixon and Laurence was their suggestion that to "truly reveal physiological correlates of hypnosis" an alert, rather than relaxation-based hypnotic induction, would be required. It is precisely this sort of scientific rigor brought to us by many serious and dedicated researchers of hypnosis that ensured that such important issues were addressed in recent research.

Before focusing on data relating to the key points highlighted, we must debunk the "special process" myth started by Nick Spanos 15 years ago. Contrary to Ernest (Jack) Hilgard's controlled research and clinical findings from Herbert and David Spiegel showing hypnosis to be a part of everyday life for those with hypnotic capacities, the "special process" label caught on. As pointed out by Kirsch and Lynn (1995), the labels "state" and "nonstate" were largely dropped in favor of "special process" and "social psychological" by those of the sociocognitive persuasion when Spanos (1982) coined the term "special process" as a label for E. Hilgard's (1977) neodissociation trance-state conceptualization of hypnosis. The "special process" mislabel has been confusing for those new to the field as well as to those endeavoring to understand hypnotic phenomena ever since. The "special process" label wrongly implies a state unachievable in everyday life under normal conditions, thus misleading researchers as to the need to address the occurrence of spontaneous hypnosis when testing the effects of hypnosis or suggestion. The need to obtain subject "state reports" (see Hatfield, 1961; LeCron, 1953; Tart, 1963) has been ignored far to often. Such depth of hypnosis reports were so fruitfully employed in the clever hypnosis studies of the 1960s era and has recently reemerged in a more sophisticated form, developed by McConkey, Wende, and Barnier (1999).

The E. Hilgard and Tart (1966) experiment showing the significant effects of a hypnotic induction on responsiveness to suggestion, versus suggestion alone in relaxation, is just one brilliant example. State reports made it possible to assess hypnotic responding on a 0-3 scale. Participants are told to respond "0" to the question "State" if they felt in their usual, normal, wide-awake state; to respond "1" if they felt very relaxed or were drifting off, as in going to sleep; to respond "2" if they were in a mildly hypnotic state; and to respond "3" if they were more deeply hypnotized. Because depth of hypnosis often fluctuates within a session, these reports were frequently called for repeatedly within a session, typically before and after a test suggestion. For example, in the E. Hilgard and Tart (1966) study, if participants were in the waking condition and reported "1" they were aroused until the report returned to "0."

The latest approach to measuring hypnotic depth developed by McConkey and his colleagues (McConkey, Szeps, & Barnier, 2001; McConkey et al., 1999) asks participants to turn a dial to indicate their hypnotic depth, in terms of variations in strength of their experience during the progression of hypnosis at the test item level. Participants turn the dial as they progress in hypnosis. Because data is available for the induction, suggestion delivery, participant's response to the suggestion, release from the test item, and awakening from hypnosis the potential to index variations if physiological reflections of the hypnotic experience exists. This clever and promising technique is currently in use in our (A.F.B.) lab and elsewhere. At last, we are beginning to attempt to quantify, biologically, the complexity of hypnotic responding.

Of course, clinicians have far too frequently been routinely obtaining some measure of assurance of adequate hypnotic depth before calling on the participant for difficult responses, such as might be needed for a medical procedure. Unfortunately, state reports and strength of experience indexing and spontaneous hypnosis have been ignored by researchers drawing conclusions about the equivalence of suggestion with veridical hypnotic responding.

Jack and Josephine Hilgard, Herb and Dave Spiegel, Erika Fromm, Ron Shor, Jack and Helen Watkins, Michael Nash, Marianne Barabasz, and I (A.F.B.), as well as many others, have consistently accredited continuities between hypnotic trance and everyday experiences. For example, simple dissociations such as absorptive imagery and the more complex phenomenon of spontaneous hypnosis have long been known to exist and have been repeatedly verified in the lab and in everyday applications by those of us involved in clinical hypnosis. The fact that hypnotic-trance experiences can and do occur in everyday life should not be construed as implying that hypnotic trance is not in some way uniquely differentiable from nontrance or what is often termed "waking states." Plentifulness of alternative conscious states does not mean they are the same, no more than a cornucopia of apples and oranges makes them alike.

Several recent experiments shed new light on Kirsch and Lynn's (1995) assertions that (a) hypnosis is nothing more than social influence, (b) there are no physiological markers of hypnotic responding, and (c) the structure of hypnotic communications is unimportant in determining hypnotic responsiveness. First, it is important to underscore the point that the focus of contemporary research on responses of the brain to hypnosis is not to attempt to uncover some simplistic unidimensional EEG "signature" of the hypnotic state, per se. The complexity of hypnosis is such that instead we must consider both saliency and individuality in responding to hypnosis. Kilhstrom (2003), citing A. Barabasz et al. (1999), explained that very similar hypnotic effects can be achieved by very different neutral means. The structure of the hypnotic suggestion modulates the precise psychophysiological correlate of the effect.

The notion of a unique brain signature of hypnosis is like the special process notion, a construction of a straw man by those who wish to reconceptualize hypnosis as a social construction. The need to see such a unidimensional signature trivializes the range and complexity of hypnotic-state responses. E. Hilgard (personal communication, ca. 1989) wondered whether they (Chaves, Kirsch, Lynn, Spanos) expect to see a light flash on one's head when experiencing hypnosis. Surprisingly, EEG and brain imaging techniques have shed light on this issue. The question that has been answered convincingly in the affirmative is whether physiological indices directly reflect the subjective state sensed by the individual responding to a hypnotic induction, whether it is formally induced by an operator, self-induced, or spontaneously experienced.

The EEG line of studies from the Barabasz research group, reflected the interests of Dave Spiegel, Jack Hilgard, and others, refines our point of convergence on the determination of whether hypnotizable individuals exposed to a hypnotic induction, with depth sufficient for the demands of the specific task, can show EEG brain ERP changes that correspond to their subjective experiences that can be physiologically differentiated from the effects of suggestion, relaxation, and expectancies.

Recently, we (A. Barabasz et al., 1999) culminated 20 years of event-related EEG hypnosis research by dispelling the original concerns about nonreplication (Dixon & Laurence, 1992; Spanos & Coe, 1992) of physiological markers of hypnosis. The data revealed that apparent inconsistencies in the ERP-hypnosis literature could be accounted for by the wording of the hypnotic suggestions. Once accounted for, the physiological markers of trance are interpretable consistently, logical, and robust. The effects of positive obstructive and negative obliterating instructions on visual and auditory P300 ERPs were tested (A. Barabasz et al., 1999). Participants were selected for hypnotizability using the *Harvard Group Scale of Hypnotic Susceptibility* (Shor & Orne, 1962) and the *Stanford Hypnotic Susceptibility Scale*, Form C. Attempts to maximize or plateau participants' hypnotizability before individualized testing and between hypnotizability testing sessions were made using repeated hypnosis. To adequately test for potential differences between hypnotic and nonhypnotic responding, researchers must carefully differentiate high- and low-hypnotizable individuals. Little can be said about hypnotic responding by studies operationally defining highs and lows by median splits particularly when only group or psychometrically weak individual measures of hypnotizability are used. Simple high-low scoring splits pose a special problem for hypnosis research because hypnotizability in the general population is clustered about the mean (average hypnotizability). Thus, such simple splits will likely produce groups of high- and low-hypnotizable individuals that are not significantly different from each other. This situation leads the unwary to falsely conclude mere suggestibility, and expectancies rather than hypnosis might account for the apparent findings.

After our participants were stringently selected, both groups were requested to perform identical tasks during balanced conditions of waking suggestion only and alert hypnosis (A. Barabasz & Barabasz, 1996, 2000). An alert hypnotic induction was chosen in contrast to a traditional relaxation induction to preclude EEG effects that might be attributed to relaxation alone. High-hypnotizable individuals showed significantly greater EEG ERP amplitudes while experiencing negative hallucinations and significantly lower ERP amplitudes while experiencing positive, obstructive hallucinations in contrast to the low-hypnotizable individuals (who were trying to mimic hypnotic responses to the suggestions) and their own waking-imagination-only conditions. The data clearly revealed that when responses are time locked to events, rather robust physiological markers of hypnosis emerge. Rather than producing a unidimensional signature of the hypnotic state, these bidirectional ERPs varied consistently by type of suggestion after a hypnotic induction to directly show alterations in consciousness that corresponded closely to participants' subjective experiences of perceptual alterations. These effects were not produced by the low-hypnotizable individuals, by social influence (trying to mimic responses to the suggestions), or by the highs in a waking condition. These findings have been fully replicated in separate studies by Calvin (2000) and Jensen et al. (2001). The next investigation was intended to bring even further stringency to the A. Barabasz et al. (1999) investigation.

The study (A. Barabasz, 2000) completely separated hypnotizability testing (completed 6 to 9 months earlier) from the context of the experiment. How could the high-hypnotizable individuals be holding back their best efforts in the suggestion condition (Zamansky, Scharf, & Brightbill, 1964) when they had no knowledge that this was a hypnosis experiment or that hypnosis was to be used, until after the suggestion-only data were collected?

The data showed that only the hypnotic induction, with efforts to ensure adequate hypnotic depth, made it possible for the high- but not the low-hypnotizable individuals to significantly attenuate their ERPs in response to the hypnotic induction plus suggestion condition, in contrast to the identical suggestion alone's disproving one the sociocognitive notion that suggestion alone accounts for all that can be wrought with hypnosis.

Although it would seem that adequate hypnotic depth should be produced before expecting a participant to complete a difficult task with hypnosis, as reviewed elsewhere (A. Barabasz & Barabasz, 1992), one highly hypnotizable partcipant in the this study (A. Barabasz, 2000) produced almost identical responses to the two conditions. During the postexperimental inquiry he noted, "When I got the instruction to make like there were ear plugs in my ears, I just did what I learned to do when I was a kid." "Tell me more," replied the independent postexperimental inquirer (who was uninvolved in any other aspect of the experiment). "Well, when I'd get spanked by my Dad for something, I could turn off the pain like just going to another place, so that's what I did with the suggestion too — same as the hypnosis part too." This response appears to be a classic example of spontaneous hypnosis with apparent dissociation as first elucidated by E. Hilgard and Tart (1966) nearly 40 years earlier. Clinicians who use hypnosis regularly with difficult cases frequently observe that hypnotizable patients spontaneously evoke the hypnotic state in their own idiosyncratic ways, rather than slavishly responding to the practitioners' instructions.

The findings reveal that suggestion-expectancy was insufficient to produce a difficult response without hypnosis. Only those who had demonstrated their ability to become hypnotized were able to produce such changes showing robust physiological markers of hypnosis that directly reflected alterations in consciousness that corresponded to participants' subjective experiences of perceptual alteration.

The EEG studies, regarded as breakthroughs by a number of national awards, have nonetheless been superseded by brain-imaging technology (positron emission tomography) that provides even better brain-region localization to determine more precisely the state effects of hypnosis.

Positron emission tomography has illuminated our understanding of the hypnotic state, showing that trance effects are reflected in neural activity in the brainstem, thalamus, and anterior cingulate. It has been consistently shown that hypnosis reduces the activity of the anterior cingulate cortex but does not affect the somatosensory cortex, where the sensations of pain are processed, showing that the analgesic effects of hypnosis occur in higher brain centers (Rainville, Duncan, Price, Carrier, & Bushnell, 1997; Rainville, Hofbauer, et al., 1999; Rainville & Price, 2003; Ray & De Pascalis, 2003; D. Spiegel, 2003; Szechtman, Woody, Bowers, & Nahmias, 1998). The findings support H. Spiegel and D. Spiegel's (1978–1987, p. 23) conceptualization of hypnosis as "a response to a signal, a state of attentive, receptive intense focal concentration with diminished peripheral awareness ... a function of the alert individual who utilizes their capacity for maximal involvement with one point in space and time and thereby minimizes their involvement with other points in space and time." Consistent with E. Hilgard's (1977) neodissociation theory, the changes that take place in hypnosis occur at the executive level of functioning. The anterior cingulate is involved in the type of executive functioning that allows one to focus or pay attention to one set of cues (Aston-Jones, Rajkowski, & Cohen, 1999). For example, a person fully absorbed in listening to a lecture, watching a movie, or reading a book maybe be dissociated from distracter cues that might otherwise trigger arousal (A. Barabasz, 1982; J. Hilgard, 1974, 1979).

The data from the EEG ERP studies (A. Barabasz, 2000; A. Barabasz et al., 1999; A. Barabasz & Lonsdale, 1983; D. Spiegel & Barabasz, 1988; D. Spiegel et al., 1985) showing that ERPs after a hypnotic induction to hallucinate a block to visual and auditory stimuli show alterations in consciousness that corresponded closely to participants' subjective experiences of perceptual alterations (see Figure 3.1). This discovery converges with the Szechtman et al. (1998) research implicating the anterior cingulate in the hallucination but not the simple imagining of external stimuli only for participants who could experience hypnosis. Furthermore, the Rainville et al. (1997) anterior cingulate findings showed that its activity closely paralleled subjective experience, reflecting the emotional component but not the sensory component of experimentally induced painful stimuli.

The color-perception positron emission tomography research by Kosslyn et al. (2000) is perhaps one of the most elegant examples of research on the physiology of hypnotic responding. Only in hypnosis were color areas of the left and right hemispheres activated when asked to perceive color, whether they were actually shown the color or a gray-scale stimulus. Unlike a number of other brain-imaging studies, the Kosslyn et al. study analyzed only the areas of the brain hypothesized to be regions of interest *a priori*. The point was that if the hypnotized participants perceived the hypnotic hallucination as real, the blood flow in the color-processing region of the brain would be affected consistently with the hypnotically suggested hallucination. Just as in the A. Barabasz (2000) ERP study of an auditory-blocking hallucination, Kosslyn's color-hallucination suggestion to perceive differently occurred only after the hypnotic induction. The positron emission tomography effects were different for the mental-imagery instruction, using the same suggestion in the no-hypnosis condition. The only difference in both studies was the use of hypnosis; the suggestions and social demands for performance were identical, yet the brain showed us different affects that reflected the subjective perceptions of the participants. The color-hallucination suggestion (to perceive differently), after a hypnotic induction consistent with our ERP findings observed changes in subjective experience achieved only during hypnosis, were reflected by changes in brain function. It was concluded that hypnosis was a psychological state with distinct neural indices and is not just a result of adopting a role (social influence).

It is important to recognize that all of these highly consistent findings do not contradict the notion that social influence, expectancy, and context may be useful in maximizing treatment outcomes with patients. The point is simply that hypnosis per se can make certain responses possible that go beyond and are different at basic physiological levels from those that might be wrought by social influence; more simply put, "suggestibility." Hypnosis is obviously much more than simple or even complex socially influenced expectancy responses to suggestion. Killeen and Nash (2003) reminded the scientific community of the data showing that responses to hypnosis do not correlate with most types of suggestibility and that those who respond to hypnosis are not usually gullible and they are not more responsive to placebos, social pressure, or authority figures. The belief that suggestibility can account for all that can be wrought by hypnosis does not meet the tests of science. We can recognize the reality of the trance state while still doing all we can for our patients in the artful realm of maximizing the appropriate use of social influence, expectancy, context, and numerous other variables to bring about the most optimal outcomes.

In the light of the overwhelming neurophysiological data now extant, the "nonstate" conceptualization of hypnosis must, like the elephant of fable, drag itself off to some distant jungle to die if hypnosis is to be credible to science in general, to psychology, and to medicine in particular. Killeen and Nash (2003) concluded that we should now see the "hypnotic situation" to mean the "hypnotic state (HS) in which the subject's responses are characteristic, and different than without the state." The state versus nonstate argument must give way to the study of the "different combinations of necessary causes that will bring about the phenomenon" (Killeen & Nash, 2003). The most efficacious use of hypnosis in the treatment of our patients will probably always involve a complex interplay of multiple domains, including those unique to hypnotic states and to social influence and other causes.

Notes

1. In a personal observation, J. Watkins reported that he applies this principle of "creative regression" when writing scientific contributions, poems, or short stories (Watkins, 2001). On rousing from sleep, instead of getting out of bed at once, he lies in a half-wake state for an hour or two; during that period new ideas and more succinct phrases often become consciously available but are forgotten if not recorded shortly.
2. We acknowledge that Kirsch (2003) altered his theoretical perspective in the light of the new data recognizing "states" of hypnosis. Similarly, Lynn (2003) stated, "Of course there are altered states of consciousness."

Chapter 4
Hypnotizability

If patients walked into your office and requested hypnotherapy, how would you know whether they were hypnotizable? Would it be necessary for you to spend long and frustrating sessions only to conclude that they were so highly resistant to hypnosis as to require an alternative intervention (J. Watkins, 1987)?

Differences in participants' hypnotic talents have intrigued workers in the field for many years. Numerous attempts have been made to correlate hypnotizability with some measurable psychological trait. If only we could know in advance just who is hypnotizable and who is not, a great deal of wasted effort, humiliation, and impaired status would be saved the practitioner. Patients, who had read about the "miracles" of hypnosis and sought treatment with it could be spared subsequent disappointment and disillusionment with the therapist.

Hypnosis as a Matter of Degree

As we discussed in the earlier chapters, hypnosis is not a special process with a one-dimensional EEG brain signature where, when experiencing a hypnotic state, a light bulb of sorts flashes on the participant's forehead. The research (discussed earlier) now shows clearly that rather than a simple matter of "either-or," reliable physiological correlates reflect the various subjective states perceived by the participant. Hypnosis is also a matter of degree. Some individuals apparently can enter a deep state and exhibit very bizarre behavior such as regression, time distortion, and hallucinations. Others seem to reach a plateau where they will carry through simple suggestions, but not unusual ones involving major distortions of perception, whereas others might become more relaxed or slightly more alert only with minimal involvement. We are, therefore, concerned not only with the question as to whether given participants or patients are hypnotizable but also to what degree of depth they can be expected to respond. Some hypnotherapeutic techniques and experimental research responses require rather deep states; others can be effectively employed with the participant only slightly hypnotized. The first question to be answered is the participants' level of hypnotizability, and next their depth capability. It is a frequent mistake among researchers and clinicians, we have observed, to assume that because participants have shown a high score on a reputable standardized scale of hypnotizability, once hypnosis is induced, they are somehow automatically at an adequate hypnotic depth to complete demanding responses to hypnosis. Such is not the case at all. Given such faulty reasoning on the part of the researcher or clinician, it is no surprise to see that the scales of hypnotizability, useful as they are, only predict responses to hypnosis about half of the time (E. Hilgard, 1979). Efforts should be made to ensure adequate depth, which will vary throughout the period of hypnosis, depending on the receptivity of the individual to the induction and deepening procedures. Depth may also vary for dynamic reasons according to the demands placed on the individual by specific suggestions. We recommend that when a matter of depth is an issue, such as might be required to achieve a response to a demanding suggestion, that the E. Hilgard and Tart (1966) method reviewed in chapter 3 be employed. Pending further research, the McConkey, Wende, and Barnier (1999) "dial" method may be shown to be even more useful. Ideally, one should become comfortable with using both methods to the point of their becoming second nature in your inductions so they do not interfere with the responses of the participants or your ability to observe them.

Informal Tests of Hypnotizability

Prior to using hypnosis with a patient or research participant, it is advisable to familiarize the individual with hypnotic-like experiences to reinforce your debunking of myths about hypnosis and ameliorate potential underlying fears about the modality, which will also help build rapport and trust. These informal clinical tests are generally useful in screening suitable individuals for hypnosis practice, and later in evaluating patients for possible hypnotherapy. Not only do the following tests serve to screen and evaluate but their very administration also can establish a positive psychological set and make easier later induction of hypnosis.

Chevreul's Pendulum

The response to the Chevreul's pendulum test is an indicator correlated with hypnotizability. It presents an excellent opportunity to reveal anxieties about hypnosis denied or left unstated in the initial interview with the patient when myths about hypnosis were debunked and the participant's questions answered. It is a good nonthreatening demonstration of the effect of how the participant's thinking about something can affect his or her behavior without the ceremony of the initial hypnotic induction. A small object, such as a Lucite or crystal ball, a plumb bob, or simply a bolt attached to the end of a string, can be used. When using this test in the first research on hypnosis conducted in Antarctica, my (A.F.B.) personal identification dog tags swung from the neck chain to the same effect (A. Barabasz, 1980c). Ideally, the participant is standing up, feet close together, with elbows away from his or her sides, with the object suspended over the intersection of two lines drawn on a blank sheet of paper. The first line is horizontal, running the length of the paper and labeled "A" at one end and "B" on the other. The second line is vertical and is labeled "C" and "D." The participant is simply instructed to relax and just make his or her eyes and thoughts go back and forth across the A-B line. The instruction is repeated. If the participants have fears about hypnosis not previously mentioned, they will frequently be anxious enough to deliberately interfere with the tendency of the body sway to produce the back and forth motion. This is an easy test. Typically, the object will, within moments, swing back and forth across the line. Once the back and forth motion is established, the therapist switches the instruction to indicate that the motion is changing: "Now it can move up and down from C to D."

Alternatively, the participants can be seated at a desk or table and be given instructions as follows (see Figure 4.1): "Put your elbow on the desk and hold this string between your fingers so that the weight at the end [ball, plump bob] just misses touching the desk." This means that the distance from the fingers to the desk will be about one foot. The suggestions are now continued: "Stare at the weight and concentrate all your attention on it. As you look at it you will notice that it has a tendency to move." Movements, even though slight, are almost certain to appear. The therapist watches carefully, and when the movements begin to stabilize in one direction, the therapist capitalizes on this movement.

"You notice that the weight is beginning to swing back and forth, back and forth, back and forth" (or whatever direction it is swinging). The therapist permits this movement to continue and enhances it until it is clear to the participants and to all observers that this movement is indeed taking place. The therapist then suggests a change in the direction of the move-

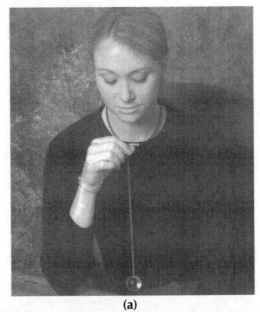

(a)

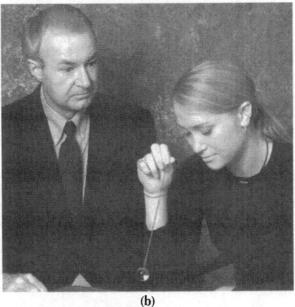

(b)

Fig. 4.1 Chevreul's Pendulum. (a) The object is suspended from a chain just above the tabletop. The therapist suggests that the participant move her eyes from side to side and the pendulum will begin to swing. (b) The pendulum appears to automatically swing back and forth.

ment: "Now, as you watch this weight, you will notice that the direction of movement begins to change. There is now a tendency for it to move from side to side." After the side-to-side movement has been established, the therapist may notice that the movement becomes a bit circular. The operator immediately takes advantage to suggest, "The weight is now beginning to move round and round in a clockwise [or counterclockwise] direction. Round and round it goes swinging in an ever larger arc."

Finally, the therapist suggests a change in the direction of rotation by indicating, "It is now slowing down and beginning to turn in an opposite direction. Notice the tendency for it to move counterclockwise (or clockwise), round and round in an ever-increasing arc. That's fine." Then the therapist says, "Were you making the weight perform those movements or were they just happening? Were you aware of any movements on your own part that caused it to swing back and forth, then side-to-side, then clockwise, and finally counterclockwise?"

In almost all cases, the participants will state that they were not aware of any voluntary action to cause these movements to occur. Many will show considerable surprise, thus helping to create an accepting attitude toward future positive responses. A few will even mention that they tried consciously to resist the movements, but that they occurred in spite of their efforts.

This test makes a good demonstration of the effects that can occur as a result of hypnosis per se without the participant's expecting to feel particularly unusual. Such nonhypnotic responses to simple suggestion, whether it is direct or indirect, may be closely related to the suggestive aspects of once commonly accepted practices such as water witching.

Many years ago, when John Watkins was a high school science teacher, he lived in a community in which all the wells had been located by witching. One of his students was the son of a local "witch" and volunteered to give a demonstration, because he "had been taught how to witch" by his father. Louie came to class the next day bringing his forked peach branch, and the entire class proceeded to the fields, which surrounded this rural high school. As he came to one spot, the branch turned downward. A peg was driven into the ground at that point, and Louie approached it from another angle, and then another. In each case, it turned down near the peg; Louie, with an air of considerable confidence, then stated, "There's where the water is located." No attempt was made to contradict him, but instead he was asked, "Louie, are you sure that you aren't doing this yourself with little muscle movements?" Louie insisted that the stick had turned down by itself, that he had held it loosely, and that he had no part in its movement. Then he was asked, "If it is the stick doing the movement, you will not object to performing the experiment again blindfolded?" Louie, with some surprise but still with confidence, indicated he was willing to do the experiment. After he was blindfolded, he was led all over the field, including several times by the point where the stake was driven. Never once did the stick turn down twice at the same location. Finally, Louie was led over an area where the water pipes entered the school building. Again, the stick failed to turn down. When confronted with this evidence, Louie regretfully threw his peach branch away with the remark, "It doesn't work, but I sure never could convince Dad of that."

At the end of the term, the instructor asked a final (noncredit) question on the exam: "What do you think of water witching?" Twenty-nine students indicated they no longer believed in it, but one wrote, "Louie just ain't a good witch." Such simple yet apparently dramatic responses to suggestion, without induction of the hypnotic state, has served to mislead many professionals in the healing arts into thinking hypnosis is nothing more than response to suggestion.

The Arm-Drop Test

It is generally unwise to ever base an assessment of a person's ability to enter hypnosis on a single item (A. Barabasz, 1982). However, a clinically urgent situation may impose time constraints, which limit us to a single test item. In our opinion, the arm-drop test is the single, most valuable test in that it can be applied in a very short period of time and it also creates an advantage for the therapist. The word *hypnosis* need not be mentioned to the patient. It provides an easily administered rapid indicator of a patient's probable response to hypnotherapy. Although an item from the *Stanford Hypnotic Susceptibility* Scale our clinical experience shows, it is one of the most sensitive of the screening techniques. A positive response on this test typically means that the participant or patient is capable of responding favorably to the induction of hypnosis to a significant degree. Furthermore, with a simple extension it can be turned into an actual induction procedure.

Perhaps one of its greatest advantages is that it permits the therapist, especially one who is relatively inexperienced and not secure in his or her ability to induce hypnosis, to determine, at least to a small degree, the patient's hypnotizability before committing to the use of hypnosis.

When the therapist is uncertain of the chances for success in inducing hypnosis with certain patients, this lack of certainty is often initiated in such patients, who becomes resistant to the induction procedure, not because they are unhypnotizable but because a lack of confidence in the therapist has been perceived. When the test is favorable, the therapist, knowing that the participant is probably hypnotizable, begins the induction procedures with an air of confidence, that then transmits itself to the participant and increases the likelihood of responsivity. Accordingly, we recommend that students of hypnosis learn this procedure and practice it on their first participants.

The therapist tells the participant simply, "I would like to test your reflexes. Would you please sit up straight in your chair and extend both arms straight out in front of you, palms down. Don't let them touch each other. That's right. Now close your eyes and imagine that I am giving you a bucket to hold in your right (or left) hand. Please close your fingers around the handle of the bucket." (Note that the therapist now treats the imagined bucket as a reality by asking participants to close their fingers around the handle.) "Now I want you to visualize what it would be like if I were standing in front of you pouring water into your bucket from a pail of water that I am holding. Your bucket can hold over two gallons, and I am now pouring one quart into the bucket. Observe the stream of water flowing into your bucket. Now, I'm pouring more and more water into your bucket. There are now two quarts in it, and you can feel the increase in weight. Three quarts. More and more water going into it. Four quarts, now five quarts, and your bucket is half filled. You are becoming increasingly aware that more and more water is being poured into your bucket. I shall continue to pour water into it. Six quarts, seven quarts, eight quarts, and the bucket is beginning to fill up. Notice how heavy two gallons of water are? Now nine quarts, and the bucket is almost full, almost full. There now. I shall pour the tenth quart into it, and the bucket is full right up to the brim. Two and a half gallons of water and the bucket is completely full." The therapist allows another 10 to 20 seconds and carefully observes the movements in the participants' arms (see Figure 4.2).

Hypnotizability is indicated by the following movements:

1. The hand gradually lowers while the therapist is suggesting that more quarts are being poured into the bucket. The degree of lowering of the arm is significantly related to the hypnotizability; that is, if the hand goes all the way down until it rests on the lap, or on a desk or table in front of the participant, then it is probable that the participant is highly hypnotizable and can either enter hypnosis rapidly or may even be capable of entering deep trance states, which will make possible the initiating of such phenomena as regression and hallucinations.

2. If during the period of the test the hand lowers somewhat but does not go all the way down, the inference is that the participant is responsive to hypnotic suggestions but may be resistant, a slow

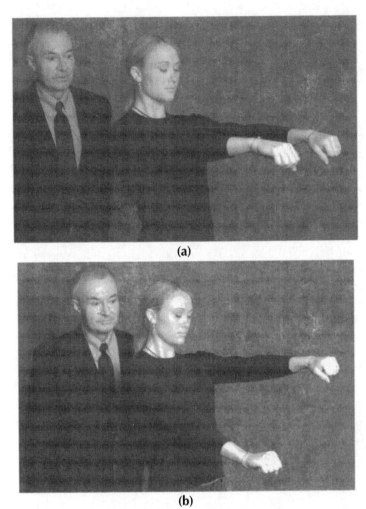

(a)

(b)

Fig. 4.2 Arm Drop Test. (a) The therapist asks the participant holding the imaginary bucket to notice the weight of the bucket pulling the right arm down. (b) The participant's right arm begins to show evidence of fatigue as the imaginary quarts of water are poured in.

responder, or capable of reaching only a light or medium trance, not a deep one. However, in our experience, the individual who responds in this way eventually may become a very good hypnotic participant after his or her initial doubts and anxieties have been resolved and a better relationship has been established with the therapist. The slowness of response may only be a way of saying, "I don't completely trust you yet, and this situation is disturbing to me." The extent of one's response is related to one's hypnotizability at this

(c)

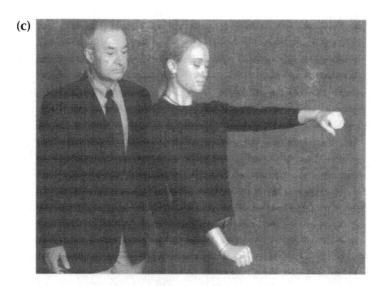

Fig. 4.2 *Continued.* (c) The imaginary bucket, "filled to the rim with water," is so heavy that the participant's right arm is pulled completely down.

point in time. Thus, if the right hand is some 6 or more inches below the left at the end of the test, then the participant shows a substantial degree of hypnotizability, even if it has not come all the way down. If the hand has slowly moved downward, at least 3 inches, then the participant shows a positive response even if it is not strong. Such an individual indicates to the therapist at least an ability to become hypnotically involved to some degree, and with proper handling may be able to achieve an even more significant response level. Because it is not necessary that a deep degree of hypnosis be induced in a client for the effective use of many hypnotherapeutic techniques, this individual should certainly not be rejected as a possible candidate for hypnotherapy. Occasionally, some participants' right hand will not drop downward at all, but they will manifest a considerable struggle to keep it level with the left one. There may even be slight tendencies for it to drop, followed by slight corrective movements designed to pull it up, level with the left hand again. These actions might be interpreted that such individuals are responsive to hypnosis but do not think that they should be, or that they are fearful of losing control, that the situation is one in which they are in competition with the therapist, one in which they must demonstrate strong willpower. When this occurs the therapist should not let it deteriorate into a struggle for control. Participants might be approached as follows: "I noticed that you seemed to have some difficulty. It was as if the arm felt like dropping down as the bucket became heavier, but you did not want it to do so and wished to show that you were capable of resisting this tendency. You obviously are quite capable of resisting it, like I said when we were talking about what hypnosis is and I mentioned that you, not the therapist, are always ultimately in control. But it might be interesting to see what would happen if you did not fight such tendencies; simply let happen whatever occurs naturally, don't make it happen, just let's see if it happens by itself, without interfering."

3. Perhaps the response that is most related to lack of hypnotic talent is no response whatsoever. The hand does not go down, it does not rise, and its position parallel to the other hand seems to be maintained without any effort. In this case, it is often useful to ask participants about their response and feelings concerning it with such questions as "Could you visualize the bucket when I described it to you?" or "Could you experience the water being poured into it?" Often the nonresponsive individual will say, "I was not able to imagine the bucket" or "I could see the bucket, but I didn't feel as if any water was being poured into it." Further questioning might be continued as follows: "Did the bucket feel heavy?" "Did you notice any difference in the feel of your two arms?" "Do your arms feel tired now?" These questions often elicit a positive response, even in the resistant individual. Holding one's arms out for a minute or more naturally creates physiological fatigue. The normal person admits it. A complete denial of feeling any fatigue suggests individuals who are very fearful of hypnosis and are determined to show that they can be strong. If such participants admit that the arms feel tired, they may then be asked, "Which arm feels the most tired?" The response that both arms feel equally tired usually indicates considerable resistance to hypnosis, either because the individual does not possess any hypnotic talent or because of fear and a strong determination not to be controlled. When there has been no overt movement of the hand downward but participants state that the right arm feels more tired than the left one, they are showing, at least to some extent, that they are capable of responding, but the influence is at a perceptual level, not at the motor level. With such individuals, the possibility of using hypnotherapy is still open.

In case the matter of employing hypnotic treatment techniques has already been explored, and the patient is not completely ignorant of this possibility, then the therapist and patient might discuss the matter. If the patient says "Doctor, does this mean that I am not hypnotizable?" a good response would be, "Not necessarily. Some people respond easily to hypnosis. Others have more difficulty and are slower to react. This simply means that it might take a little longer to teach you how to respond. If hypnosis seems to be a possible treatment for your problem, we can work on it more intensively. It may well be that you are a bit nervous, tense, or that you have some fears about hypnosis. Tell me how you feel about the matter." This may lead into an airing of the patient's fears, doubts, and preconceptions. However, let us leave a fuller discussion of how to handle these patients in later chapters on induction procedures.

As Ernest (Jack) Hilgard once explained (personal communication to A.F.B., November 8, 1990), one should never qualify or disqualify an individual for hypnosis on the basis of responses to a single test item, no matter how predictive it usually may be. There are a number of other tests that can be administered, and we describe these shortly. Nonetheless, the arm-drop test appears to be the single most sensitive one and is the technique of choice, especially if only one test can be given.

The Postural Sway Test

This test is also positively correlated with hypnotizability and has the advantage that in the case of a strong favorable response, it can be turned into an actual induction technique. The therapist asks the participant to stand up straight with his or her heels and toes together. This distributes his or her weight over the smallest area and maximizes minor signs of unsteadiness. A chair is placed about 6 inches behind the participant. Preferably, this chair should be large and cushioned, with arms and a high back. The therapist gives the following instructions: "Close your eyes and take several deep breaths. That's good. Now I want you to imagine that your feet are hinged to the floor and that your body extends upward. You may feel a bit unsteady, but don't worry. If you should fall I will catch you." (If you think that the participant is highly hypnotizable, a little more leverage can be gained by saying, "When you fall I will catch you," instead of "if you fall." In the first case, the suggestion of a possible fall is implanted; in the second, a conviction that this will happen is inculcated.) Because the therapist's conviction that a hypnotic suggestion will be carried out is an important part of its success, the choice of wording may depend on one's own certainty and clinical judgment regarding the particular individual with whom one is working. If the second hypnotic suggestion is given by an insecure and doubting therapist, it will most likely fail. It is no surprise to experienced clinicians, who annually use hypnosis successfully with large numbers of patients, that some university research studies conducted by inexperienced graduate students or disbelieving researchers seem to achieve comparatively few of the phenomena produced routinely in a clinical setting.

In all hypnotic work, whether it is hypnotizability tests, induction techniques, deepening procedures, or therapeutic interventions, the manner, confidence, and precise communications of the clinical experience of the therapist are paramount. Weaknesses in any of these critical prerequisites determine why one operator is successful with a given individual whereas another is not.

The therapist should now be positioned at the side of participating individuals in order to have in sight the side of participants' noses or the back of their heads, so as to detect slight movements in relation to the opposite wall. Successful hypnotizing requires that we align our hypnotic suggestions as closely as possible to reality during the initial stages of a hypnotizability test, or an induction. Accordingly, it is wise to wait for a brief period while observing any signs of swaying movement by the participant. In general, inductions begin with the use of the future tense. For example the therapist might say, "The longer you stand there, the more unsteady you may [will] feel yourself becoming. Don't worry. Just remember that I will not allow you to fall and hurt yourself. I am here and will catch you. This unsteadiness will increase, and you may develop a swaying feeling."

The therapist should wait a little while longer while observing carefully signs of movement as determined by a sighting of the participant's nose or back of head projected onto the wall. Time and the implementation of these suggestions will tend to increase the feeling of unsteadiness. Because the participant's feet are placed together heel to heel and toe to toe, slight swaying motions along with adjustments of posture are almost certain to appear in any individual. Once the therapist observes that signs suggested in the future tense have begun to occur, he or she then builds on these by using the present tense as follows: "You notice that you are now drifting forward." After saying the word *drifting*, the therapist pauses and observes the movement again. As soon as it has been ascertained as forward, it is labeled "forward." If the movement were backward, it would be described accordingly. The point is that some swaying has almost certainly been initiated. The therapist then calls it correctly, immediately after its direction has been determined. This may continue for some time as the therapist reports the natural movements of the participant.

Floating and *drifting* are good words for the therapist to use at first: "You are now drifting backward. Now you are floating forward. Forward, backward." Later, as the movement becomes more pronounced, and more obviously in response to the therapist's suggestions, the wording can be changed to *swaying*. The therapist will notice in most cases that the participant's back and forth movement soon ends, like the swinging of a pendulum; rhythmical and evenly spaced. The individual sways through a specific arc that may be 3 or 4 inches forward, then 2 or 3 inches backward. During this time the therapist has been following these movements and reporting them, now in a firm and even more confident voice. His or her credibility rises in the mind of the participant. It is almost as if the patient were thinking, "The doctor says I am swaying forward, and I am. Then when I am swaying backward, that's called correctly also. The doctor knows what he is saying, and it's always right. I can believe it."

At this point, the therapist moves from following the movements to leading them. If the therapist has been following and correctly reporting the area of movement, he or she might be saying, "Swaying forward, swaying forward, swaying forward — now swaying backward, swaying backward," and so on. Now the therapist can make an attempt to interrupt this cycle in midpoint. When participants are swaying forward and have reached the center of the arc — before they have completed all of the normal forward swaying motion — the therapist in the same confident voice reverses the suggestion to "Swaying backward, swaying backward," and so on. If the participants have by this time become hypnotically involved (absorbed, not just following simple suggestions), they will interrupt the normal pattern of forward movement in midpoint and reverse the sway. After this, the therapist can lead the swaying movements rather than simply follow them. The participants are then likely following suggestions at a hypnotic level. At this point, the therapist can conclude that the test has been positive and that the individual will be hypnotizable at least to some degree.

What we have done so far constitutes another test of hypnotizability. In a later chapter on advanced induction techniques we return to this point and describe how this postural sway procedure can be continued to initiate an induction of an actual hypnotic state, sometimes a very deep one, in which various hypnotherapeutic techniques can become successful. A slightly different form of this procedure is found in the *Stanford Hypnotic Susceptibility Scale* (Weitzenhoffer & Hilgard, 1959) in which the therapist stands behind the participant and gives suggestions to induce falling backward. The therapist then catches the participant.

The Hand-Clasp Test

This is a somewhat more aggressive procedure that culminates in an actual hypnotic challenge to the participant. It is useful as part of a group screening procedure, but it may have less value in the clinical situation, where the object is to work therapeutically with a patient. It relies to some extent on suggested intimidation of participants to precipitate a hypnotic response, hence pulling on transference relationships to a dominating parent figure, if that had characterized their childhoods. It is similar to what Ferenczi (1926) called "father hypnosis" (see chapter on theorizing about hypnosis for a discussion of Ferenczi's conceptualization).

The therapist instructs the participant or group of participants as follows (see Figure 4.3): "Please clasp your hands tightly in front of you and look carefully at my clasped hands at the same time." The therapist demonstrates by interlacing his or her own fingers so that the hands grip each other very tightly. The suggestions to the participant are now being given verbally by the commands of the therapist and visually, as the focus is on the clasped hands of the therapist, which are clasping tighter and tighter. "Now make those hands tighter and tighter. Imagine they are like fingers of steel encased in a block of concrete, which is shrinking or a vice that is being screwed down and locked. The hands get tighter and tighter and tighter." The therapist raises his or her voice, making it ever more strong and firm. At the same time, the therapist's fingers dig into each other so that the muscles and blood vessels stand out. Notice how the colors change in those fingers. (Note that the term "those fingers" rather than "your fingers" is used to facilitate dissociation of the hands from the participant as if they are involuntarily acting on their own.)

The therapist might say, "That's it, tighter, tighter, tighter. In fact, so tight that it doesn't seem as if they could come apart. It seems as if the more you try to take them apart, the tighter they stick together. The more you try to take them apart, the tighter they stick. They are sticking so tightly they will not come apart. They will not come apart. They are tightly stuck together. Try to pull them apart. Try to pull them apart. You see, they are so tightly stuck together they cannot come apart. The harder you try to pull them apart, the tighter they stick together."

At this point, a challenge has been issued, and a substantial number of participants will be unable to pull their hands apart if a hypnotic response has been truly elicited by a competent practitioner. The participants are now observed as they struggle to pull their hands apart. Then, within no more than 3 to 5 seconds, the therapist releases his or her own hands and places them around the participant's clasped hands, moving them up and down gently and reassuringly while saying, "Your hands are relaxing, they are normal and can now come apart." He or she then gently assists the participant in performing the release. Alternatively, the therapist still holds his or her hands tightly clasped together, and then immediately pulls his or

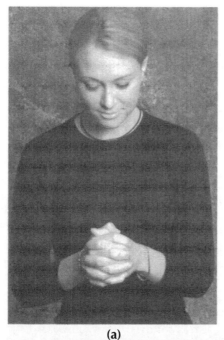

(a)

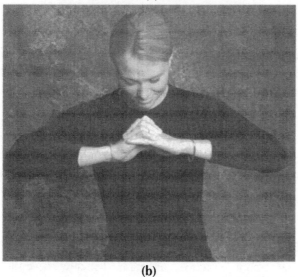

(b)

Fig. 4.3 The Hand-Clasp Test. (a) The participant is instructed to interlace her fingers together. (b) Transitioning to hypnosis, the participant is told that her hands are locked together. She is asked to pull her hands apart, but they will not come apart. She is astonished by her inability to release her hands.

her own hands apart, as if with difficulty, and says, "Now you can pull your hands apart. See! They will come apart now."

If only one individual is being tested and seems to be succeeding in pulling his or her hands apart — that is, the individual is showing signs of loosening — the therapist quickly intervenes before the hands are apart with a cessation of the challenge and permission to pull them apart. Such participants are then left with the recognition of how tightly their hands were stuck together and with doubt as to whether they would have been successful in pulling them apart if they had continued to try. The test is considered to be successful if participants, after 3 to 5 seconds of struggling, are unable to separate the hands.

The therapist uses the principle of the reversed effect toward the end of the test. He or she suggests, "The harder you try to pull them apart the tighter they will stick together." Hence, the participant's trying to pull the hands apart becomes the stimulus cue for being unable to separate the hands. This principle can be used in many different ways as a part of an induction and therapeutic procedures, which we describe later.

Some participants will resist this test by not making the grip tight to begin with. This resistance can be observed, and the therapist can then urge the participant as follows: "Okay now, that's a start. Now really tighten your hands." If little further tightening is then observed, the therapist says, "Just relax your hands now — bring them apart," and then asks the participant about the half-hearted response to the request to tighten the hands. Others will respond to the challenge by pulling their fingers apart easily. The amount of hypnotic talent of participants may be inferred by the degree of difficulty they experience in pulling the hands apart at the time of the challenge. In this test we are, of course, enlisting normal physiology on our side. By "freezing" the participants' tightly clasped hands together, we make it much more difficult physically for them to draw the hands apart. The good therapist uses normal muscle physiology to enhance the psychology of induction procedures.

Arm Levitation

This procedure is especially good in screening the more hypnotically talented individuals from a group of volunteers. It is not to be confused with the induction technique of the same name, which we describe in the next chapter. The therapist asks the participants to sit up straight, close their eyes, and hold out one arm. He or she then gives the following visualization: "I want you to imagine that a balloon filled with helium gas has just been connected to your wrist with a cord. It is large and of your favorite color. It is floating above the wrist. As you observe it, you will notice that it is pulling strongly upward on the wrist. Watch it as it floats higher, higher, higher. With each passing moment, the lifting sensation becomes stronger and stronger, and the balloon is floating up, up, up, higher, higher and higher."

A balloon, a typical remembrance of childhood, is deliberately chosen to facilitate at least a partial regression. Notice that the attention is centered on observing the balloon as it floats upward. The rising of the hand then becomes a consequence of the balloon's upward movement and is suggested indirectly. By indicating that the balloon is "of your favorite color," the feeling of participation is encouraged. As the participants visualize the balloon in their favorite color, they become more personally and imaginatively involved. The participants exercise free will in the choice, and what happens afterward can then occur on a more involuntary basis. Again repetition is used, a technique that is commonly a part of all induction procedures, to intensify the hypnotic suggestion. The therapist continues the wording previously discussed and repeats it for a minute or so, until a number of the participants show substantial lifting of the arm. Very talented hypnotic participants may finally have their arms lifted almost straight up. In a large group, they are easy to spot. Your volunteers for further hypnotic study now have raised their hands.

Head Nod Forward

Although the experienced hypnotherapist usually becomes sensitive to many slight signs of hypnotic involvement, for the beginner in the field, it is desirable that hypnotizability tests show some overt movement as a positive signal. Accordingly, if the eyes have become closed during one of the foregoing procedures, the following test is useful. A positive response confirms the hypnotizability that the participant has demonstrated so far. Consistent with the principle that the carrying out of hypnotic suggestions is frequently hypnotizing, its successful accomplishment by an individual will tend to deepen whatever hypnotic state is now present. If an eye closure was part of a group screening, but not all have yet closed their eyes, they are now all simply instructed to do so. Then the operator proceeds as follows: "Now that your eyes are closed you will notice a tendency for your head to nod forward as if some force were pushing on the back of it. The head will tend to move forward and the chin to drop down toward your chest. The head is becoming heavier and heavier and heavier." Notice, again, to facilitate dissociation, the therapist said "the head" not "your head." This wording has a tendency to remove the head from voluntary control so that "it" is responding; "you" are not bringing your head down. The head is dissociated from "subject" and designated as "object." Objects are elements outside the self, over which we have no voluntary control.

They are controlled by outside forces for which we have no responsibility. They just happen to us.

Inability to Push Hands Together

This test can now be conveniently administered to participants whose eyes are closed and who have indicated some nodding forward of the head. It is similar to one of the items in the *Stanford Hypnotic Susceptibility Scale*. The participants may be given the following suggestions: "Hold both hands in front of you, facing one another, about a foot apart. You will notice if you try to bring the hands closer together that there is a force that seems to push them apart. It is like trying to push in on the two sides of a pillow. The harder you try to bring them together, the stronger becomes the force holding them apart. It is almost impossible to bring them together so closely that they touch each other. Try to bring them together."

This test, like the finger lock, consists of a challenge. However, if participants have responded favorably to the previous tests, such as the eye-closure and the head nodding forward tests, they are likely to be involved hypnotically. Accordingly, the participants may manifest a positive response by struggling to bring the hands together and discovering that they are unable to get them closer than about 6 inches apart.

By now, in this series of hypnotizability exercises, many participants will be quite hypnotically involved. In fact, a true hypnotic state may have been induced. As the therapist proceeds in hypnotic technique, he or she will note that the tests, with a little extension, turn into trance-induction procedures, and induction techniques, when continued, become methods for deepening the hypnotic state. They are all part of the psychological process of restricting attention, concentrating on minor movements first, and then spreading the involvement to larger areas of the person, psychological and physiological. They include the elements of narrowing the perceptual field and regression to earlier modes of response, which characterize the hypnotic condition. Many of the participants may now be capable of responding to suggestions of a hallucination.

Hallucinations of Warmth

Those participants whose eyes spontaneously closed, whose heads nodded forward, and who were unable to push their hands together in the previous tests may now evidence an actual perceptual hallucination when suggestions such as the following are administered: "I wonder what is wrong with the furnace. The thermostat must be stuck, because it's getting hotter and hotter in this room. The air is becoming stifling. It's getting so warm that it's very hard to breathe. What I wouldn't give for a breath of fresh cool air. It certainly is getting warmer and warmer. Makes one sweat. What can we do in the face of all this heat?"

At this point, the participants who are rather deeply involved hypnotically will make some movements indicating they are experiencing the intense heat. These movements may include breathing heavily, fanning themselves, wiping the forehead, and so forth.

As the hypnotic involvement becomes greater, the therapist approaches that stage that has been called somnambulism. Participants have now passed beyond the point of perceptual restriction and the performance of minor motor movements. They are now, typically, capable of walking about and behaving in many complicated ways, while still remaining in a deep hypnotic state, one that is often so dissociated from their normal condition that they manifest a complete amnesia for it on being removed from hypnosis; that is, the participants cannot even remember what they did while in the hypnotic state.

The earlier tests of hypnotizability should have indicated that a participant was, or was not, likely to be able to respond to hypnosis. The initiation of hallucinations and the following test, which involves decisive motor action, may indicate those participants who are capable of entering a fairly deep hypnotic state.

Compulsive Rising

Let the therapist continue to assume that he or she is screening those individuals with good hypnotic talents from a group (although the following suggestions similar to those given previously can just as well be applied to a single individual). The therapist now tells the participants the following: "As you sit there, you begin to be aware of a strong need to stand up, to rise from your seat. This tendency is becoming stronger and stronger. Feel that need to stand up. The need is becoming so powerful that if you remain seated you will feel increasingly uncomfortable. Your inner tension gets stronger and stronger, and you know that if you could stand up, you would immediately feel relieved. It seems that only by rising from your seat could you get rid of this uncomfortable tension and feel at ease."

Such hypnotic suggestions are continued until some members of the group rise from their chairs. Others may put up quite a struggle, whereas some sit passively and manifest no tendency to stand up. They may have felt the need to rise and wanted to rise for some time, but felt embarrassed to be the first ones to do so. As those who are still seated (with their eyes closed) hear the sound of others standing up, there is a strong group suggestibility effect. Do not make the mistake of assuming that these later-rising suggestion-responsive participants are also hypnotically involved. They are likely responding to social influence.

Finally, all or almost all of the individuals will rise, even though some of them are not at all hypnotically responsive, but feel the need to conform. Accordingly, the early risers tend to have better hypnotic talents. This test, too, involves a kind of challenge. It is therefore better adapted to the selection of good hypnotic participants for research, demonstration, or practice purposes rather than for the evaluation of the hypnotizability of patients with whom one may wish to develop a sensitive, therapeutic relationship later.

Standardized Tests of Hypnotic Responsivity

The obvious benefits of a systematic method of measuring hypnotizability can be traced as far back as the 19th century (Perry & Laurence, 1980), when Braid attempted to define stages of hypnotic depth. However, serious and exhaustive research on the measurement of hypnotic responsivity did not begin until the 1950s, at Ernest (Jack) R. Hilgard's Laboratory of Hypnosis Research at Stanford University. By 1959, the *Stanford Hypnotic Susceptibility Scale,* Forms A and B (SHSS:A, SHSS:B, respectively) had been fully developed. The *Stanford Hypnotic Susceptibility Scale,* Form C, now considered the "gold standard" (A. Barabasz & Barabasz, 1992) of hypnotizability measurement, was published in 1962 (Weitzenhoffer & Hilgard, 1962). The SHSS:C, frequently referred to by researchers as simply "the Form C," eclipsed the Forms A and B, because the Form C included a range of more difficult test items to determine whether the participant could manifest dissociative responses. Like the Forms A and B, the Form C consisted of 12 items of progressively greater difficulty and required about 1 hour to complete the administration. At last, investigators of hypnosis had a uniform yardstick with excellent psychometric properties against which studies and clinical trials among different researchers and clinicians could be assessed. Shor and Orne (1962) developed the *Harvard Group Scale of Hypnotic Susceptibility* (HGSHS:A) was developed by on the basis of the SHSS:A. Although far inferior to the use of the individualized Form C, it provides a relatively easy method of obtaining a "first cut" for researchers needing to tease out those with particularly high or low hypnotic capacity.

The SHSS:C and HGSHS:A have become the most widely used scales in hypnosis research conducted since their introduction, except by a minority of researchers who held a nonstate view of hypnosis. These sociocognitivists have preferred to use their own tests, which have fewer items and psychometric properties that can wrongly classify low-hypnotizable individuals as medium-hypnotizable individuals. The tests include the *Barber Suggestibility Scale* (T. Barber & Glass, 1962), which takes 10 minutes to administer, and the group scale the *Carleton University Responsiveness to Suggestion Scale* (CURSS) (Spanos, Radtke, Hodgins, Stam, & Bertrand, 1983). The aptly named CURSS attempts to measure "suggestibility" in 11 minutes, including a 5-minute induction, followed by seven items of 50 seconds each, then indices of susceptibility are given. Not including self-scoring by the participants, this test is completed in about 25 minutes. As might be expected, the CURSS and the gold standard SHSS:C show relatively good agreement in identifying high- and low-hypnotizable individuals, as these individuals are at extreme ends (Spanos et al., 1983). Unfortunately, most of the individuals classified as having medium or average hypnotizability by the CURSS were classified as lows on the SHSS:C (Perry, Nadon, & Button, 1992; Spanos, Salas, Menary, & Brett, 1986). All studies using the CURSS to obtain a pool of "average hypnotizables" would then, in all likelihood, have low-hypnotizable individuals wrongly labeled as medium-hypnotizable individuals. As we know, low-hypnotizable individuals respond to suggestion and placebo but are incapable of true hypnotic responses that could be produced by trance states that can be experienced by true medium- and high-hypnotizable individuals (McGlashan, Evans, & Orne, 1969). Studies using the CURSS to obtain "average" hypnotizables then are preloaded to produce effects consistent with sociocognitive conceptualizations of hypnosis as suggestion–role-play response.

Summarily, the Form C (SHSS:C) includes comprehensive pretest instructions aimed at maximizing rapport, alleviating anxieties about the test, and maximizing the probability of obtaining the most accurate measure. Next, a nonscored lengthy set of eye-closure hypnotic induction instructions are provided, which provides opportunities to move on to the test upon eye closure, without the necessity to complete the full induction. Thereby, different speeds of participants' responses to the induction are taken into account while still maintaining a standardized procedure.

Briefly, the SHSS:C items are as follows:

1. *Hand lowering.* The therapist asks the participants to hold out their right arms at shoulder height, attend to feelings in the hands, and imagine holding something heavy, maybe a heavy baseball. The therapist gives suggestions about the hand feeling heavy and slowly but surely going down. The item is scored plus if the hand has lowered 6 or more inches after a 10-second wait.

2. *Moving hands apart.* The therapist asks the participants to extend their arms to the front, with palms facing each other, close together, but not touching. Then the therapist administers suggestions, calling for imagination of a force pushing the hands apart. The item is scored plus if the hands move at least 6 inches apart 10 seconds after cessation of the suggestions.

3. *Mosquito hallucination.* This is the first test item to call on a more difficult response requiring dissociative processing, taken from the SHSS:A. It is essentially the only item calling on dissociation in the earlier test. The therapist suggests that the participant may not have noticed a mosquito that has been buzzing around the room. The participant should to try to listen to its high-pitched buzzing; the therapist suggests the mosquito is landing on the participant's hand, it tickles a little, it might bite, and the participant does not like it and wants to get rid of it, brush it off, and so forth. A plus is recorded if there is grimacing, movement, or acknowledgment of effect.

4. *Taste hallucination.* This more complex dissociation suggests developing a sweet taste in the participant's mouth then changing it to a sour taste, such as lemon or vinegar. A plus is recorded if both tastes are reported as experienced, if either is experienced with overt signs such as lip movements or grimacing, or if one is reported as strong.

5. *Arm rigidity.* Returning to a motoric measure shared with the SHSS:A, this response to hypnosis is a more difficult response than those called for in Items 1 and 2. Here, the therapist asks the individuals to hold their right arms straight out and to think of them as becoming stiffer and stiffer, as though tightly splinted and unbendable. Then the participants are asked to test how stiff they are and to try to bend them. The item is scored plus if in 10 seconds the bend is less than 2 inches.

6. *Dream.* Calling on dissociation again, this item explains that the operator is interested in finding out about hypnosis and what being hypnotized means to people, and it states that one way to do so is through the dreams one has while hypnotized. The therapist then asks the participants to rest and tells them that they will "sleep and have a dream." After 2 minutes have passed, the participants are told the dream is over, but that they can remember every detail. The therapist asks the participants to describe the dream. A plus is scored if an experience comparable to a dream, not just vague or fleeting experiences, is reported.

7. *Age regression.* This two-part dissociation item is still more demanding. First, participants are asked to go deeper and deeper into the

hypnotic state and, as this takes place, they are given a pad and pencil in a manner to facilitate writing. Participants are asked to write
down their names, ages, the date, and so forth. Then, using further
deepening techniques and using a 1 to 5 counting method, the therapist tells the participants that they are getting younger and smaller,
going back to the fifth grade, and that they will actually be there.
The therapist asks the participants' age, where they are, what they
are doing, and so on; the therapist then asks the participants to write
their names and ages, the date, and the day of the week on the pad.
The therapist uses a two count for deepening and regression and
tells the participants they are no longer in the fifth grade but are getting still younger, back in the second grade. Again, similar questions
are asked, as is the request to write on the pad. Once this task is
completed, the participants are told to grow up again, and the therapist carefully brings them back to the present date, time, and locale.
The participants' reorientation is confirmed before moving to the
next item. A plus is scored if there is a clear change in the handwriting from the present age to one or both of the regressed ages. (It is
important to understand that the ability to pass this item need not
depend on the identicality of the writing samples with those that
might have been retained by the participant from that age; the point
is to determine whether a dissociative response was possible. The
actual memory traces may have been lost, but the participant's dissociative capacity is unlikely to be affected. In such a case, the participant constructs the age regression, yet nonetheless it can be a true
response to the hypnotic state [A.F.B.].)

8. *Immobilization of the right arm.* This item is also taken from the
   SHSS:A. The therapist gives suggestions that the participants' arms
   have become heavy and that they will not be able to lift them. The
   therapist ends the item with a challenge to "try to lift it." The item is
   scored plus if the arm rises fewer than 1 inch within 10 seconds.

9. *Anosmia to ammonia.* When properly administered, this rather dramatic dissociation item is difficult to pass by nonhypnotizable role-
   playing or hypnosis-simulating participants brought into various
   research studies as controls. The therapist tells the participants that
   in a moment they will not be able to smell any odors, they can smell
   odors less and less, and so forth. Then the participants are told to
   take a good sniff of an odorous substance placed under the nose to
   demonstrate that they are incapable of smelling any odors. The therapist holds an opened bottle of household ammonia under the participants' noses and they are instructed to take a good sniff. The

therapist gives suggestions for the participants to return to their normal state of smell, and the ammonia is reintroduced with the test suggestion. The participants are asked to compare the two odors and are reassured that all is again normal and that there will be no more odors. A plus is scored if the ammonia is denied and overt signs were completely absent. (In actuality, the response to ammonia relates to pain receptors far more than the olfactory sense.) Clinicians or researchers involved in work requiring repeated administration of odors to test responsiveness should, therefore, use stimuli that are established as purely olfactory in nature. For example, on the basis of the A. Barabasz and Lonsdale (1983) research on EEG event-related potential responses to hypnosis, we found laboratory-grade eugenol to serve that purpose.

10. *Hallucinated voice.* This demanding dissociation item begins by the therapist's telling the participants that the examiner forgot to tell them that there is someone in the office who wants to ask some questions, such as the participant's age and place of birth. The questions will be asked over a loudspeaker-microphone combination on the wall. The participants are asked to talk good and loud when answering questions and are told that "the speaker has been turned on, there's the first question." A plus is scored if at least one realistic answer is heard or if evidence of having hallucinated the answers is apparent.

11. *Negative visual hallucination.* This is an extremely difficult item, which is usually passed only by those in the hypnotic virtuoso category. The therapist tells participants that in a little while they will be asked to open their eyes while remaining deeply hypnotized and that two small boxes have been placed on the table in front of then, when in fact, three boxes (2 inch × 3 inch × 0.5 inch; colored red, white, or blue) are placed in front of the participants. The participants are then asked to open their eyes and look at the two boxes. Once confirmation is obtained, the participants are pressed with further questions as to whether they see anything else and are asked to name the colors of the boxes, and so forth. A plus is scored if the hallucination is present.

12. *Posthypnotic amnesia.* This item appears last, because of the requirements of test administration rather than that of graduated difficulty. (We regard it as less difficult than the preceding items 9 to 11.) Here participants are asked to listen carefully and are told that they will be counted out of hypnosis and will have been so relaxed that they will have trouble recalling the things that were said and what was done;

they will forget all that has happened until the therapist says they can remember everything. Once awake and completely out of hypnosis, participants are asked to tell everything that happened since the induction began. The examiner records items in order of mention and asks if there is anything else the participants remember. The release suggestion is given and the additional items mentioned are recorded. The participants are asked about the quality of the experience and so forth. A plus is scored if 3 or fewer items are recalled before the release.

The pluses are added to determine the participants' hypnotizability score. The mean (average) score in samples drawn from university student studies in the United States runs from 6.0 to 6.7, depending on the sample. The *Stanford Hypnotic Susceptibility Scale* reliability has been tested over the 25-year period from 1960 to 1985, yielding an $r =.64$ for the 10-year period of 1960 to 1970, an $r =.82$ for the 15-year period of 1970 to 1985, and an $r =.71$ for the entire 25-year period (Piccione, Hilgard, & Zimbardo, 1989).

Standardized Clinical Scales of Hypnotizability

Recognizing that the best scales we reviewed above were lengthy to administer and seldom used by practitioners, the need for shorter clinical scales became apparent if measured hypnotizability was to become of direct use with patients, rather than with primarily curious university student volunteers. The first of the clinically oriented scales were closely adapted from the parent *Stanford Hypnotic Susceptibility Scale,* Forms A, B, and C. Arlene Morgan and Josphine Hilgard introduced the *Stanford Hypnotic Clinical Scale* (SHCS) in the now classic book *Hypnosis in the Relief of Pain* by E. Hilgard and J. Hilgard (1975). The SHCS was intended to make measurement of hypnotizability more suitable for hospitalized patients who might be suffering from conditions in which pain was prominent. Reduced patient mobility was considered in drawing items from the *Stanford Hypnotic Susceptibility Scale,* and the scale was reduced to a total of five items, with a scripted relaxation hypnotic induction. It takes about 20 to 25 minutes to administer and debrief the patient. We have found it is a particularly easy scale to learn to administer for those new to hypnosis, and it is useful as an aid in guiding the selection of particular procedures to be used in therapy, as it helps predict responsiveness to hypnosis beyond the screening of pain patients. For example, A. Barabasz, Baer, Sheehan, and Barabasz (1986) found SHCS scores to correlate significantly with successful responses to hypnosis for smoking cessation at an 18-month follow-up at Harvard Medical School and Massachusetts General

Hospital, although experience of the therapist was still a better predictor of outcome.

Briefly, the SHCS items are as follows:

1. *Hands moving together.* The therapist asks participants to hold their hands straight out to the front, about a foot apart. The therapist gives hypnotic suggestions to the participants to imagine magnets in each hand attracting each other or rubber bands stretched between the wrists, to think of a force acting on the hands pulling them together, and so forth. The item is scored plus if the hands are fewer than 6 inches apart within 10 seconds. In the case of an immobile arm, the hand-lowering Item 1 from the SHSS:C is substituted.

2. *Dream.* The therapist asks participants to continue relaxing and tells them that they are going to have a real dream much like the kind they might have at night. A timed period of 1 minute is allowed, and then the patients are told the dream is over but that they can remember it very clearly. The therapist asks the patients to please tell all about the dream. The administrator probes for details as needed, and the patients are asked to assess how real they felt the dream was. A plus score is recorded if the reported experience was comparable to a real dream.

3. *Age regression.* Participants are given the choice of returning to the third, fourth, or fifth grade and are told that in a little while they will be going back to a happy day in elementary school. A count from 1 to 5, "younger and smaller," and so forth is used in the attempt to elicit an age regression response while also deepening trance. On the count of 5, the participants are told they are "now a small boy [or girl] in the [selected] grade." The therapist then asks a series of questions, such as, "Where are you?" "What are you doing?" "Who is your teacher?" "Who is with you?" The participants are told that they can grow up and come back to their present age, and so on. Care is taken to ensure the participants are fully reoriented in time and space. A 5-point scale is used for the participants' subjective rating (given after all hypnosis). The scale ranges progressively from 1 (no regression at all) to 5 (participants actually felt they were back reliving a past experience). A plus score is recorded for the item if either the administrator's rating is "good" or the participants' rating is 4 or 5.

4. *Posthypnotic suggestion.* The posthypnotic suggestion of clearing of the throat or of coughing is rather cleverly embedded within the final amnesia item. During the amnesia instructions (see the next item) participants are told that later, when the administrator taps a pencil twice on the table, they will have a sudden urge to cough or

clear their throat and then will do so. A plus score is recorded if participants do so after they are brought out of hypnosis and the pencil is tapped.

5. *Amnesia.* The therapist explains that at a backward count from 10 to 1, the participants will come out of hypnosis gradually. The post-hypnotic suggestion in the previous item is administered with the instruction that the participants will forget that they were told to cough or clear the throat, just as the participants will forget all that has happened until the therapist says that they can remember everything. After awakening, the participants are asked to tell everything that happened since closing their eyes. A plus score is recorded if they remember no more than two of the test items.

Herbert Spiegel and David Spiegel (1978) developed the *Hypnotic Induction Profile* (HIP), which takes 5 to 10 minutes to administer. It is intended to tap hypnosis as a subtle perceptual alteration, involving the capacity for attentive, responsive concentration that is inherent in the participant. The HIP provides a procedure for trance induction and a standardized measure of hypnotic capacity. Unlike the other scales, the HIP was standardized and validated on a patient population in a clinical setting, rather than on young, more fully functioning university students.

The Spiegels focused on the clinical point of view in the development of the HIP, rather than the research point of view emphasized by the *Stanford Hypnotic Susceptibility Scales.* The Spiegels saw the need for an even shorter test of hypnotizability than the 20- to 25-minute SHCS. At the same time, they wanted a scale that would facilitate the clinical-therapeutic relationship, rather than one intended primarily to meet the needs of the laboratory situations.

The Spiegels conceptualized hypnosis as a state, rather than as merely a function of social influence. They also recognized that context and motivation are key factors in any psychological measurement. Certainly, tests administered to student volunteers for the sole purpose of hypnosis experiments must measure different dimensions than those presenting themselves for clinical treatment (Frankel & Orne, 1976). University students curious about hypnosis are no doubt less motivated than clinical patients seeking help with a personal problem. The HIP was intended to overcome the difficulties inherent in the university-based scales of hypnotizability. The test consists of three major components and is the first attempt to bring a biological measurement directly into a test of hypnotizability. Considering that the HIP was developed in the 1970s and that the biological components of brain responses to hypnosis have only very recently been established, the authors' inclusion of a biological measurement in the test was remarkably foresightful. The three major components are as follows: a biological component, an eye roll that records presumed biological trance capacity; an idiomotor item consisting of hand levitation; and a subjective discovery experience, the control differential between hands. The test is intended to yield information regarding a participant's hypnotizability sufficient to make a clinical decision regarding the role of hypnosis in treatment. The scale correlates significantly with the best *Stanford Hypnotic Susceptibility Scale*, but, more important to the clinician, it is rich in predictive relationships to treatment outcomes and psychopathological factors.

Consistent with the other recognized scales, the HIP correlates significantly with the SHSS:C (Frischholz et al., 1980) and assesses a single trance experience as it progresses through the stages of entering hypnosis, experiencing hypnosis, and responding to hypnotic suggestions. The HIP also establishes a structure for the sequence, but the specific point in time in which the shift from customary waking awareness into trance varies from person to person. The SHSS:A, SHSS:B, and SHSS:C provide for this variance by moving from the eye closure to the test, but allowing for several different phases of the eye-closure experience to be experienced so that it accommodates for different participants' individual responses. Unfortunately, the SHCS has but a single relaxation induction after which participants are assumed to be in hypnosis.

The HIP punctuates the trance experience and divides it into phases by 10 individual items. Six of the items are actually used for rating the participant's trance capacity and for scoring the HIP according to the profile-scoring method. The remaining items are intended to further establish the clinical picture for entering and exiting trance and for subsequent self-reporting. However, scoring these last four items is considered optional, because they are not part of the core HIP summary score. The technique induces hypnotic trance quickly under observed and specified conditions and, as in the other scales, provides a clear shift out of trance on signal. Simultaneously, the test introduces the participants to their own individual idiosyncrasies for entering and exiting trance. The examiner measures trance capacity, and the participants learn to identify the trance experience so they can initiate it and use it independently in the form of self-hypnosis, without the need of a therapist at a later time.

The HIP is divided into four phases of measurement. As in the SHSS:A, SHSS:B, and SHSS:C, there is first a pre-trance or pre-induction phase that lasts until eye closure. The SHCS asks the participants to voluntarily close their eyes before relaxation induction instructions are given, and, therefore, much is lost from the clinical and psychometric picture of assessing the participants' response to the induction.

Briefly, the four phases for measurement of the HIP are as follows:

1. *Pretrance.* Preinduction state of customary awareness is tapped by the up gaze and is one of the optionally scored items.
2. *Induction.* Formal trance is induced by eye-closure instructions and instructions for postinduction responsivity, as well as the instructions for exiting the formal trance with eye opening. This phase includes the eye-roll sign and the instructional arm levitation.
3. *Initial postinduction.* Initial postinduction is measured in the post-formal trance with open eyes to tap postformal trance responsiveness. It includes the items of tingle (optionally scored), dissociation, signaled arm levitation, and control differential. The administrators touching of the participant's elbow end this phase.
4. *Postinduction final phase.* This phase comes after trance, once the customary state of awareness has been established. The items include amnesia (optionally scored) and float.

Briefly, items of the HIP are as follows:

1. *Dissociation.* Scoring on this item requires spontaneous response from the participant and can be scored positive 1 or 2 if the participant reports that the arm used in the preparatory levitation task feels "less part" of the body than the other arm, or if the hand feels "less connected to the wrist" than the other hand.
2. *Signaled arm levitation.* This item is scored 1 to 4 if, on the instructed signal, the participant's arm rises to the upright position. Scoring is based on the number of verbal reinforcements necessary.
3. *Control differential.* This item is also spontaneous and uninstructed. It is scored 1 or 2 if the participant feels less control over the arm in the levitation item. The administrator's questions do not indicate which arm is expected to be less controllable.
4. *Cutoff.* This item is scored positive 1 or 2 if, on the instructed signal, the participant reports normal cessation and control returning to the arm used in the levitation item.
5. *Float.* This item is scored 1 or 2 if the participant reports having felt the instructed floating sensation through the administration of the levitation item.

The HIP is an objectively scored interpersonal hypnotic interaction that obtains results comparable to standardization data established with clinical participants. The induction requires skill and experience. There must be momentum or rhythm that is established and maintained during the interaction. There cannot be long silences or pauses during the test administration, and the pace cannot be so rapid that the participants do not have a chance to attend their experiences. Administration of the HIP requires considerable expertise on the part of the administrator and complete familiarity with the test, which is not required by the *Stanford Hypnotic Susceptibility Scale*. It is for this reason that at Washington State University we generally introduce the HIP only at the very end of the advanced course in hypnosis. This means graduate students beginning to learn the scale will have already completed a minimum of 500 to 1,500 hypnotic inductions and are well advanced in their PhD programs. Even so, without considerable clinical experience and confidence, the HIP can be difficult to master. It is a scale reserved for the experienced clinician. Detailed instructions for administration of the scale appear in the H. Spiegel and D. Spiegel's classic text *Trance and Treatment* (1978) and in the second edition (2004).

The Quantification of Hypnotic Depth

A number of attempts to quantify hypnotic depth, or at least to indicate the characteristics of various levels of hypnotic involvement, have been published over the years. Charcot (1882/1888) considered that there were three types of hypnosis: catalepsy, lethargy, and somnambulism. Bernheim (1964) and Liebeault (1866) classified various levels of trance ranging from drowsiness to catalepsy (e.g., rigidity in the limbs achieved through suggestion), up to suggested hallucinations experienced posthypnotically.

Davis and Husband (1931) published a scale that differentiated five levels of hypnosis, assigned a depth score, and indicated the percentage of participants they found capable of reaching each level (see Table 4.1).

J. Watkins (1949) published an expanded version of this scale, which added the following items: 8, Hyperamnesia slight; 16, Hyperamnesia marked; 19, Regression; and 32, Negative visual hallucinations, posthypnotic.

Efforts to correlate hypnotizability with other personality traits have, in general, been unsuccessful. However, J. Hilgard (1979) showed that the ability to respond hypnotically is related to "keeping alive the imaginative involvements of childhood." Those individuals who enjoy fantasies through reading or identification seem to respond better than average.

In the *Thematic Apperception Test*, participants are asked to imagine stories about the pictures that are presented to them. One of the pictures shows a boy lying, apparently asleep, on a couch with an older man leaning over him. This picture is often perceived as a picture of hypnosis. There is some evidence that the relationship between this boy and the older man, as described by the participant, may tell something about whether the individual regards the therapist favorably and trusts him or is suspicious of his

Table 4.1 Davis and Husband's (1931) Hypnotic Susceptibility Scale

Depth	Score	Objective Symptoms	Number of Cases	Percentage of Cases
Insusceptible	0		5	9
Hypnoidal	2	Relaxation	16	29
	3	Fluttering of lids		
	4	Closing of eyes		
	5	Complete physical relaxation		
Light trance	6	Catalepsy of eyes	10	18
	7	Limb catalepsies		
	10	Rigid catalepsy		
	11	Anesthesia (glove)		
Medium trance	13	Partial amnesia	8	15
	15	Posthypnotic anesthesia		
	17	Personality changes		
	18	Simple posthypnotic suggestions		
	20	Kinesthetic delusions; complete amnesia		
Somnambulistic	21	Ability to open eyes without affecting trance	16	29
	23	Bizarre posthypnotic suggestions accepted		
	25	Complete somnambulism		
	26	Positive visual hallucinations, posthypnotic		
	27	Positive auditory hallucinations, posthypnotic		
	28	Systematized posthypnotic amnesias		
	29	Negative auditory hallucinations		
	30	Negative visual hallucinations; hyperesthesias	3	
		Total	55	100

motives and feels a need to resist. Response to this picture may be of help to therapists (who practice either hypnotherapy or other types of psychotherapy) in assessing the therapeutic relationship and the possibility of favorable response from their patient.

For successful therapeutic intervention, the therapist must translate theory into practice. Clinical hypnosis cannot be learned from reading books alone. The ability to employ the hypnotic modality in effective treatment of patients requires that the learner spend considerable time in practice, working with real, live patients. Accordingly, practicum exercises, which include some of the preceding hypnotizability tests, should enable researchers or clinicians to develop their skill at selecting suitable participants for hypnotic work.

Chapter 5
Introductory Techniques of Hypnotic Induction

Given that hypnosis is essentially a psychophysiological state of aroused attentiveness, characterized by enhanced receptive focal concentration with a corresponding diminution in peripheral awareness, there are innumerable ways by which this hypnotic state, or trance, can be initiated, such as by a formal induction in contrast to spontaneous trance that is aroused either internally (daydreaming) or externally (trauma). They differ widely in the relative emphasis on motor, perceptual, or dissociative processes. There are successful hypnotic inductions that go beyond the responses that can be wrought by mere suggestion and social influence; each contains some of the following elements. I (A.F.B.) have observed that careful attention to three basic phases of hypnotic induction (particularly among beginners with fewer than 500 successful inductions) is of critical importance, if true hypnotic responses are to be obtained from an individual who is hypnotizable.

Three Phases of Hypnotic Induction

The preparatory phase consists of descriptions of hypnotic responding, which may simply be embedded in the hypnotic induction that are presented entirely in the future tense before they occur. The participant is attentive. Wording might include suggestions such as "Your eyelids will become heavier and heavier and you will want to close your eyes, eventually your eyes will be so tired you will close them — it will be come impossible to keep them open, the pressure of your hand resting on your leg will be less and less — *that* hand [the word *that* is used to then dissociate the hand from the person] will become lighter and lighter and eventually it will begin to rise, to lift on its own, you may notice that you will get an increase in salivation as you go into hypnosis, some people have that response, you might too, it's just one of those perfectly normal responses some people have at this stage, maybe you will have it too, maybe not, but all of the time you will become more and more calm" (or more alert, if an alert induction is the plan; these are specific responses indicating what will be felt, rather than some vague call for "relaxation"). The key element of the preparatory phase is that the therapist is completely safe in suggesting responses in the future tense when there is no evidence of them in the participant. I (A.F.B.) once took nearly an hour to evoke the rising of an individual's hand from the leg. The induction response became so profound to the individual that future hypnotic rapport was ensured and deep rapid inductions took place, resulting in dramatic therapeutic gains and major positive changes in the patient's life.

The transition phase consists of descriptions in the present tense of hypnotic responding as the therapist observes them. Participants' concentration becomes effortless as they begin to dissociate and become unaware of all but the hypnotic activity. Moving on to this phase prematurely is a recipe for failure to achieve true hypnotic responding. In such cases, at best, the therapist might achieve simple relaxation and simple effortful responses to easy suggestions. The therapist should initiate this phase only when clear evidence of the participant's responses, hypnotically suggested in the preparatory phase, are actually observed. As therapists become experienced in hypnosis, they will learn to observe the participant more closely as they become less preoccupied with carrying out the specifics of the induction procedure. As a result, the therapist will be able to use these subtle clinical observations of hypnotic responding in the transition phase, regardless of whether they were suggested in the earlier phase. Clients frequently repeat their own idiosyncratic responses in the process of entering hypnosis. Wording typical of the transition phase might be as follows: Upon noticing eye flutter, say, "Your eyes are beginning to flutter, they may close soon"; then as the eyes close for an instant, say, "There the eyes closed, so much more comfortable closed than open."

The hypnotic rapport phase constitutes the true hypnotic experience. Wording involves whatever is required by the clinical demands of the situation or the research protocol. Hypnotic deepening, as we discussed in the earlier chapters, and depth checks should correspond to the difficulty of the hypnotic response required. Consider, for a moment, that the patient is regressed at least to some degree. Why would you expect to be trusted to use hypnosis in therapy any further if you were perceived to be unsure of yourself or, worse yet, to have no belief that the hypnotic state is real? No caring therapists, no matter how clever, can resonate with a patient while trying to hide disbelief in the modality they are trying to use. To obtain difficult responses to hypnotic suggestions (pain relief, surgery without anesthetic, amnesia, trauma resolution, etc.), you must absolutely expect it to work, you must know it will work. You will gain the prestige and the expertise to help your clients achieve a hypnotic state, but you must also be honest in therapy if it is to work.

Develop a series of graded hypnotic suggestions and do not interrupt the process by calling for simple voluntary behaviors. These points are key to helping your patient to achieve an altered state and not mere relaxation- or suggestion-produced responses. In this phase the patient shows (a) increased suggestibility; (b) attentional redistribution (if told to listen only to your voice, all else will be effortlessly ignored); (c) no desire to make plans, the here and now is all that you can focus on; (d) a reduction in reality testing where reality distortions are readily accepted (may uncritically accept hallucinated experiences such as petting an imaginary rabbit); (e) responsiveness to posthypnotic amnesia when so instructed and with restoration of what has transpired by posthypnotic signal; and (f) the ability to readily enact unusual roles when instructed to do so, such as reenacting behaviors characteristic of an earlier age-age regression.

Principles of Induction

To narrow the perceptual field, ask participants to concentrate on some aspect of their physical or psychological functioning: concentrate on a single aspect, remove attention from other aspects of their being. Thus, to get the patients to gaze at an eye-fixation object, say, "Please try to stare at that thumbtack up on the wall"; to get the patients to sense the feelings in their hand, say, "Just look at that hand and notice what you can notice"; or to get the patients to visualize a certain scene, say, "Imagine yourself on a tropical island."

To minimize conscious and volitional effort, tell the participants that they need not attend to the words of the therapist: "My words will enter your mind without trying to listen, do not to try to do anything, merely to let happen whatever happens."

To dissociate the hand from control of the participants and turn normal self or "subject" movements into not-self or "object" actions. Participants may be told, "*The* hand is moving toward *the* face." (Not "*Your* hand is moving toward *your* face.")

In an effort to bypass voluntary or ego participation, tell participants, "You are not really concerned about the fact that you can achieve many things without having to think about them." Statements of this type have been highly developed by Milton Erickson. They are viewed as constituting a "confusion" technique (Erickson, Rossi, & Rossi, 1976).

To induce a regression by stressing comfort, relaxation, passivity, even infantile dependency, tell participants, "You are in a soft, warm place where all your needs are taken care of, and you can enjoy this experience with every fiber of your being" (a womb fantasy).

To tie together hypnotic reactions with ordinary suggested behaviors, tell the participant, "As you sit there relaxed in the chair, you begin to notice a sensation of lightness coming into your hand."

To use repetition as an aid to creating a dissociative response, tell the participant, "You are becoming sleepier and sleepier and sleepier." (It makes no difference to the participant that the hypnotic state has nothing to do with the actual sleep state.) By contrast, the alert induction might involve wording such as "You are becoming more alert, more and more alert, more awake and completely alert."

To focus attention on tiny normal movements and expand them into behaviors involving larger segments of the body, tell the participant, "You are blinking and your eyes are getting heavier and wanting to come down, down, down, down."

To establish a set for entry into trance, tell the participant, "I will count up to 20. Your arm, which I am holding, will get heavier and heavier. At the count of 20, when I drop it, you will drop rapidly with it into a deep state of calmness." This instruction is similar to "On your mark, get set, go!" A readiness for hypnotic response is suggested. The participant waits and anticipates its occurrence.

To assist natural entry into a trance state, ask the participant to imagine a kind of fantasy or dream.

In this chapter, we describe several of the more customary and traditional approaches to trance induction in considerable detail so that through practice sessions with suitable participants the beginner can learn how to hypnotize. In the next chapter, we consider additional techniques that involve greater complexity and skill for their successful execution or that deal with specialized problems.

Introductory Induction Techniques

The Relaxation Technique

As we noted in the chapter on history, earlier workers, such as Liebeault, perceived the hypnotic state as akin to sleep, and they used the word frequently as part of their induction verbalizations. Because research has shown that the condition of hypnosis is physiologically and psychologically different from that of sleep, workers in the field now tend to avoid this term. However, in its place there is a great deal of use of the term *relaxation,* both in orienting patients to the meaning of hypnosis and in providing a set for the more effective inculcation of suggestions.

Relaxation is not at all necessary for a hypnotic induction (A. Barabasz & Barabasz, 2000); however, Meares (1961) devoted almost an entire chapter to describing a relaxation approach and specifically told his patients, "It is easier to attain the mental state of hypnotic sleep, if one lies flat on one's back." On the other hand, E. Hilgard and J. Hilgard (1975) found no difference in the response to hypnosis depending on whether the participants were seated or standing. Several techniques, such as the postural sway and certain rapid approaches, use an initial standing posture. The fact that individuals can be hypnotized when standing, sitting, or lying down is indicative of the point that hypnosis is not the same as simple relaxation. As a rather extreme example, I (A.F.B.) have hypnotized pilots while literally flying upside down in a fighter trainer, and have hypnotized airline pilots in training — in a Boeing 737 full motion simulator — in research on increasing attentiveness.

However, many induction and deepening techniques do employ some variation of relaxation, both as a process and as verbalized to the patients, and its use seems to make the induction process develop in a more gradual and natural manner. Furthermore, when hypnosis is described to patients as a form of "natural relaxation," they may lose any fears of involving themselves in it. It becomes, then, no longer a strange, mysterious experience in which their will can be overpowered, but it simply is a natural and pleasant physiological state to which they are already accustomed. Hypnosis then becomes divorced from the erroneous notion of "special process."

Before modern pharmacological treatments for hypertension were developed, Jacobson (1938) described a detailed process of "progressive relaxation" to teach patients to lower their blood pressures. He did not consider this to be hypnosis. However, the use of progressive relaxation techniques often results in an easier entry into hypnosis by a patient. These same procedures can also be employed as a preparation for hypnosis when patients are initially very tense and resistant. As they relax, they tend to relinquish rigid postures of opposition to hypnotic suggestions.

The progressive relaxation suggestions are aimed at making the patient highly aware of the difference between a state of tension and a state of relaxation progressively in different members of the body. An example might be as follows:

Lift your right foot off the floor and extend your leg straight out. Now imagine that there is a heavy weight placed on your ankle. Be keenly aware of the tensions throughout your entire leg. Think about them. Notice the pulling and the fatigue. Concentrate on all the feelings in that leg. That's it. Now let go. Let your leg drop down loose and limp until it is completely relaxed. Let all the tension and control go out of it.

The procedure is now repeated with the left leg. Similar suggestions may now be moved to the abdominal region.

Tighten the muscles across your abdomen. Make them like a tight band. Tighter, tighter, tighter. That's it. Hold that tension. Concentrate on it. Be keenly aware of every feeling in it. Good. Now let go. Let all the stiffness and tension go out of the abdominal muscles. Let them become completely relaxed.

Similar instructions are now administered to target the chest muscles, each arm, the hands, the facial muscles, the eyes, and the forehead. Each in turn is tensed, sensed, and then calmed to a more relaxed state. The patient becomes very conscious of the difference between tension and relaxation and learns how to achieve relaxation first in each part of the body and then finally throughout the entire body. The exercises, although minimally effective for their original intention of controlling high blood pressure, have been found to be very beneficial in treating many kinds of anxiety reactions and psychosomatic conditions in this day where the demands of our complex, information-overloaded society are significantly related to a wide range of physical and psychological tension disorders. If relaxation has been employed in treating such conditions, it is an easy step to incorporate it into an initial stage of hypnotic induction.

The therapist using such techniques talks in a slow and soft voice, thus modeling the state of relaxation. Meares repeated phrases such as, "Calm, easy, comfortable, let yourself go, drowsy, drifting, feel the heaviness, let the muscles loose, all of your body relax, it's all through you," and so on.

Each therapist will modify the exact wording, but the general principles involved in this induction will be the same; namely, providing continual suggestions of becoming calm, letting tensions go, drifting, picturing pleasant calming imagery, and modeling by the therapist of a state of relaxation. Although skilled operators always observe movements of their patients and attempt to coordinate suggestions with them, this approach probably calls for less attention to this factor than many others. The monotonous voice and the hypnotic-like suggestions of ever greater involvement in becoming calm have a cumulative effect that ultimately can result in the hypnotizable individual slipping into a trance state.

The Eye-Fixation Technique

James Braid (1960) is credited with developing what has become a classic induction method. Braid viewed eye fixation as key to an individual's hypnotic involvement.

The participant is seated in a comfortable armchair, and asked to rest comfortably. A pencil (or other object) is held just above the bridge of the nose, perhaps 6 to 8 inches away, and sufficiently close as to induce ocular fatigue. To focus on it the participant has to look upward and direct the eyes inward. The intention is to build on the eye fatigue so that it ultimately becomes natural to eliminate it by closing the eyes. The good therapist is extremely attentive to all tiny muscular responses and uses each to build on for the administration of suggestions aimed at inducing reactions in greater segments of the body.

Eye closure may be rapid or it may take a considerable period of time in the resistant individual. Accordingly, the arm of the therapist may become quite tired after holding it for a long time above the participant's eyes. Furthermore, in this approach it is better to stand at the side of the participant's chair rather than in front. This position is easier to maintain. If the therapist stands in front of the participant and holds his or her arm high, the therapist will become fatigued more rapidly; slow reactors might require 15 or more minutes before the eyes close. In the preferable position, the therapist's arm is resting against his or her side and his or her fingers, which are below the participant's eyes, hold the pencil.

The therapist should observe the participant's reactions carefully and time the suggestions very closely with them. For example, the remark, "Occasionally, they are going to blink," might be made immediately after perceiving a blink. What is important is that suggestions must correspond to what is observed. In the early stages of the induction the suggestions follow movements of the participant. Later, as the hypnotic involvement becomes greater, the therapist can lead or initiate such movements by appropriate suggestions. Knowing just when to change from a following to a leading is important and requires the closest attention. There are a number of variations to this approach, but a typical set of verbalized suggestions might be as follows:

Stare at the shiny part of this pencil. Fix your eyes on it. Take a few deep breaths. Just keep breathing deeply. Listen to the sound of my voice. You will find that your eyelids will get heavy. Almost as if they had a heavy weight attached to them. And the longer you stare at this, the more your eyelids will get heavy, and you blink, and they will have a feeling like something is pulling them down, as if they wanted to slowly close, and get drowsier and sleepier and heavier And you have a feeling as if they were slowly closing, slowly closing, getting drowsier and more tired, and when they finally do close, how good you will feel. Drowsy, heavy, pulling down, down, down, slowly closing, getting harder and harder to see, and you feel good. Very, very hard to keep them open, feel that very soon they will close tightly, almost tightly closing, almost tightly closing, tightly closing. Your eyes are tightly closed; you feel good; you feel comfortable; you're relaxed all over; just let yourself drift and enjoy this comfortable relaxed state. You will find that your head will get heavier, tends to nod forward some, and you just let yourself drift in an easy, calm, relaxed state.

The feeling of heaviness and the feeling of the eyes wanting to close are suggested first. Perceptions such as feeling the eyes wanting to close cannot be challenged, as can actual behaviors. If the therapist said at first, "Your eyes are closing," when in reality they were staring wide open, then their credibility would be lowered. Often in such a case, the participant structures this into a challenge. Then they become engaged in a kind of battle where the therapist is insisting, "Your eyes are closing," while the participant is fiercely resisting the eye closure. In such cases, the therapist often loses. Even if the eyes finally do close, the effort to induce the closure and that of the patient to resist has initiated a confrontive type of relationship. Obviously, this is counterproductive. There are some cases where verbal force and pressure are the only way to induce a trance state, but these should be employed minimally in therapeutic hypnosis.

Sometimes the heaviness in the eyes and the tendency for them to close can be enhanced by the therapist's passing a hand, perhaps with fingers apart, slowly downward several times between the participant's eyes and the pencil.

The induction proper is considered completed when the participant's eyes are completely and firmly closed. This may be tested by a challenge as follows:

Your eyes are tightly closed, and you will find that they want to remain closed. They are tightly stuck together, so tight that it seems as if the harder you try to pull them apart, the tighter they stick. The harder you try to pull them apart the tighter they stick together. They stick so tightly together they will not come apart no matter how hard you try. Try to pull them apart.

After the participant has tried for a moment or two the therapist may then say, "That's all right. You don't have to try any more. Now you can go down into a very deep state of relaxation, deep, deep, deep."

Experienced therapists tend to avoid challenges. Furthermore, if the individual is a patient for whom hypnotherapeutic treatment is to be administered, challenges may have an impairing effect on the relationship. Challenge suggestions tend to establish a dominant-dependent type of relationship, which may be contrary to the aims of the therapist. However, in some cases the therapist may feel it necessary to test the extent of hypnotic involvement before proceeding further. At this point deepening procedures are usually employed, or if the doctor feels that the patient is sufficiently involved in hypnosis, therapeutic suggestions or other treatment procedures may be applied.

Variations of the Eye-Fixation Technique. It may be inconvenient to hold an eye-fixation object, such as the pencil, in front of the participants' eyes. Accordingly, they can be asked to fix the gaze on some object across the room, preferably one that requires them to look upward. Some practitioners, such as those who use an analytic couch, may place a thumbtack in the ceiling at which the patient is asked to look. By having patients fixate on an object across the room, the eye-fixation procedure can be used to hypnotize simultaneously a number of members of a group. Group hypnosis is quite feasible (as in the group hypnotizability tests), and hypnosis is also being employed by a growing number of group therapists.

However, the difficulty is that the hypnotic suggestions cannot be timed as precisely to participants' eye movements or other postural indicators of hypnotic involvement. Accordingly, some participants will have achieved eye closure in a few minutes, whereas others are still staring with wide-open eyes at the fixation object. Group therapists obviously have to adapt their verbalizations to such a general situation.

Sometimes therapists place his or her fingers on the participants' foreheads and asks them to fixate on the end of the thumb. This, too, can be tiring and may also create other matters for consideration because it involves touching.

Patients who wear contact lenses should be asked to remove them before beginning an eye-fixation induction.

The Eye-Blink Method

This eye-closure method has the advantage of requiring little vocal effort on the part of the therapist. It is also quite easily administered to a group.

Participants are asked to sit back comfortably in their chairs, to close their eyes, and to take a few deep breaths. This, of course, is fairly standard procedure for many different inductions and simply establishes a responsive set and a feeling of security. Instructions may then be given as follows:

> I am going to count some numbers starting with one. Each time I say a number I want you to blink your eyes open for just a fraction of a second and then immediately close them. Continue doing this, responding to each number I speak by a rapid and momentary opening and closing of the eyes, until such time as your eyes become so tired and heavy they no longer wish to open. You may then just keep them closed and relax deeply.

It is desirable for the therapist to demonstrate the eye-blink counting behavior before beginning the induction to show what is expected.

The therapist then begins counting at 5-second intervals. The therapist closely observes the participants' eyes to see that they are carrying out the instructions, making only a very quick blink open and instantly closing again each 5 seconds.

After about 20 counts the therapist begins to put longer spaces between each count, perhaps a transitional period of 7- to 8-second intervals while counting from 21 to 30. After that, the intervals are systematically increased by about 5 seconds each for 10 to 20 counts. Hence, from 30 to 40 or 50 each number may be separated by a 10-second interval; from 50 to 60 or 70 separated by a 15-second interval. By the time 20-second intervals are reached, as many as 15 minutes or more has been spent in the induction. It is recommended that the therapist speaks the early numbers in a clear, firm voice, and that the therapist's voice becomes softer and more gentle as the induction proceeds, until by the time the therapist is counting with 20-second intervals, his or her voice is almost a whisper.

This procedure draws on natural physiological tendencies. As participants become increasingly relaxed, they find it less and less desirable to open the eyes. Each time they do they are confronted with a visual perception of reality to which the organism must adjust, but that is so momentary that they really do not have time to readapt to the normal awareness of the unhypnotized state. We tend to repeat behaviors that result in the cessation of feelings of unpleasantness. We also avoid behaviors that bring about unpleasantness or punishment. Opening the eyes creates a feeling of unpleasantness; closing them reinstates the pleasant state of calmness. So, in time, it is much easier simply to keep the eyes closed and continue on in a "deep state of relaxation" that the therapist has not only given permission to enjoy but also suggested would occur.

The Direct Stare

This technique was used widely by Bernheim and is described in much greater detail by Meares (1961, pp. 195–204) than we describe here. It is an extremely aggressive approach, which for its success relies on the domination by the operator of the participant. It is especially suited for emergency situations where the participant has, for example, just suffered physical or emotional trauma. I (A.F.B.) have used it in hospital emergency rooms, where immediate hypnosis to help the patient cooperate with treatment or a medical test procedure is required. One case involved a bouncer from a local bar who had been stabbed in the back. This rather huge fellow still had the knife stuck in his back, but because of pain and agitation, he was unable to keep still long enough for the urgently needed X-ray. This is not the time to measure hypnotizability or attempt a long drawn out relaxation induction. The direct stare induction produced a deep trance with great rapidity.

Because it is quite forceful in manner, there are certain specific indications for its most effective use and certain precautions and contraindications. It establishes the rather traditional dominance-submission relationship described in the Svengali-Trilby story (du Maurier, 1941) and thus is not advised for a long-term treatment situation, which can involve analytic or other similar types of psychotherapy. This does not create the type of relationship that is normally considered to be therapeutic.

However, as in the previous case example, when it is essential that a trance state be rapidly induced, especially for the purpose of relieving an acute pain (such as might occur on a battlefield or following a severe accident), it can be the method of choice. The therapist must initiate it only with the greatest air of confidence and boldness, and must use a firm commanding voice. It is an approach that would be infrequently used. The presence of paranoid trends in the patient is contraindicative, because such patients may incorporate the therapist into his or her delusional system as a possessor of the "evil eye." There is also the possibility of traumatizing timid patients and developing in them a lasting fear of hypnosis or of that specific therapist. Still, when it is necessary that immediate, firm action be taken to quiet a hysterical individual or to administer immediate and effective hypnoanesthesia (perhaps when chemoanesthesias or analgesias are not available or are contraindicated) the practitioner should be prepared to use this procedure.

The patient should be lying down or sitting and facing the therapist directly, and the eyes of the therapist are fixated on a point between the patient's eyes and at the bridge of the patient's nose. The face and eyes of the therapist should be quite close, in fact can be so close that the therapist's eyes cannot actually focus on the nose bridge, but stares through it, as if fixed on some distant point on the other side of the patient's head. This staring through the bridge of the patient's nose, rather than at it, will greatly relieve feelings of eye tension in the therapist, but will be just as effective to the patient. Grasping the shoulders of the patient the therapist might then give suggestions such as the following in a commanding voice:

> Stare into my eyes. Look, don't take them away. You have to look into my eyes even though you would like to turn them away. Your eyes are becoming very, very heavy. They cannot stay open. There is an irresistible force pulling them down. Down! Down! Down! Heavier. They blink [spoken immediately after the patient has blinked]. They are closing, closing tightly shut. The eyelids are sticky. Struggle if you like. You cannot keep them open. The harder you try to keep them open the more irresistible is the force pulling them down. Your eyes are tightly closed, and your body is growing numb.

Suggestions of this type are continued for 2 or 3 minutes, by which time those participants who can respond favorably to this approach will have achieved a firm eye closure. Occasionally, a participant will enter a deep hypnotic state with eyes staring, wide open. This will be noted because hands passed in front of the eyes will evidence no response. The eyes will not adjust to fixate on them, and the individual will react as if not seeing the therapist's passes. Such an "awake" trance state can often be very deep. It involves catalepsy of the eyes but with them wide open rather than tightly closed. It may be useful then simply to close the lids by pulling them down while saying, "There, they are now tightly closed and need not open. You can now go down into a very, very deep state."

This technique is often used by stage therapists. It typifies that manner described by Ferenczi (1926), as the "father hypnosis," in which transference reactions involving fear of early authority figures are mobilized as a motivation for entering the hypnotic state. One must decide whether the covert fear, which is engendered toward the therapist by this procedure, is offset by the advantages of rapid induction and immediate receptivity of the patient to powerful suggestions, such as might be necessary to counteract acute pain.

The Arm-Drop Induction Method

This approach in some ways resembles the arm-drop test of hypnotizability (see Figure 5.1). However, it is different and begins with a variation of eye fixation. The therapist asks the participant to raise an arm so that the hand is slightly above the head and gives suggestions as follows:

Stare at one of the fingers, either the index or the middle finger. You may continue to look at it, or, if you wish, close your eyes and visualize it in your mind's eye. As you fixate your gaze on it you will notice that the other fingers tend to fade out of focus and that your entire arm begins to feel heavier and heavier. The longer you concentrate on that finger the heavier and heavier your arm becomes. But you will not go into a deep state of relaxation until the arm has come all the way down. Keep concentrating on that finger while the arm gets heavier and heavier and heavier. [Say when downward movement becomes apparent.] Notice that as the arm is getting heavier it is slowly coming down, down, down. But you will not relax into a deep and profound state of relaxation until the arm is all the way down and touching. Going down, down, down, deeper, deeper, deeper. [The hypnotic instructions must be timed with the actual movement of the arm.]

There are a number of aspects of this induction, which are worthy of special notice. First, the arm is placed in such a position that fatigue will eventually bring it down. The downward movement is tied into going "down" into a "deep state of relaxation." The harder the individual keeps fighting to hold it up, the more one is committed to the proposition implied by the statement that, "You will not go into a deep state of relaxation until the arm is all the way down." This means, of course, that, "You will go into such a state when the arm comes all the way down."

Quite often, the eyes also come down as the arm does and they close when the arm is all the way down. Notice that the participants are given a number of choices in which they feel that they are exercising conscious volition. However, none of these choices imply the freedom to avoid going into a deep state of relaxation. The participants can choose which one of their fingers to fixate on. They can decide whether to stare at it or visualize it in the mind's eye, and the therapist gives them the option of not going into a deep state simply by preventing the hand from coming down. But normal physiology works against such conscious volition. Sooner or later, the fatigue and sense of discomfort will be so great that the arm must come down. The participant's resistive energies have been spent fighting internally, rather than fighting the therapist.

This is a pressure technique. Trance can be avoided only by a complete refusal on the part of participants to be drawn into the dilemma that confronts them. Sometimes the individuals will simply lower the arm rapidly and voluntarily, then open the eyes and decline to "play the game." This is a good opportunity to remind participants that in doing so, they are demonstrating ultimate control, but that when experiencing real hypnosis the

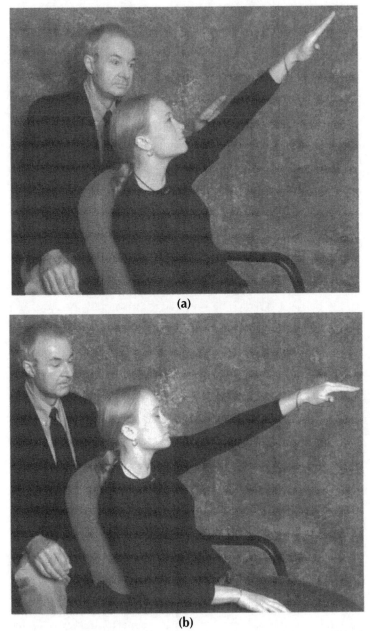

Fig. 5.1 Arm Drop Induction. (a) The participant is in the initial position of arm-drop induction. (b) The participant's arm begins to lower.

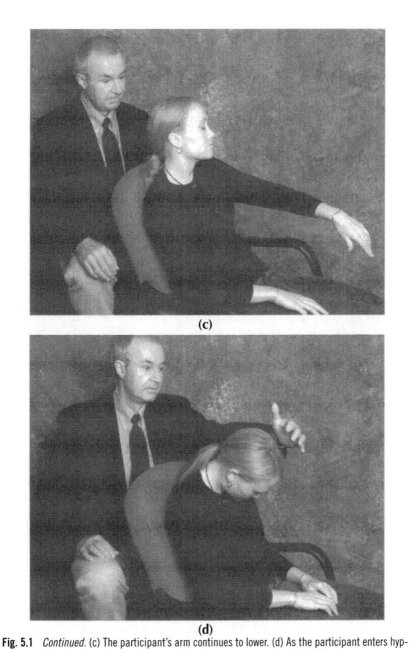

(c)

(d)

Fig. 5.1 *Continued.* (c) The participant's arm continues to lower. (d) As the participant enters hypnosis, the therapist's hand passing downward reduces light to her closed eyelids, giving the message, "Down deep."

idea is not to "make it happen" but rather merely "not keep it from happening": "Please just think about the things I suggest and let's see how we can make hypnosis work best for you, I need to learn what works best and that is accomplished by seeing which approaches are most acceptable to you (or acceptable to your subconscious) and work best for you."

No technique will hypnotize all individuals, but this one is frequently effective, combining as it does the principles of eye fixation, physiological fatigue, and apparent choice, restriction of perception, reversed effect, and repetition.

The Arm-Levitation Technique

In this approach, the therapist suggests the reverse movement, so it does not use the physiological fatigue factor. In fact, it operates in the opposite direction and must overcome such fatigue. However, it does start aroused focal concentration with a corresponding, diminution of peripheral awareness. Attention, directed perception, and tiny movements are then spread to larger ones. At each stage of the induction, there are overt movements that indicate the extent of hypnotic involvement so that the therapist is continually receiving cues from the patient. This makes it possible to continue each step with further repetition until it is successfully executed before proceeding with the next stage (see Figure 5.2).

So that we can analyze each step and the principles involved, we numbered the following verbalizations (the numbers are not part of the verbalization):

[1] Put your right hand [or left hand if the left is the dominant hand] on the table. [2] Please concentrate all your attention on that hand. You can look at it and see if you can be aware of all the sensations and feelings in the hand. [3] For example, you are aware that it is sitting on the table. There is weight there. You are aware of the texture of the table; you can keenly sense the position every finger has toward every other finger. [4] Notice the temperature of that hand, and as you look at that hand with this concentration, you will begin to notice that one of the fingers in that hand will feel different from the others. [5] Now, it might be the thumb or the little finger or perhaps the index finger, or the big finger or the ring finger, but one of them will feel distinctly different from the others. [6] And that feeling may be that it's a little more warm or that it's a little cold. It could be that it kind of stings a little or that it's numb. It could feel lighter or heavier, [7] but if you concentrate well, you will be able to know which finger it is that has the different sensa-

tion from the others [8] and as you pay close attention that particular finger will lift itself a little bit from the table over the others. Now concentrate on that, and you will notice that one of the fingers will tend to lift itself up from the table a little. [9] It's that [little?] finger. [10] Now please concentrate and you may find that finger becoming kind of numb; it's sticking straight out; it's almost as if it were made out of wood [11] and that wooden feeling will start spreading to the other fingers around close to it, and they too will begin to lift themselves and straighten. And you will find that next the finger will come up. And you will find that same lifting feeling coming into the [big] finger, and it sort of stiffens and straightens itself. And there is a light feeling, a woodenlike feeling, and then it moves into the [little] finger, and that, too, gets light and feels like it's floating, and then it gradually spreads into the hand. [12] And the hand begins to feel like it is made out of wood or cork and like cork it sort of wants to float as if it were in water and wants to come up. [13] Or perhaps you can imagine there is a balloon attached to the wrist and this hand keeps wanting to float up [14] in the direction of your face and it gets higher and higher and higher. [15] And you feel a drowsy sensation as it comes closer to the face. [16] It's about 12 inches away, then it's about 11 inches, [17] and the higher the hand comes, the drowsier you feel, [18] and you begin to think that when the hand touches the face you will go into a deep and profound relaxed state. [19] Now, it's only 5 inches away. And now, it's 4 inches away. Coming, closer and closer. It's going to touch pretty soon. Three inches away. [20] And when it touches you will go into a very deep state. [21] Almost touching, almost touching, almost touching. An inch away. Coming closer and closer. [22] Touching, touching. [23] And you just feel a sense of relaxation, [24] and as your hand goes down, you go down, too, into a deep, deep, deep relaxed state. And you feel yourself go down to a deep, comfortable, relaxed state.

Let us go through this induction again, indicating the purpose and principle involved in each suggestion or set of suggestions:

1. "Put your right hand on the table." This is a specific, directed instruction, and not contestable.
2. "Please concentrate all your attention on that hand. You can look at it and see if you can be aware of all the sensations and feelings in the hand." This involves concentration and directed attention.

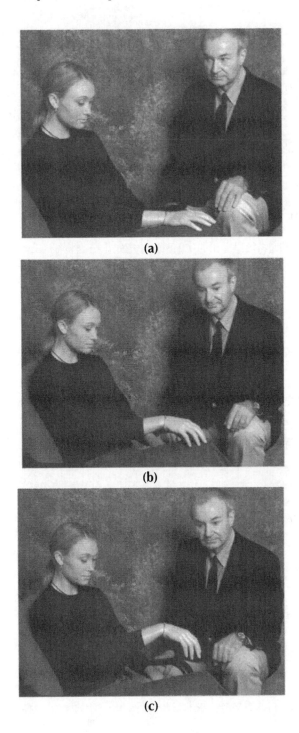

(a)

(b)

(c)

Fig. 5.2

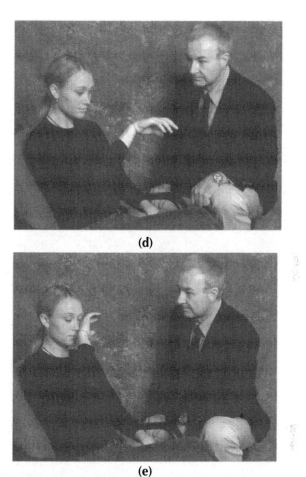

(d)

(e)

Fig. 5.2*Continued.* rm Levitation Induction. (a) The participant is in the initial position of arm-levitation induction. (b) The participant's arm begins to rise while the tips of her fingers remain in contact. (c) The participant's arm is now clearly levitating. (d) The participant's arm levitation increases.
(e) The participant's hand touches her face and she enters a state of hypnosis. The therapist is ready
to guide the hand down to provide a nonverbal message for deepening.

3. "For example, you are aware that it is sitting on the table. There is
   weight there. You are aware of the texture of the table; you can
   keenly sense the position every finger has toward every other finger."
   This involves highly specified perceptions, one after the other; there
   is no time to think and criticize each.
4. "Notice the temperature of that hand, and as you look at that hand
   with this concentration, you will begin to notice that one of the fingers in that hand will feel different from the others." This involves
   concentration on one part of the body; tying together the act of

attention to first perception of an unusual, and hence suggested feeling; no specification as to the nature of that "different" feeling.

5. "Now, it might be the thumb or the little finger or perhaps the index finger, or the big finger or the ring finger, but one of them will feel distinctly different from the others." The participant is given a choice of fingers, but no choice of not having this "different" feeling.

6. "And that feeling may be that it's a little more warm or that it's a little cold. It could be that it kind of stings a little or that it's numb. It could feel heavier or lighter." Again the participant has a choice of feelings but not a choice to have no such unusual feeling. Participants feel that procedure is extremely permissive, which it is, in the manner in which they go into hypnosis.

7. "... but if you concentrate well, you will be able to know which finger it is that has the different sensation from the others..." The difference in feeling is presented as fact. It is the participants' responsibility to perceive this by demonstrating their ability to concentrate.

8. "... and as you pay close attention that particular finger will lift itself a little bit from the table over the others. Now concentrate on that, and you will notice that one of the fingers will tend to lift itself up from the table a little." If it does not lift it is because the therapist has not paid close enough attention. A tendency to lift is suggested first, not that it is lifting.

9. "It's that [little?] finger." Slight movement is seized upon by the therapist and verified, thus increasing his or her credibility.

10. "Now please concentrate and you may find that finger becoming kind of numb; it's sticking straight out; it's almost as if it were made out of wood." The therapist makes suggestion from movement back to perception, this time of anesthesia and rigidity, and makes comparison to the insensibility of wood.

11. "... and that wooden feeling will start spreading to the other fingers around close to it, and they too will begin to lift themselves and straighten. And you will find that next the finger will come up. And you will find that same lifting feeling coming into the [big] finger, and it sort of stiffens and straightens itself. And there is a light feeling, a woodenlike feeling, and then it moves into the [little] finger, and that, too, gets light and feels like it's floating, and then it gradually spreads into the hand. The paraesthetic feelings, the stiffness, the rigidity, and the lifting movement is spread from one finger progressively through all fingers and the entire hand. More and more of the body of the participant becomes hypnotically involved. By using such a phrase as "you will find," the thera-

pist places participants in the position of being a passive observer of the finger behavior that is happening. They are not doing it; it is perceived as "object," not within voluntary self action. "It" happens; the participants are not doing it. A dissociation between the participants' hand movements and the perception of their own voluntary processes is being established.

12. "And the hand begins to feel like it is made out of wood or cork and like cork it sort of wants to float as if it were in water and wants to come up." The wooden feeling is spread to the entire hand and then the therapist makes the comparison from wood to cork so that the next suggestions of floating in water will be facilitated.

13. "Or perhaps you can imagine there is a balloon attached to the wrist and this hand keeps wanting to float up..." This is another image the therapist can suggest to facilitate floating upward tendency. Notice "the" wrist, not "your" wrist — treating it as object, not part of the self. Note also that it "keeps wanting" to float up; hence, independent of self, "it" is making the choice of movement.

14. "... in the direction of your face and it gets higher and higher and higher." The specific direction of movement is suggested with repetition.

15. "And you feel a drowsy sensation as it comes closer to the face." The involvement in hypnotic "sleep" is being tied to upward movement toward "the" face, not "your" face.

16. "It's about 12 inches away, then it's about 11 inches, ..." The therapist suggests approaching movement of the hand toward the face but keeps close to the actual position of hand. Do not lead too much.

17. "... and the higher the hand comes, the drowsier you feel, ..." Increased sensations of hypnotic "sleep" are tied directly to hand movement.

18. "... and you begin to think that when the hand touches the face you will go into a deep and profound relaxed state." Participants have anticipation that they will enter profound hypnosis at the moment of touching.

19. "Now, it's only 5 inches away. And now, it's 4 inches away. Coming closer and closer. It's going to touch pretty soon. Three inches away." The therapist makes further suggestions of movement and anticipation of touching.

20. "And when it touches you will go into a very deep state." The therapist offers repetition of anticipated touching and ties it again to entry into a very deep state.

21. "Almost touching, almost touching, almost touching. An inch away. Coming closer and closer." The therapist offers repetition and urging of movement.
22. "Touching, touching." The therapist provides confirmation at moment of touching.
23. "And you just feel a sense of relaxation, ..." The therapist makes this a moment of personal achievement for the participant, who is rewarded with pleasurable positive reinforcement.
24. "... and as your hand goes down, you go down, too, into a deep, deep, deep relaxed state. And you feel yourself go down to a deep, comfortable, relaxed state." The participant has achieved touching; now the consequence of entry into a deep relaxed state can take place. The therapist offers repetition with firmness. The participant verifies this by his or her own "comfortable" feelings. Note repetition of word *down* with more than one meaning.

A variation of the arm levitation technique preferred by the first author does not involve a table as the initial resting point of the participant's dominant hand. Instead, it begins with the hand on the participant's leg. This allows the doctor to focus the participant's attention rather differently. After drawing attention to small finger movements, as in the previous protocol, you might proceed with "[1] Notice the warmth generated between the hand and the leg," the warmth and pressure of the hand on the leg can then more easily be reframed as "[2] a kind of special tension will form between the hand and the leg. I don't know when and you don't know when it will happen, but it will be a kind of tension, ... perhaps its already there, I do not know, and you might not know but the tension will mount, the tension will grow and grow, [3] now as that tension grows between your hand and your leg it will push the hand up from the leg the hand and the arm become lighter and lighter." Once some very minor confirmation that the hand is lifting, usually the fingers at first keep contact with the leg as the hand rises from the center of the back of the hand, say, "[4] Yes, there it goes lifting, lifting up, rising up. [5] Now, I do not know exactly where that hand is going, but it is rising up, moving in some way toward your face"; if the hand lifts about 1 foot high or more, follow-up and persist with "[6a] It continues to rise up, rise up toward your face, all the time watching it move on its own, fascinating it is to see your hand move up toward your face, and when it touches your face you will go down into a deep state of hypnosis as deeply down as you ever wished, to help make hypnosis work best for you." If after 20 or more minutes the hand has barely risen from the leg, continue with "[6b] Amazing isn't it how the hand has moved up like that, all by itself, up off your leg — and now it's finally OK to let yourself go into a deep state of hypnosis as deeply down as you ever wished, but try to keep from going too deeply into hypnosis like that until the hand falls back on to your leg."

Remember, the participant has no clue as to how high the hand might have gone up. Even a slight effortless rising of the hand as a prerequisite to 6b might be all that is necessary to help the participant reach a very substantial depth of hypnosis. Also, remember to be patient and completely confident throughout the induction; there is no time limit and no reason to rush. I (A.F.B.) once took nearly an hour to obtain some rather minimal lifting of the hand with a very skeptical and untrusting patient who had been to several other therapists who "used suggestive techniques." A slight effortless rising of the hand was all that was necessary to allow the patient to obtain a depth of hypnosis sufficient for pain relief. Subsequently, use of pain medication ceased entirely within a few weeks. The patient was proud to have a new skill and to have overcome more than 1 year's use of dependency-producing pain relievers. The patient also returned to a normal work schedule, much to the satisfaction and amazement of the referring physician.

To awaken hypnotized individuals therapists can give a suggestion such as, "As I count from 10 to 1 you will gradually come out of hypnosis; when I reach 5 open your eyes [assuming eye closure was part of the induction] but you will not be completely out of hypnosis — fully alert and feeling just fine until I reach the count of 1. When I reach 1 you will be completely out of hypnosis feeling just fine." Once therapists reach 1, they ask the participant how they are feeling. If the participant indicates feeling groggy, say, "That happens sometimes when a person goes rather deeply in hypnosis, so let's go back into a light state as I count from 1 to 3: 1, 2, 3. [Typically the participants' eyes will close but it is not necessary.] Now this time as I count you out of hypnosis you will be completely awake, alert, fully normal feeling. [Count firmly with a commanding voice.] 3! 2! 1! COMPLETLY OUT OF HYPNOSIS NOW — GOOD that's fine now." At this point, the participants can be questioned about feelings, behaviors, and sensations as to how deeply hypnotized they might have felt and so on.

Repetitive Movement — Wagging Hand

A much simpler induction technique involving hand movement is that of repetitive movement, sometimes facetiously called "hand wagging." It combines eye fixation and concentration on a moving object, repetition, a gradual change of the movement from subject to object, and a tying of this action to eye closure. Less skill is required of the therapist than in the arm-levitation approach. It is one of the best techniques for a beginner to use.

Meares (1961) described this approach in considerable detail and reported it was especially effective in working with resisting individuals who were unable or unwilling to relax completely. Instructions to be given to the patient are as follows:

Repetitive Movement.
"Place your elbow on the table with your forearm up like this. Now I want you to stare at that hand while I move it up and down. Up, down, up, down, up, down. As you stare at that hand, you will notice a tendency for your eyes to become heavier and heavier, as if they might want to close. Keep staring while the hand continues to go up, down, up, down, up, down!" The therapist positions the participant's elbow on the table with his or her own fingers on the back of the participant's hand and his or her thumb on participant's palm just above the wrist.

2. "You will also notice that the movement in this hand is becoming more and more automatic. It is as if the hand itself wants to move up and down without your doing anything about it. Up, down, up, down, up, down. Your eyes are getting so very heavy that they are gradually closing. It doesn't seem as if they could be held open." The participant's hand is wagged up and down in time with the verbal suggestion of "up, down." The hand is increasingly dissociated as it is referred to as "the" hand, not "your" hand. The hand is becoming an "it."

3. "You are relaxing deeply all over while the hand is moving more and more by itself. Up, down, up, down, up, down. Now, the movement of the hand is so automatic that it keeps going up, down, up, down, up, down all by itself and it doesn't need any more help from me to continue its movement. Up, down, up, down, up, down." The therapist now gradually loosens hold of the participant's hand until only lightly touching it by the thumb and forefingers. As soon as the therapist is convinced that the participant's hand movement will continue automatically the therapist removes his or her hand entirely.

4. "It is now becoming so automatic that it continues to move all by itself without any control by you. Up, down, up, down, up, down. It seems to be almost outside you with a will to move up and down independently of you. It controls its own actions. You do not control them." The therapist continues to reinforce the movement with "up, down" as long as necessary to ensure automatic action.

5. "As it goes automatically up and down it seems to be saying to you, 'Deep, relax, deep, relax, deep, relax. Up, down, deep, relax, up, down, deep, relax.' You are going more and more into a deep and profound state of relaxation. Your eyes are closed. Your head is

heavy. It is nodding forward, and you are going deeper and deeper and deeper." The "up, down" movement is now tied to the suggestion of "deep, relax," keeping the same timing and coordination.

6. "I will take the hand now and stop its movement. As I bring the hand down you will go down with it, deeper and deeper." The therapist now stops the movement and brings the hand down to the table, emphasizing both "downs."

7. "Deep, deep, deep, deep, deep." The therapist says the "deeps" strongly and rapidly as the hand comes down. For emphasis, the therapist presses the participant's near shoulder down slightly.

Summary

The methods of induction we described in this chapter represent those that probably have the widest use. They are well validated and will show a high percentage of success when employed skillfully with hypnotizable individuals. Many of the principles of hypnosis are employed although no single technique described previously comprehensively focuses on all aspects. The prestige of the therapists and their sense of confidence are critical to successful inductions that produce true hypnotic trance responses that go beyond those that can be wrought by mere suggestion or relaxation.

At one time, when I (J.G.W.) was first hypnotizing, a group of student volunteers were waiting (in a colleague's office) to be screened for hypnotizability. Buzzing with curiosity they inquired of him, "Can Dr. Watkins really hypnotize us?" My associate replied, "Of course, I have seen him hypnotize dozens of people. You'll be in a deep trance state in no time at all." This was a gross misstatement of fact. However, the effect of the social influence of the friend's "recommendation" was that almost all the volunteers became quickly and easily hypnotizable. It is no wonder that professional hypnotherapists display their qualifying certificates and that stage therapists assume mysterious and awe-inspiring titles. Yes, hypnosis is an altered state of consciousness and an intensive interpersonal relationship experience.

There is nothing wrong with professional prestige, as long as it is used in the service of the patient's needs, not for personal aggrandizement or the satisfaction of power needs in the therapist.

Chapter 6
Advanced Techniques of Hypnotic Induction

Siddhartha informed the eldest Samana of his decision to leave him. He told the old man with politeness and modesty fitting to young men and students. But the old man was angry that both young men wished to leave him and he raised his voice and scolded them strongly.

Govinda was taken aback, but Siddartha put his lips to Govinda's ear and whispered: "Now I will show the old man that I have learned something from him."

He stood near the Samana, his mind intent; he looked into the old man's eyes and held him with his look, hypnotized him, made him mute, conquered his will, commanded him silently to do as he wished. The old man became silent, his eyes glazed, his will crippled; his arms hung down, he was powerless. ... Siddartha's thoughts conquered those of the Samana; he had to perform what they commanded. And so the old man bowed several times, gave his blessings and stammered his wishes for a good journey. The young man thanked him for his good wishes, returned his bow, and departed.

On the way, Govinda said: "Siddartha, you have learned more from the Samana than I was aware. It is difficult, very difficult to hypnotize an old Samana." (Hesse, 1951, p. 23–24.)

Despite numerous studies concerning the trait of hypnotizability, almost no empirical evidence seems to be available directly comparing one induction procedure with another upon the same or comparable populations. Earlier studies published by E. Hilgard (1965) implied that hypnotizability was a fixed trait inhering in the participant. Accordingly, little variability would be expected between different therapists and different induction techniques. If an individual were hypnotizable, almost any technique applied by any therapist would be successful.

Most clinical workers, however, are convinced that there is a great deal of difference between the effectiveness of different techniques and between the skills with which they are applied by different practitioners. Few studies have focused on this issue, perhaps because the vast majority comes from university academicians, more often than not with little or no full-time clinical experience with challenging cases, or simply because the majority of those collecting data in university settings are graduate students, learning about hypnosis. The problem is ignored by the few clinicians who take (or have) the time to do and publish research.

Clinicians are not usually well placed to do comparative experience studies, and the interest in doing so is attenuated by their rather well-founded perception that "obviously experience and a proper induction makes a great difference in the ability to produce a trance state sufficient for therapeutic change [effects]" (Fromm, August 16, 2002, personal communication to A. Barabasz). The hypothesis of hypnotizability as a constant state denies psychodynamic aspects of the hypnotic relationship as being significant.

Much more research is needed in this area, but experimentally controlled investigations have addressed the experience-induction issue with consistent findings. At Harvard Medical School and Massachusetts General Hospital, A. Barabasz, Baer, Sheehan, and Barabasz (1986) obtained follow-up data on 307 patients completing a two-session treatment for smoking cessation. Clinical psychology interns produced the least effective rates (4% to 13% abstinence at 4 months), whereas experienced clinicians achieved far better abstinence rates (28% to 47% at 10 to 19 months follow-up). More recently, A. Barabasz et al. (2003) tested experience and tailored versus scripted inductions in a controlled study of age regression and focal point dependency. Nonhypnosis-related research has established that, unlike adults or younger children, those children of about age 5 years show an ability to determine whether an abstract figure is right side up or up side down. Twenty university student participants who had passed the regression item of the *Stanford Clinical Scales* and had a total score of 3 to 5 (out of a maximum of 5) points were seen by either graduate students or licensed clinicians with decades of clinical experience with hypnosis. Both a scripted induction and a tailored induction were tested to produce age regression to the age of 5 years. Analysis revealed that (a) the use of the scripted induction failed to show significant focal point dependency as a regression indicator for either group, (b) the tailored hypnotic induction failed to show significant focal point dependency for the 10 participants in the student therapist group, and (c) the tailored induction administered by the experienced clinicians showed significant focal point dependency (regression) in 5 of the 10 participants in that group. The findings suggest caution about studies reporting results based on the use of scripted inductions administered by inexperienced research assistants. Experience and inductions tailored to the participants' responses were of critical importance in this research.

On the basis of these findings and, perhaps more important, the fact that most practitioners believe that induction techniques are an important part of their modes of operation, we describe in this chapter a number of additional ones, particularly some that differ from those discussed so far in being rather unusual, more complex, requiring greater skill, or being better adapted to certain specialized cases or problem patients.

Advanced Techniques of Induction

The Postural-Sway Technique

In chapter 4, we described a hypnotizability test termed "postural sway." We noted that this approach could not only serve as a test of hypnotizability but also be extended into an actual induction. This procedure has the merit of being very different from the types of eye-fixation hypnotic inductions that are frequently characterized in movies and television, involving the swinging of a watch or other object before the participant's eyes — often depicted as the unwilling victim of some villain. Individuals who have observed such films may have developed anxieties about eye fixation and accordingly are able to respond with less fear to something entirely different, such as this postural-sway method.

Because the induction is simply an extension of the hypnotizability test, we do not need to repeat the initial stages of the procedure (see Figure 6.1). We refer the reader back to chapter 4 in which the verbalizations for taking the participant or patient up to the point of some significant hypnotic involvement have already been presented. Continuing from this point, the amplitude of the swaying arc is increased and swaying suggestions are further repeated so as to allow time for the participant to shut out opposing stimuli and focus on the hypnotic involvement.

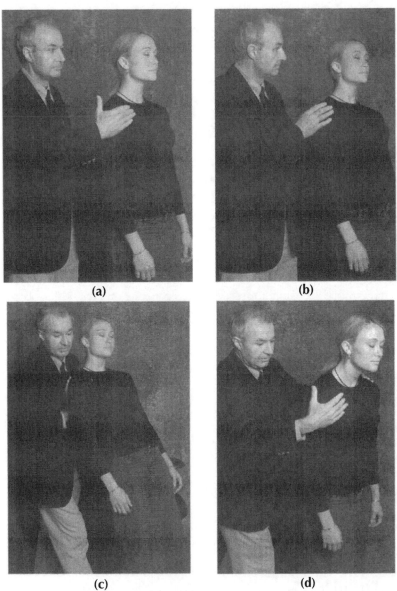

Fig. 6.1 Postural-Sway Test and Induction Technique. (a) The therapist tells the patient to roll her eyes up. She begins swaying back and forth, back and forth. (b) The therapist tells the patient to begin to drift backward, and reassures her that he will not let her fall. (c) The participant is prevented from falling forward by therapist's hands on her shoulders (d) First swaying forward, the therapist then tells the patient she is falling backward into a huge haystack. She is supported in the midfall position by the therapist's hands on her upper back.

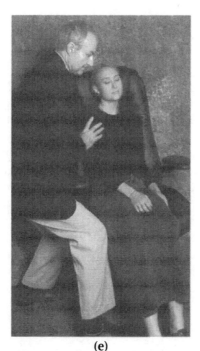

(e)

Fig. 6.1 *Continued.* (e) Falling backward, the patient is eased slowly into the chair by the therapist.

To induce a deeper trance the therapist's voice tone is now much firmer, and he or she gives the swaying suggestions somewhat more rapidly. "Swaying forward, swaying backward, forward, backward," the volume of the therapist's voice growing stronger and stronger. Finally, the therapist makes an attempt to induce the patient to fall over backward into a deep trance. The therapist increases the emphasis on "backward" and diminishes the emphasis on "forward" and changes the verb from "drifting" or "swaying" to "falling, falling backward, falling forward, falling backward, falling forward, falling over backward, falling, falling, falling, falling" rather rapidly and in a higher pitched and more emotional tone. If a deep trance has been induced, the patient will increase the amplitude of the sway until he or she can no longer stand erect. The patient will then fall over backward in a deep trance state and is then caught by the therapist and eased into a waiting chair.

If patients are in a light trance only, they might start to fall backward but catch themselves by placing one foot back or attempting to sway sideways or to steady voluntarily in some manner. This indicates to the therapist that a deep trance has not yet been induced. The therapist can then do one of two things: (a) continue the monotonous repetition of "falling forward, falling backward," and so on, to induce a deeper degree of trance; or (b) reassure patients that they will not fall by placing a hand lightly behind the patient's shoulder. This allays fears that might arise and interrupt the hypnotic process. After patients realize that they will not be permitted to fall and be injured, the tendency is to lose the signs of anxiety that might have begun to appear. A patient may then fall back against the therapist's arm, whereupon the therapist continues the suggestions "falling over backward, falling backward, falling back into a deep sleep, back into a deep sleep, deep sleep, deep sleep," and then eases the patient gradually over into a chair. An armchair should have been placed behind the patient. The patient can also be gradually lowered back on a couch that has been located conveniently nearby.

If patients are placed back on the chair either in a completely limp or in a stiff cataleptic posture, the therapist should consider this is evidence that a fairly deep level of trance has been induced. However, if the patients take steps backward or put their hands on the armchair as a help to sitting down, then, at best, only a light or hypnoidal trance has been induced. Or, worse yet, they are merely responding to the social demands of the situation rather than hypnosis.

Several very important postural reactions on the part of the therapist will enhance the effectiveness of the procedure. Because the participant is standing with the eyes closed, he or she must rely entirely on a kinesthetic sense to verify swaying backward and forward. This feedback can be enhanced by the therapist if he or she holds one hand behind the participant's back just below the neck and the other hand on the participant's shoulder, near the blade in front. The hands of the therapist will be about 18 inches apart, leaving room for the swaying of the participant back and forth between them such that when the forward part of the arc is reached the shoulder blade just barely touches the hand of the therapist. Likewise, when the back part of the swaying arc is reached, the participant's back just touches the therapist's hand. Such touching at each extreme of the arc provides a tactual cue that validates the swaying in addition to the kinesthetic feedback. When the participant is female, it is advisable to hold the hand in front sufficiently high that it is the shoulder and not the breast that is contacted.

After the participant's body has touched either hand, a slight push is given to suggest swaying in the reverse direction, but the hand does not follow the contrary movement of the body and continue the touching. To do this would simply mean that the swaying would be caused by the nothing more than the nonverbal suggestion given by the therapist's hands pushing the participant back and forth, not by the potential effect of actual hypnosis.

There is another value to this touching. The therapist has already assured the participant that "I will not let you fall." The touching, because it involves the entire flat of the hand on the back and on the shoulder blades, gives further validity to that assurance. In fact, as the swaying increases in amplitude, the point will be reached where if the therapist's hand were not restraining the participant, he or she would fall over. As this point is approached it is wise for the therapist to extend the arm around the back until, when the participant is falling back, support will be provided by the therapist's arm curved around entire upper back region. It will be noted that restraint from falling forward does not require that the forward arm be extended further than just enough to place the hand on or near the shoulder. If both arms had to be all the way around, the therapist would have to be standing very close and embracing the individual. (This is not a good idea if you value your license to practice!)

Because the terminal point in this induction is assumed to be reached when the participant falls back (often in a cataleptic condition) into the easy chair placed behind, it is imperative that one be gently lowered into that chair, not dropped into it, which could jar the participant out of the hypnotic state. The individual must have no fear of letting go and sinking back into the chair, hence no anxiety about being permitted to fall and be injured.

Clearly, it is important that as the swaying backward increases in amplitude, the therapist gradually moves farther back so that one foot is about level with the patient's feet and the other foot is 2 or 3 feet back, perhaps behind the front legs of the easy chair. This makes it possible for the therapist to support the individual who is falling backward and gradually, very gradually, ease him or her into the chair. Sometimes patients will become so cataleptic throughout their entire body that they fall backward completely rigid, like a board, and their hips even have to be pushed down to conform to the chair. If the patient is either rigid or completely limp, the therapist considers the induction proper to have been completed at this point. Deepening techniques may be applied, or perhaps the participant is ready now for research or therapeutic procedures. Some participants react to this postural-sway method with entry into a profound trance; others may be resistant or unresponsive to the procedure.

A variation in the technique can be employed with the resistant individual who manifests very little sway. When the therapist is saying, "You are drifting forward, forward, over forward," and so on, the therapist follows by swaying further to the rear of the patient, putting his or her weight on the leg that is behind the individual. Thus, as the therapist starts the suggestions of swaying forward, the mouth (and hence the voice) of the therapist might normally be about level with the individual's ear. But as the individual sways slightly forward, the therapist has swayed in the opposite direction so that the patient hears the therapist's voice as it emanates from a position one or more feet behind. The response can be further enhanced by the Doppler effect (note the apparent change in pitch of a train whistle as a train goes by) on the perception of the sound waves if the therapist continues to speak as he or she moves behind the patient.

Then, suggestions are changed to "You are now swaying backward, backward, over backward," and so on, and the therapist moves in the counterdirection. As the participant drifts backward, the therapist's mouth (and hence the source of his or her voice) is a foot or so forward of the participant. The therapist's weight is now on the forward foot. Because individuals orient themselves in space and determine direction by the angles at which sounds enter their two ears, the participant's illusion of swaying backward and forward is substantially enhanced. In fact, sometimes an unresponsive individual who is standing quite still and not drifting at all will get the feeling of a great arc of swaying because of the changing locus of the therapist's voice. The therapist should make use of the Doppler effect to further create the illusion of much greater sway. The procedure frequently serves to help the participant experience greater hypnotic responsiveness.

Obviously, the postural-sway procedure is contraindicated for patients who are weak or bedridden, suffer pain on standing, or are much larger than the therapist. A heavy person is very difficult to control when falling backward, especially by a small therapist. Women wearing high heels should be asked to remove their shoes. In our book *Psychoanalytic Techniques* (in press) we explain the underlying psychoanalytic processes that may be initiated by this approach.

A Rapid Induction

Although this technique is not well suited to use in a clinical setting, it may be used to demonstrate to a class that the trance state can often be initiated in a hypnotizable individual in a very short period of time. Lengthiness of the induction process is not necessarily related to depth of involvement. The ability of individuals to enter trance rapidly is not predictive of the hypnotic depth they are capable of achieving.

The therapist asks the participant to stand. To ensure safety and to establish a set, the therapist stations two assistants at the participant's side and tells them to catch him or her upon falling. This method should not be attempted unless the therapist is certain that it will be successful as suggested by the participant's previous strong positive responses on hypnotizability tests. The therapist instructs the participant in a firm, confident voice as follows:

> I am going to count 1, and you will remain wide awake and free from any hypnotic trance. Then I will count 2, and you will continue to remain awake. When I count 3, you will still stay awake, but the moment afterward, when I clap my hands you will fall instantly, in a fraction of a second, into a deep hypnotic state. My assistants will catch you when you fall.

The therapist counts 1 and then asks the participant, "Are you awake?" The affirmative reply is frequently accompanied by smiling. The count of 2 is given, and then the count of 3 is given; after each count the same question is asked. The therapist then claps hands, and the good responder usually slumps immediately. As an additional precaution, a chair should be in place behind the standing individual so the assistants can ease the slumping and deeply hypnotized person into it.

Rapid Rehypnotization

If the participant has already been hypnotized at least once by the therapist and has clearly demonstrated the ability to enter a deep trance state, a long induction procedure may be quite unnecessary. This is especially true if patients have been brought out of hypnosis to inquire about their reactions while in the state and if the period of conscious interview was brief (5 minutes or less). The rapid rehypnotization may be accomplished as follows (see Figure 6.2):

> Extend your arm upward and out. Focus your eyes on the hand while I take your wrist. I am going to bring your arm down, and as I do you will go back into a deep state of calmness like that from which you have just emerged.

The therapist takes hold of the participant's wrist and brings the arm down gradually until it is all the way down, usually on the lap or leg. While doing this, the therapist says in a strong, commanding voice, "Here we go. Down, down, down. Deep, deep, deep," and so on. If the individual is highly hypnotizable, has been hypnotized before by this therapist, and has recently been brought out of hypnosis, he or she usually sinks rapidly back into a hypnotic state. This is due to a condition typically termed "the aura," which probably is simply the fact that when first brought out of

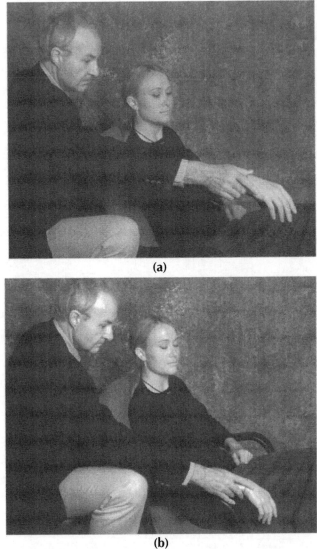

(a)

(b)

Fig. 6.2 Rapid Re-Hypnotization. (a) The therapist grasps the patient's right wrist and informs her of what will happen as the arm is lowered. (b) The therapist brings the patient's arm down while saying "Let yourself go down deep into hypnosis."

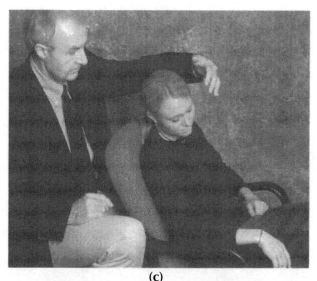

(c)

Fig. 6.2 *Continued.* (c) Recognizing the behavioral signs of the patient's entering the hypnotic state, the therapist further deepens the state nonverbally by passing his hand downward in front of her face, progressively blocking light to her already closed eyes.

hypnosis vestiges of the trance state linger. In fact, it can take 5 or more minutes until the patient is fully out of hypnosis, and therefore the patient requires a more lengthy induction to reenter trance.

The Coin Technique

This is another direct and rather authoritative but rapid approach. Different variations are advocated by different writers. Crasilneck and Hall (1985) suggested that the coin should be placed in the palm of the participant's hand (see Figure 6.3). As the therapist gives suggestions so the participant's hand slowly turns, there comes a moment when the coin falls off. The participant has been told that when he or she hears the clink of the coin striking the floor the (note the use of the word *the* to dissociate the eyes from the person and to imply the patient's eyes will act on their own) eyes will close and he or she will be deeply relaxed.

Kroger (1977) is most detailed in his instructions, and he began the induction with the participant's eyes closed. In Kroger's approach, participants are instructed to clasp coins tightly in their hands. The therapist then gives suggestions to the participants to relax the hands, sometimes to the point of a count for each finger, which then comes unclasped. The goal is the same, that when the coin falls the sound of it striking the floor will induce an immediate, deep hypnotic response.

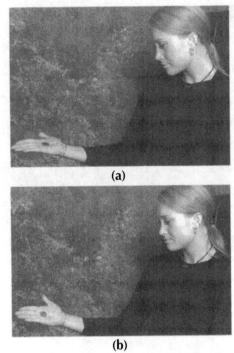

(a)

(b)

Fig. 6.3 The Coin Technique. (a) The patient stares at the coin that has been placed in her hand. (b) The patient's hand gradually tips until the coin falls off. She enters a hypnotic state.

The coin technique uses the sociocognitive principles of set and expectation to facilitate the individual's transition into a true hypnotic trance, just as in the previous rapid induction method. It should be remembered that such approaches are quite directive and have advantages and limitations. Generally, far less authoritative procedures are preferred by most participants, but these rapid inductions have a place in the armamentarium of hypnotherapeutic techniques.

Because it is the nature of hypnosis that things appear to happen to the participant, apparently without his or her conscious control or willing of it, the experience of an involuntary action can be administered by a simple situation known as the Kohnstamn phenomenon. Students are advised to experience this phenomenon themselves if only to acquaint themselves more intimately with the kind of feeling hypnotized participants have when they are responding to suggestions while in the trance state.

The Kohnstamn Phenomenon

The therapist instructs the participant as follows:

Stand near the wall, facing perpendicular to it, with your feet about a foot from the wall. Now, with your arm hanging at your side, push the back of your hand against the wall. That's it. Now harder. Do not lean your body toward the wall. Just push the back of the hand against the wall as if you were trying to push it harder, harder even harder. Now, I want you to continue this for an entire minute. A minute will seem like a long time while you are doing this. [The therapist may announce 15-second intervals but keeps on urging the participant to push harder with all his or her might against the wall with the back of the hand.]

At the end of 1 minute the therapist give the instruction "Now turn and face me." In most individuals (and to their great astonishment) the arm will slowly rise as if automatically. Of course, the phenomenon is not a hypnotic effect but is based on muscle fatigue. By tiring one set of muscles in the arm, the opposing muscles simply contract and lift the arm. Although this is not hypnosis, the experience is close to that felt by individuals who are responding to hypnotic suggestions in the trance state. Something is happening to them; they are not doing it.

Barabasz's Verbal-Nonverbal Induction for Resistant Individuals

The verbal-nonverbal dissociation technique (A. Barabasz, in press) builds on the Kohnstamn phenomenon as a bridge to hypnotic responding. Although it is applicable to any individual physically capable of performing the demands of the technique, it is especially well suited to resistant patients or research volunteers (see Figure 6.4). It is worth attempting even with those who have scored in the lowest ranges of the *Stanford Hypnotic Susceptibility Scale* or the *Hypnotic Induction Profile,* because in a small but significant number of cases it overcomes underlying resistance to hypnosis that may be due to variables other than lack of innate hypnotizability. The therapist instructs the individual as follows:

Okay, if you're ready, please stand with your left [or right] shoulder about a foot from the wall, here let me help. [The therapist shows participant exactly how get into the correct proximity to the wall consistent with the basic Kohnstamn requirements.] Okay then, please just simply press the back of your hand against the wall, just your hand not your body, pretty much as hard as you can press it. Are you pressing hard now? [Presumably the individual says "yes."] Good, press a little harder if you can. This takes a whole minute to do but you can do it. [The therapist watches clock behind the indi-

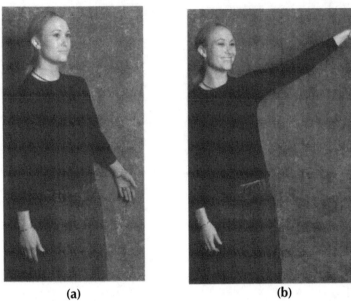

(a)   **(b)**

Fig. 6.4 Kohnstamm Phenomenon. (a) Pressing her hand against the wall, the patient demonstrates the initial position of the Kohnstamm phenomenon. (b) The patient is astonished to find her arm rising involuntary.

vidual, having noted the start of the hand pressing thus allowing the constant contact with the participant's eyes, actually looking at the participant's bridge of the nose.] Okay that's already 30 seconds, just 30 more seconds to go, just keep pressing and pressing that hand harder and harder against the wall, pressing, pressing, pressing nearly as hard as you can. The rest of your body calm and at ease, but that hand, pressing against the wall can feel it pushing harder. Just keep pressing harder. Now just 10 seconds to go, keep that hand pressing against the wall, real hard now. Almost there [at about 1 minute elapsed time]. Okay good, now just step away from the wall a few feet.

The therapist continues staring directly at the participant's bridge of the nose. As the individual moves away from the wall, the therapist uses peripheral vision to note the typical hand-rising effect, but at the same time ever so subtly leads the participant's arm float by lifting his or her own arm while continuing to look directly at the bridge of the nose (see Figure 6.5). The therapist should lift the opposite arm as that used by the participant, so he or she is providing a mirrorlike image to the participant

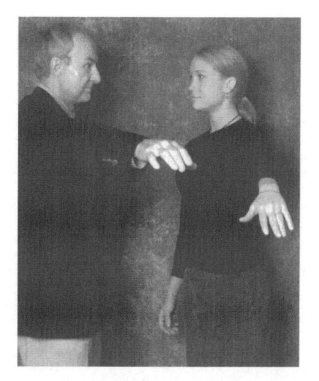

Fig. 6.5 The therapist nonverbally suggests the arm raise, and he leads the patient by raising his arm. First he stares into her eyes, and then he focuses on an object behind her to distract her conscious interference with her potential natural hypnotic talent. The perception, on her part, is as if he is looking through her.

with a nonverbal hypnotic induction cue. As the participant's arm rises, the therapist says,

> Your arm [so it is not misunderstood to be that of the therapist] is just floating up by itself, great! But it can relax too and be calm and as it goes back down, you too, can go down into a deep pleasant hypnotic calmness and when it's all the way down, your eyes can close too, but please try to keep them open until your arm is so calmly down, down, down, and you are seated in that chair behind you. Please try not to go any deeper into hypnosis until you are in the chair.

Once the arm is all the way down, the individual is seated, and the eyes are closed, the therapist may proceed to test hypnotic suggestions or further deepening according to the research protocol or therapeutic intervention. The entire procedure requires practice and experience so it can flow with calm confidence. The therapist must exude the confidence that he or she knows these suggested reactions will happen despite the fact that he or she might be surprised with little expectation that a known resistant individual will actually respond. Contrary to notions promulgated by certain research findings, the therapist's expectation, based on the low hypnotizability score or other beliefs about the individual, will not affect the outcome of the induction, so long as the therapist conducts the session with professionalism. This is but one feature that separates the more effective therapist from the second-rate one who is limited to reliance entirely on participants' most easily elicited hypnotic talents, such as mundane easily achieved responses to suggestion, rather than being able to help individuals to unleash their dissociative hypnotic-state capabilities.

Opposed-Hand Levitation

This approach is designed for the participant who shows a great deal of overt resistance to the induction of hypnosis. Occasionally, a therapist will have a patient who obviously perceives the hypnotic situation as one of confrontation between the patient and the therapist. This resistance may be manifested by such remarks as, "You can't hypnotize me because I have too strong a willpower." Sometimes this tendency will be demonstrated in the arm-drop hypnotizability test by a rising instead of a lowering of the arm that is carrying the suggested weight. This phenomena has been described as "countercontrol," and it represents a kind of reverse reaction to the demand characteristics of the situation.

The procedure involves the acceptance by the therapist of the participant's interpretation of the induction as a contest. In fact, the therapist specifically builds it up as a conflict situation between them. However, he or she then subtly restructures the hypnotic suggestions until they imply that the therapist is actively opposing the participant's efforts to achieve a deep relaxed state, hence that the participant's "natural" desire to enter a hypnotic state is being deliberately counteracted by a physical conflict between the therapist's hand and the participant's hand. After a considerable struggle, the participant finally can enter the state of hypnosis by overpowering the therapist. The participant's needs to triumph over the doctor are mobilized and enlisted in the induction process.

The technique starts out the same as the traditional hand-levitation procedure we described in chapter 5. However, instead of suggesting a differential sensation in one finger, the therapist immediately gives the suggestion that the hand is getting lighter and lighter and wants to float up off the desk or chair arm (see Figure 6.5). This is continued for some time, and the amount of resistance to bringing the hand up is noted. At a certain point, the therapist abruptly changes his or her voice into a more demanding and challenging manner as follows:

> Even though your hand is getting lighter and wants to lift up into the air, I will not permit it to do so. I am putting my hand on it, and I will hold it down so that it cannot rise.

The therapist then places a hand firmly on top of the hand of the participants' and presses down. The participants' reaction at this point is usually one of surprise and sometimes one of anger. Their freedom of movement is now being specifically and physically restricted. This acts as a challenge and tends to mobilize their will to resist the therapist's suggestions. Accordingly, the therapist continues as follows:

> I am holding your hand so strongly that even though your hand wants to rise up it cannot do so. My hand is stronger than yours, and yours is too weak to push back against mine.

The therapist then alternates slightly between pushing down on the back of the participant's hand and relaxing that pushing. If the will to resist is being stimulated in participants, they will soon feel a tendency to push back. This will become evident as their hands slightly rise and maintain contact with the therapist's hand each time the doctor has raised his or her hand slightly.

The therapist continues with strong challenging remarks to the effect that the participant's hand is not as strong as the therapist's, that it must accept being held down, and that it will not be able to rise. Notice that the "contact" is described as being "my hand" versus "your hand," not between "you" and "me." Of course, participants inwardly interpret it as between themselves and the therapist. However, the therapist's describing it as a conflict of the hands allows the participant to feel freer to engage in the battle. Moreover, the hands are being treated as "object," hence outside the self, not as "subject" or within one's volition. The rising of the participant's hand, therefore, constitutes a victory over the therapist for which one has no control and no responsibility. ("Look what my hand does to yours. It can beat yours.")

While continuing the challenging remarks, the therapist relaxes the downward pushing from time to time, permitting the hand of the participant to push back and begin to rise. When this occurs, the therapist changes remarks to take notice of the progress of the patient's hand as it rises against the therapist's own:

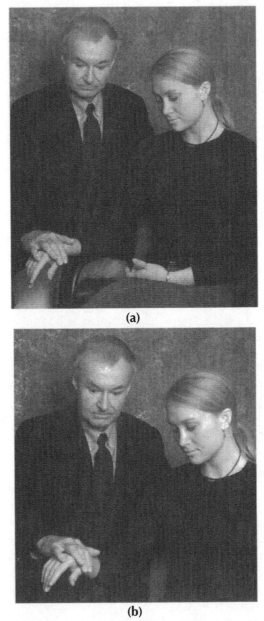

(a)

(b)

Fig. 6.6 Opposed Hand-Levitation Technique. (a) The therapist is pushing his hand against the patient's hand. (b) The patient raises her hand against the therapist's. He applies varying pressures against her hand.

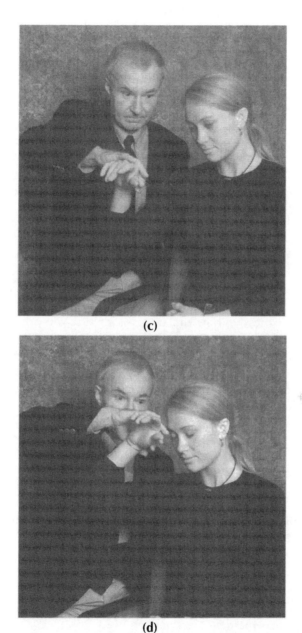

(c)

(d)

Fig. 6.6 *Continued.* (c) As the therapist slowly gives way, the patient's hand rises ever upward. (d) When the two hands are getting close to the patient's face, the "struggle" becomes intense as she triumphantly achieves the goal of touching her face in spite of the therapist's opposition. She can then enter a hypnotic state with the feeling of success.

> I shall push down against your hand with all my might, and even though yours seems to be pushing back a little it cannot be strong enough to overcome my hand. Your hand seems to be rising a bit, so I shall redouble my efforts to hold it down. It must be held down; it must not be permitted to rise any higher. Your hand is getting closer and closer to your face. It seems as if some very strong magnetic attraction between the hand and the face is drawing it closer. So I will push it back down all the harder.

Of course, the therapist is slowly giving way. Whenever the participant's hand slows in its rise upward, the therapist pushes down again. This is usually sufficient to cause it to resume the participant's pushing back again and consequent further rise. Finally, when the two hands are getting close to the face, and the struggle is quite intense, the therapist begins to include such suggestions as the following:

> Your hand seems determined to reach your face in spite of my strongest opposition. And if it achieves a victory over my hand, you can reach your goal of a wonderful state of relaxation in spite of all my opposition. I know you are thinking that you can reach this goal and enter a very deep comfortable state by proving that your hand is stronger than mine, and by it finally succeeding in touching your face in spite of my best efforts to stop it. Now it's getting closer, closer, closer. It's almost touching, almost touching, touching. The hand has been able to reach your face in spite of my best efforts to prevent it from doing so. It won out, and you can now go into the deep state of relaxation feeling completely triumphant in that my best efforts were not strong enough to prevent you from achieving this comfortable state.

Obviously, this procedure involves a certain measure of deception as the entire situation is restructured into a contest between therapist and participant whereby the participant triumphs over the therapist by entering a hypnotic state in spite of the therapist's "strong opposition." The technique is not frequently used; however, we have found it successful with certain hostile, or even paranoid, patients who could not be hypnotized by any of the other methods.

The Progressive Anesthesia Technique

This method is much more gentle and less aggressive than the opposed-hand levitation. It does involve touching and stroking the patient with all the meanings related to such contact, positive and negative.

The therapist asks the participant to sit at a desk or table and to place both arms on the table (see Figure 6.7). Attention is directed to one finger on one hand (the hypnotic narrowing of the field of perception) as follows: "Focus all your attention on this finger. As I stroke it, you will notice that it begins to feel numb." (The therapist strokes the finger.) "As the numbness increases the finger gets stiffer. It tends to lift and become stiff, and it feels like a wooden peg." (The lifting and straightening of the finger is a motor sign of its involvement.) "Now I will stroke the next finger and it, too, will become numb and stiff like the first one. Both of them become numb and stiff. Now the numb stiffness flows into still another finger," and so on, until all the participant's fingers are straight, stiff, and slightly lifted. The numbness is then suggested into the whole hand. Each time the part of the body to become numb is lightly touched and stroked by the therapist. Gradually the numbness is moved up into the wrist, to the forearm, through the elbow, into the upper arm, and into the shoulder. While this is being suggested, the entire arm, like each finger before, should become stiff and straight to signify the movement of the numbness through it.

Because the entire induction takes a few minutes, it is a good idea to support the stiff arm by letting the hand rest on the table. This avoids the undue fatigue that can result from holding the arm straight out for a considerable period of time.

From the shoulder, the numbness is passed over to the other shoulder by the therapist's stroking across the back of the participant's neck. It is then transferred down the other arm as the therapist continues the stroking while simultaneously describing the movement of the numb feeling, first into the other upper arm, through the elbow, the lower arm, the wrist, the hand, and each of the fingers. Both arms are now stiff and numb, with the participant's hands resting on the table.

At this point, it seems wise not to continue the physical stroking on other parts of the participant's body because of the sexual suggestiveness that it would entail. Accordingly, we simply describe the continued flow of numbness: "Down from your shoulders into your chest, then into your abdomen. Now your right [left] leg is beginning to get numb" (usually on the same side as the first arm that became numb). "The leg is getting straight and stiff down through the knee, the lower leg, your ankle, your feet, and your toes," and so on. The participant's entire leg may at this point be sticking straight out and suspended off the floor; a posture that will result in fatigue if continued too long.

The same suggestions are now implanted as relating to the numbness flowing down into the other leg. At this point all of the participant's body

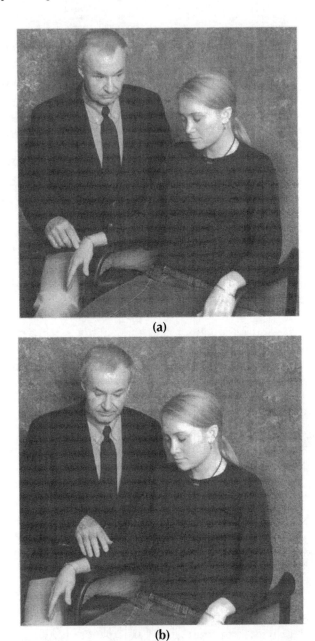

Fig. 6.7 Progressive Anesthesia Procedure. (a) Initially, the patient is asked to focus on her hand, which is being stroked by the therapist. Her hand is becoming stiff and numb. (b) The numbness and stiffness in the patient's hand are now transferred up the arm as the therapist strokes it.

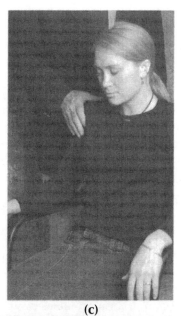

(c)

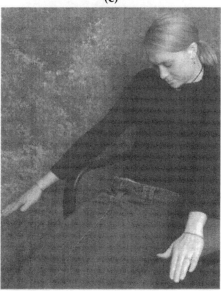

(d)

(Fig. 6.7 *Continued.* (c) The numbness is now transferred from the patient's right arm to her right shoulder, the back of her neck, her left shoulder, and her left arm. (d) The numbness and stiffness have now moved down the trunk of the patient's body to her legs.

below the shoulders should be stiff and numb. Of course, it is essential that the suggestions closely follow the responses of the participant. The therapist should not be rushed and should permit plenty of time and repetition to occur so that each member of the participant's body is clearly affected before proceeding to the next one.

Finally, the therapist suggests that the numbness is moving up through the neck, the face, the lips, and the forehead. If it is still necessary, the therapist suggests closure of the eyes, and follows that with suggestions of the participant's entering a deep comfortable sleep or state of relaxation. The participant's stiffness may be removed, and the therapist tells the participant to relax his or her muscles but to retain the loss of feeling. Depth of trance will be related to the extent and depth of the numbness. This depth can be tested by pricking the participant's skin. This induction can be useful in preparing a patient for some painful surgical procedure in which some other anesthetic is to be further applied, or if hypnoanalgesia is to be the only pain suppressant.

Nonverbal Method

On rare occasions communication problems can make it difficult, if not impossible, to use the typical induction procedures. Perhaps the patient is deaf or speaks a foreign language that is not known by the therapist. This technique can also be particularly useful with children, who are frequently more responsive to postural suggestions than to verbal ones.

The therapist seats the participant in a chair and instructs him or her to hold both arms out in front and upward so that the hands are above the eye level (see Figure 6.8). The arms should be parallel, and the hands should be about 2 feet apart. The therapist now moves back and forth in front of the participant from one side to the other, making a small postural change in the patient's right arm first, then over to the other side to make a similar change in the left arm.

First, the patient's right arm is bent at the elbow so that the hand comes a bit inward and downward (the right elbow simultaneously extending more outward). The therapist then moves over to the left side and repeats the movement of the patient's left arm in the same way. After each movement the therapist pauses a few seconds and observes the posture. This permits observation of the patient's reaction and allows time for adjustment to the new change in posture.

Once again, the therapist moves to the patient's right side and adjusts the right arm again slightly downward. This position is then matched in a few seconds with a similar adjustment to the left hand. The postural adjustments of the arms and hands are constantly transmitting the message of "inward and downward," inward into the patient's self, downward toward a more unconscious level of awareness.

Finally, when the patient's hands are almost together and are barely above the lap, the therapist grasps both arms firmly by the wrist and forcibly lowers them rapidly all the way down. At this point, the patient's eyes will usually close and his or her head slump forward on the chest. If this does not happen, the therapist can pull the patient's eyelids down and, by a push on the back of the patient's head, administer the final forceful suggestion that implies, "Go inward and downward, close your eyes and enter a deep, relaxed, hypnotic state!"

No words have been spoken, but the induction has been accomplished by the series of progressively spaced changes in posture. To remove the hypnotic state that has been achieved, the therapist simply reverses the movements. First, he or her lifts up the patient's head. Then the therapist lifts up the patient's arms to the position that was held just prior to the forcible lowering of them. Next, the therapist reverses the movements of one arm and hand at a time. The movements are now outward and upward: "Come up out of yourself and back into the conscious state" is the message. Finally, the patient's arms are back in their original position, the eyes are fully open, and the head is up. The therapist smiles at the patient and gently brings the arms down to the sides from which they had been originally raised.

The Rehearsal Technique

A simple way to hypnotize a patient who has experienced hypnosis from some previous practitioner is to repeat or "rehearse" exactly the procedure used earlier (see Figure 6.9). The therapist inquires of the participant what the other therapist did with hypnosis and in what order the suggestions were administered. For example:

You say that when your dentist, Doctor X, hypnotized you, she had you lie back in the dental chair and relax? All right. Please lie back on the couch and relax in the same way. Now what did she tell you to do first? She said to hold up your hand and focus your eyes on it? OK. Do that. Hold up your hand and focus your eyes on it just like you did in the dental chair. Then what did the doctor say? She said to take three deep breaths. OK. Take three deep breaths. One, two, three! Good! Now what did the doctor say? She told you to focus your eyes on the index finger and let yourself relax all over. All right, then focus your eyes on the index finger and start relaxing all over. What came next? She told you that your arm would get very heavy. Let your arm get very heavy now. Then what? She told you that as your arm slowly came down, you come down with it into a deep state of

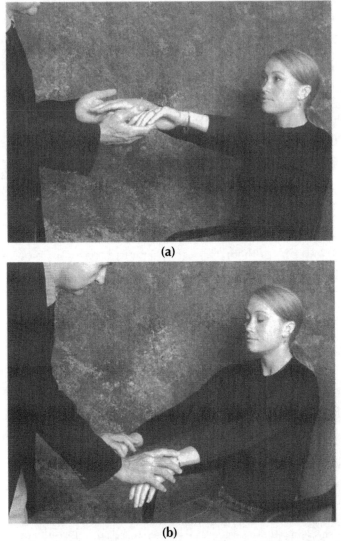

(a)

(b)

Fig. 6.8 Nonverbal Induction. (a) Initially, the therapist lifts the patient's hands into position and then gently withdraws his hand while providing nonverbal communication for her to keep her arms extended. (b) After ensuring the patient received the message, the therapist gently presses her hands and arms downward. The message to her is "Go down deeper and into yourself."

relaxation. Good. Now as your arm comes slowly down you will experience it just as before. You will come down with it into the same state of relaxation pleasantly hypnotized.

This procedure is then continued until participants are completely involved hypnotically. It can be used with almost any technique and has

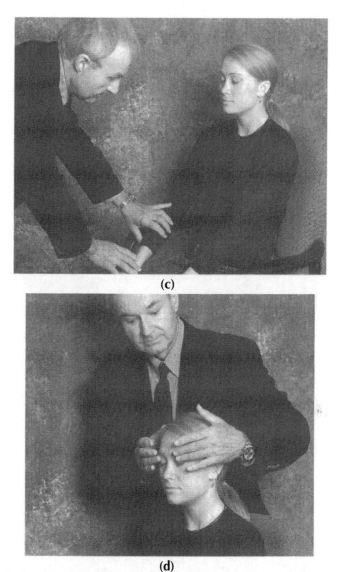

(c)

(d)

Fig. 6.8 *Continued.* (c) Gently pressing the patient's arm all the way down, the therapist gives the message to go still deeper. (d) Putting gentle pressure above the patient's eyelids, the therapist gives the nonverbal message, "Your eyes will remain closed."

the advantage that patients are simply repeating step by step a procedure that has already been found to be effective for inducing a state of hypnosis in them. We assume that the patients' relationship with the previous therapist was constructive and that they left at that time with a good feeling. Some inquiry might be undertaken before beginning this procedure.

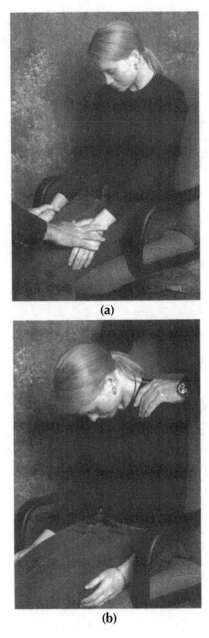

(a)

(b)

Fig. 6.9 The Rehearsal Technique. (a) Pressing the patient's hands all the way down, the therapist gives the very forceful nonverbal message to go down deeper. (b) The therapist's pressing the patient's shoulders down further reinforces the hypnotic suggestion for depth. Her head drops and she slumps into a hypnotic position.

Assess whether the patients felt angry with the previous therapist or if the practitioner had not been helpful. The patients' underlying resentment can operate as a resistance, making their rehypnotization by the same technique difficult or impossible. In such cases, considerable attention to building rapport and trust in the relationship with such patients is a pre-requisite to the therapist's success or failure in treating them.

Sleep Variation of Rehearsal Technique

An interesting variation of the rehearsal approach can be used to hypno-tize individuals for the first time, using their customary behavior in going to bed. The therapist asks the patients simply to relive the steps they go through in retiring for the night. The therapist says, "Imagine that it is bedtime and you are ready for bed." It may be best for the therapist to avoid suggesting the steps of removing clothing because this could be interpreted by the patient as a sexually seductive move by the doctor or could provoke erotic transference reactions. However, the therapist can suggest, "Imagine turning out the lights, pulling the bed covers back, crawling between the sheets, snuggling down, and then feeling the warm, relaxed feelings pouring through your muscles, your eyes getting heavier and heavier, your thoughts becoming less and less and a deep, relaxing, sleepy feeling." The procedure is the same as in the typical rehearsal of a previous induction, except here the therapist must rely on the patients' report of their customary retiring behavior. It is possible to make errors in this approach, because the therapist might say, "You feel your head sinking back into the comfortable pillow," when the patients do not generally sleep on a pillow. Suggestions that are contrary to reality tend to alert the patients and operate in the reverse direction from helping them activate a true state of hypnosis rather than merely a relaxed condition.

Jet to Hawaii and Other Fantasy Techniques

These methods employ suggestions aimed at getting participants involved in rich imagination. The methods usually begin with the therapist's asking the participants to close their eyes and then visualize something like the following:

> Just imagine that you are going to take a trip to Hawaii. You have your luggage in your hand and are in the airport getting ready to board the plane. You have your tickets, and you can see yourself now going through the hand luggage inspection. Everything is OK, and you walk toward the boarding area. You can see many of the

other passengers around you, some older people and a few children. You are now boarding the plane and finding your seat. You sit down, buckle on the safety strap, and relax. The plane's engines start; you can hear their sound and feel it when the captain applies the brakes every now and again as you taxi to the runway. The sound of the engines increase, and you feel the thrust pushing you back into your seat as the plane roars down the runway and lifts off the ground. How exhilarated you feel about this wonderful vacation. You look down from the plane's window and see the tiny houses and cars way below you. You settle back in your seat. Perhaps a flight attendant brings you some coffee or a drink. Now you reach the ocean shore. The beaches slip behind you, and all you can see is the great blue sea with a few tiny, white-capped waves below. It is so pleasant, and you are relaxing deeper and deeper, perhaps into a drowsy nap. Hours pass, and as you look out the window again, you see ahead some little dots of islands. You are coming in over Hawaii. Soon the features of Diamond Head with the beaches surrounded by many palm trees become visible below. You are feeling very excited about reaching your destination and getting to do all the interesting things you have been dreaming you will do when you get to Hawaii.

The fantasy can be made short or long. However, the important point is that the therapist must picture each step in the most vivid language possible, using descriptive adjectives. In this way, he or she induces patients to halt their own inner, distracting thoughts and to exclude contact with outer reality other than that in the relationship with the therapist. The therapist and the fantasy he or she is elaborating become the universe of experience for patients. Once this relationship has been established, participants are most likely to follow other suggestions, including therapeutic ones. Fantasy techniques like this one can serve as an induction method and as a deepening procedure once initial induction has been completed. In fact, hypnotizability tests, induction techniques, and deepening procedures (to be discussed in the next chapter) are all on a continuum. The extension of one leads into the other.

Other fantasies might involve going to see a movie, descending in a diving sphere to the bottom of the ocean, traveling on a train, going to a department store, or participating in an archaeological expedition. The choices, of course, are unlimited and restricted only by the therapist's ingenuity at providing the kind of fantasies with which the participant can identify. Occasionally, a fantasy produces resistance or a negative response in the patient, perhaps manifested by suddenly shaking off the state and self-alerting. The therapist should simply and confidently inquire what it was that induced this reaction. I (A.F.B.) apologize and say "Sorry, sometimes that can happen" and then start again by deleting the negative item in the fantasy that disturbed the patient, initiating another fantasy, or trying an entirely different induction technique.

Subject-Object: An Intricate, Complex, Indirect Technique

This is a rather unusual approach because it involves a manipulation of the locus of the patient's self-perception. There seems to be considerable variation in individual's ability to respond to it. Some individuals enter rapidly into a very deep state with this procedure; others find that they cannot throw themselves into the psychological alterations that it requires. Here is one example, assuming a female patient:

> Imagine that you are coming to my office like you did today. You are in your car and driving from your house along the streets you need to pass to get here. You can visualize the various buildings, the people walking on the sidewalk, the other cars. You experience yourself in the driver's seat with your hands on the steering wheel and making all the little turns required to maneuver your car in the traffic. You turn into the driveway and stop your car in this building's parking lot. You turn the keys to turn the engine off and open the car door, preparing to get out.
>
> At this moment a change seems to occur in you. You are now standing a few feet behind your car in the parking lot and watching a person get out of your car. She is wearing your clothes and has your color of hair. You follow her as she walks to my office and opens the door of the waiting room. She sits down for a few minutes and then is ushered into this office sitting down in the easy chair beside mine. You are standing just inside the doorway watching her. You notice that she is wearing a brown suit with a green scarf just like yours, that she has your red hair, and that her face looks just like what you see when you look into a mirror.
>
> Notice how she is reacting to my talking to her. I am starting to give her some hypnotically inducing suggestions, and it occurs to you as you watch her, the one who looks like you and is wearing your clothes, that she is beginning to get rather drowsy. Her eyes look very heavy. They blink and are beginning to close. You keep watching and observe a deep relaxation passing through all her body. Her

arms relax. Her chest relaxes. Her legs relax, and you think to your-self, "My, that person who looks like me is relaxing into a very deep state of calmness." Notice how deeply she is going. You keep observ-ing her as she sinks deeper and deeper, and as you hear my voice droning on you think that you, too, would like to achieve the same deep relaxation as she has achieved. You decide that you would like to join her, and accordingly you walk across the room and stand just in front of her chair. You turn around and back down into her seat merging your body with hers until your head coincides with hers. Your arms and hers are the same. Your body fuses with hers, and your legs and hers are the same. As you take on her entire body, you are aware that you are also taking on her feelings. You sense the deep calmness she had achieved pouring through your own self, and you enjoy the profound sense of security and warmth that she had reached. You and she are now one and the same, and you are involved in a most deep and comfortable state of relaxation.

Notice how the subject and object have been manipulated in this pro-cedure. The patient first gets involved in rehearsing the trip to the office. This image is vivified with many suggestions as to the buildings, people, and cars the patient has encountered along the way. They should be described as specifically as possible but not so specifically that they do not represent reality; hence, the therapist should not tell the patient she is driving along 9th Street if she actually came to the office along 10th Street. Up to the point of parking the car, the suggestions must coincide with reality.

Ego states have boundaries, and so we use boundaries to shift from one state to another. Walls can symbolically represent boundaries, and doors are passages from one state to another, hence, passing from one room in one's "ego house" to another. Accordingly, we used the moment of leaving the car to make a change of self-perspective. The self (subject) is now moved to a position behind the car, and the "driving ego state" is changed from subject to object. The patient now "sees" the driver of the car emerg-ing from it, whereas before the patient was experiencing being the driver. The state of being the driver of the car is now no longer subject. It has become object ("her" instead of "me"), and the patient perceives her body as a "not me." To keep the identity clear, the person who is emerging from the car is described as having the patient's clothes and hair, and later as having the same features that the patient sees when she looks in the mir-ror. When we look into a mirror we see ourselves as "object," hence, as oth-ers see us.

This change, which is really a kind of temporary dissociation, is continued as the woman who looks like the patient enters the office and sits down in the chair next to the doctor. It is that image (object) that is then hypnotized, while the patient's self views the process from a different location near the office door. Finally, the observing ego state is fused again with the experiencing ego state, and the patient resumes the experiencing of her own body again. However, as she takes on the body she must also take on all the feelings that that body has. Accordingly, if her "body over there" has been hypnotized, and she returns to it, she must also assume the hypnotic state, which the body includes.

This is an intricate, complex, and sophisticated induction technique, but it is often effective when other more direct approaches have failed. The subject-object manipulations that are involved can also be used in a number of therapeutic techniques that we describe in later chapters.

Self-Induction Procedure

Many of the techniques that have been described can be adapted to self-hypnosis if this is indicated. We have some reservations about teaching individuals self-hypnosis. Many people request it, and there is no doubt that at times it is a valuable approach. The doctor may not always be available, and the patient may suffer from intractable pain and is in need of immediate relief. People can use self-hypnosis to improve study habits, teach themselves to go to sleep, improve their golf games, and so on.

However, there are many individuals who seek hypnosis as a new kind of thrill. Indeed, the research has shown repeatedly that some of the most hypnotizable persons are by nature sensation seekers. They wish to experiment with their own states of consciousness. Some have tried various drugs; they want a new and cheap way of "turning on." Nishith, Barabasz, Barabasz, and Warner (1999) experimentally showed that in a group of university student sensation seekers, brief hypnosis could substitute for Xanax (alprazolam). Still others are already given to too much dissociating. These people include borderline psychotics or others who are increasingly living their lives in fantasy rather than facing up to the realities of adapting to a world of people and challenges. Such individuals may be more harmed by hypnosis, especially of the self-induced type, than helped by it. They employ it as a way of avoiding life's problems, rather than solving them. Also, some people will use self-induced hypnotic analgesia to suppress every pain, even pains that should serve as warnings to consult their doctor or dentist. For these reasons, one should be conservative about teaching self-hypnosis and should consider carefully the purposes to which individuals intend to put the hypnotic modality, their inner motivations, and the condition of their own inner integration, ego strength, and maturity.

For those for whom such a procedure is indicated, either for self-treatment or as an adjunct to be used between sessions with the doctor, Helen Watkins developed an adaptation of the arm-drop approach that can be easily taught and practiced. She proposed the following steps:

1. *Finger concentration with hand drop to relaxation.* Initial induction by hypnotherapist involves instructing the patient to stare at the patient's index or middle finger with eyes either open or closed. The hypnotherapist suggests that the other fingers will fade into the periphery of the patients' vision and that as they continues to stare, the hand and arm will become heavy; the more they stare the heavier the arm becomes. The suggestion continues that as the arm and hand become heavier, the hand begins to move down, and as the hand moves down the patient begins to move down into a state of relaxation, but will not enter a deep state of relaxation until the hand is all the way down.

2. *Muscular relaxation head to toe.*

3. *Internalize distractions.* "With every bit of noise I hear, I can go deeper and deeper."

4. *Concentrate on breathing.* "With every breath I exhale, I will become more and more relaxed."

5. *Deepening.* "Going down now deeper to the room with the soft, plushy couch, 1 going down, 2 going down, 3, 4, 5, half way there, now going deeper and further down, 6, 7, 8, 9, 10, you are now there, settling down on the couch."

6. *Repeat mentally.* The following is spoken by the hypnotherapist during initial induction: "Relax deeply ... relax deeply. ... As I relax deeply ... I can go to a deep state of concentration ... I won't be asleep, I can be alert ... and I can learn to use these procedures in my own style and my own way ... so that I can become the kind of person I wish to be, the kind of person I can be. ... I can learn to use this technique to rest and relax more deeply. ... I can use it to go to sleep at night. ... I can use it to study or to concentrate more ... or to gain more self-understanding and more self-control.

7. *Meditation.* Patients should meditate for a minute using personalized sentences that state positive ideas about themselves, or use meditation for whatever purpose self-hypnosis is initiated.

8. *Self-arousal by counting backward from 5 to 1.*

Self-hypnosis has received increasing interest among experimental and clinical workers. The entire July 1981 issue of the *International Journal of*

Clinical and Experimental Hypnosis is devoted to this topic. Fromm et al. (1981) pointed out that the experience of absorption and the facing of the general reality orientation is found in hetero-hypnosis and self-hypnosis. However, age regression seems to be easier in hetero-hypnosis. Self-hypnosis is much richer in imagery. Johnson (1981) analyzed the findings of the Chicago group (Fromm et al., 1981) and pointed out that self-hypnosis opens a new and rich field that has as yet been relatively unexplored. Perhaps the chief value in self-hypnosis is in establishing a physiological state related to relaxation (Kahn & Fromm, 2001). Sacerdote (1981) held that there is no pure self-hypnosis and described a number of difficulties encountered by individuals during self-hypnosis. Orne and McConkey (1981) compared research and theoretical viewpoints relating self- and hetero-hypnosis. Shor (1978) published an *Inventory of Self-Hypnosis* designed to evaluate self-hypnotic performance (see J. Smith, Barabasz, & Barabasz, 1996, for a discussion of self-hypnosis with children). Of course, because most people who have the capacity to enter the hypnotic state will often go into a trance spontaneously, all hypnosis can be conceptualized as self-hypnosis (H. Spiegel, 1998; H. Spiegel & Spiegel, 2004). In general, the area has been far less researched than hetero-hypnosis, but it promises to open new approaches to effective clinical treatment.

The Approaches of Milton Erickson

Milton Erickson (Haley, 1967; Zeig, 1982) was a widely known practitioner in the field of clinical hypnosis who contributed broadly to its literature. His approach to the hypnotic modality was so unique and substantially different from that of other workers in the field that specific analyses that aim at a theoretical explanation of his techniques have been published (Erickson et al., 1976).

Erickson apparently had considerable success in hypnotizing relatively resistant individuals. However, contrary to clinical lore, he could not hypnotize everyone. On a long visit to Ernest R. Hilgard's Laboratory of Hypnosis Research at Stanford University, Erickson admitted he could not produce a single legitimate hypnotic response in a number of student volunteers who had scored at the bottom of the *Stanford Hypnotic Susceptibility* Scales However, Erickson did develop many innovative therapeutic strategies within the hypnotic context. We do not attempt here to present a detailed description of his procedures, and we refer readers who are interested to his original publications (see Haley, 1967) for a compilation of many of these. However, a brief coverage of some of his basic concepts and illustrations of how he translated these into hypnotherapeutic manipulations is in order.[1]

Erickson believed that hypnosis is primarily an intrapsychic process and, hence, induction techniques should not rely on apparatus, such as crystal balls, metronomes, and so on. Rather, the therapist should introduce the patient to imagining the crystal balls, to hearing imagined music, or to sensing the touch of a therapist's hand that is visualized in the patient's mind's eye. This movement from attention to outside stimuli into concentration on inner images can have a profound influence in drawing the individual into a hypnotic state.

Erickson held that many failures in hypnotic induction are the result of the therapist's spending too little time with the patient. He (1952) stated that he often devoted several hours conditioning a patient before securing a trance state. Our clinical practices, and those of the late Helen Watkins, typically involve intensive contact with the patient, consisting of several hours per day and consecutive days of regular contact. After years of conventional treatment contact, 1 hour per week, I (A.F.B.) was stunned by the dramatic improvements in the level of trance that could be achieved by shifting my practice to one that was largely intensive. Clinical outcomes and their lasting effects improved dramatically as well. After many hours of contact, Erickson recognized that when it is suggested to patients that they hallucinate, visual images may be reported. However, if the patient readily accepts these images as real, during prolonged sessions, they may remain simply at a conscious image level. The time and continued suggestion — which began as an "as if" — becomes real. The patient becomes deeply involved in the trance experience and therapeutic results far greater than those that could be manifested by suggestion alone are enduring.

Another principle Erickson emphasized is that of pacing. By that, he meant ensuring that each hypnotic suggestion given to patients is within their ability to execute and is fully carried out before the next and more challenging suggestion is administered. Amateur therapists attempt to jump rapidly from a simple suggestion, perhaps the lifting of a hand, into an extremely demanding one, such as distorting perception into a positive or negative hallucination. The induction process must proceed stepwise, with ample time for the patient to become increasingly involved in the hypnotic state.

Perhaps one of the most important principles emphasized by Erickson is the protection of the integrity of the patient. In one case, he described an incident involving automatic handwriting in which the patient agreed to permit the reading of that which she would write, but Erickson continued to protect her right to secrecy, even after her apparent permission to break it. The result was her involvement shortly in a very profound trance. Similarly, he would suggest to patients who were in a light trance that they can dream a dream then forget it, that there will be no recall until it is so desired. Or he would instruct patients to withhold some item of information from the therapist. Strong appreciation of all of a patients' responses is exuded. Erickson emphasized what was happening experientially within the patients rather than what the therapist was doing to them. Erickson often issued his induction suggestions in the form of a challenge. For example, when a patient asked if hypnosis could be induced while standing, Erickson's response was, "Why not demonstrate that it can be?" He held that one should accept resistance that is offered and work with it rather than trying to overcome it. When resistance shows that a patient is ambivalent about entering hypnosis, a suggestion might be given that fails. The patient is pleased at defeating the therapist and becomes less resistant to future suggestions. Erickson often employed a technique suggesting the repetition of dreams with different content but the same meaning. He reported that the trance is deepened with each dream.

A perceptual approach suggested by Erickson, which seems to be effective, involves having patients move their attention from one object to another in the room and then close the eyes and visualize them again.

A trance may be induced or deepened by asking patients to speculate and describe what their behavior and experience would be like if hypnotized. This is a variation of the rehearsal technique. Erickson often made a series of requests that could hardly be avoided, but compliance would gradually induce the patient to enter hypnosis. The following is an example.

> Are you willing to cooperate with me by continuing to pace the floor as you are now doing? Will you please turn toward the chair in which you can sit. Now please turn away from the chair in which you can sit. Now please turn again toward the chair in which you will shortly find yourself comfortably seated. [Note the implication here of involuntary activity; for example, "in which you will shortly find yourself comfortably seated."] Now you can sit in the chair and go deeply as you relate your history.

By complying with each request, the patient has committed to settling into the chair and "going deeply" into trance once seated there.

I (A.F.B.) use a slight variation of this technique in my hypnosis classes and workshops to demonstrate how dramatically effective this induction can be with a patient of known moderate or better hypnotic capacity: "OK, I wonder if you would mind just closing the door over there, and now please put the CD in the player, please try to keep yourself out of deep hypnosis until you are comfortably seated in that chair there, just please keep your eyes open until then if you can, until you are seated." Typically, patients enter trance upon seating themselves, the eyes close immediately, and I can go on to deepening or test hypnotic suggestions. Obviously, rapport must have been well established in previous contact with the patient but the effects are rather noteworthy.

Summary

Several approaches to hypnosis are legendary. Individual practitioners learn to develop specific techniques that are effective and fit their personal style. It is impossible to become a photocopy of one of the masters. Learn to develop your own style under the guidance and supervision of your mentor (the guru, if you like). Many of the techniques we described may have different results, depending on whether the therapist has used an authoritative or permissive manner in administering them. Most of them, however, will be found similar to one or more of the foregoing. It is advised that you learn certain ones well. Practice them a great deal, with volunteers if possible, before using them on patients. Professional hypnotherapists will usually find that a few approaches in which they are sensitive and highly skilled will serve the needs of most of their patients. Familiarity with some of the other more advanced approaches can be valuable in specialized instances. Confidence, skill, and clinical experience with patients are far more important for the induction of hypnotic states than the techniques. Hypnosis is an altered state of consciousness, but for clinical practice, it is equally an intensive interpersonal relationship experience between the therapist and the patient.

Note

1. For a complete bibliography of Erickson's publications from 1929 to 1977, see Gravitz and Gravitz (1977).

Chapter 7
Deepening Hypnotic Trance

It seems obvious to even the most casual observer that various levels of response to hypnosis requires varying levels of hypnotic depth. Little hypnotic depth, if any, is needed, for example, to achieve a relaxation response to suggestions to achieve calmness, ease up, and let go in contrast to the level of depth essential for painless surgery without an anesthetic.

Such criticallity of hypnotic depth has been recognized since, if not before, Charcot (1889) proposed three basic levels: catalepsy (rigidity in limbs achieved by hypnotic suggestion), lethargy, and somnambulism. Ten years later Liebeault (1866) classified a range of depth levels from drowsiness to catalepsy to hypnotically suggested halllucinations that could be experienced posthypnotically. The Davis and Husband's (1931) 30-point *Hypnotic Susceptibility Scale* gives the negative visual hallucination the highest score. So J. Watkins (1949) published a more comprehensive, refined, and expanded version of this scale, grading, for example, hypermnesia slight to marked, levels of regression, and hypnotic to posthypnotic negative visual hallucinations. As you will recall from your reading of chapter 4, the posthypnotic suggestion for a negative hallucination (suggestion of only two boxes on the table, when actually there are three in front of the participant) is, for example, considered the most demanding item of the 12-item *Stanford Hypnotic Susceptibility Scale*, Form C (SHSS:C) (Weitzenhoffer & Hilgard, 1962).

Perhaps because of the important impact of the well-researched *Stanford Hypnotic Susceptibility Scale* (Forms A, B, and C), used widely since the 1960s, and the *Hypnotic Induction Profile* (HIP) of Herbert and David Spiegel (1978–1987) the criticality of hypnotic depth sufficient for the task at hand has largely been abandoned in the research literature in favor of hypnotizabilty test scores.

The problem with substituting hypnotizability scores that measure the patient's capacity or ability to enter hypnosis does not imply that high-scoring individuals are somehow magically at their maximum capacity or depth after any sort of credible hypnotic induction. As editor of the *International Journal of Clinical and Experimental Hypnosis*, I (A.F.B.) remain amazed to see the number of articles submitted from major authors in the field, most frequently from university settings that make just that assumption.

Why would anyone assume that just because a person had a capacity for responding to difficult hypnotic suggestions that he or she would be adequately hypnotically involved to accomplish feats such as negative hallucinations or painless surgery after having been read a brief scripted hypnotic induction?

If hypnosis were simply an "either-or," we could at this point proceed directly to treatment. However, its induction appears to be a continuous process, starting with the first responses to hypnotic suggestion and gradually developing into an increasingly profound involvement in the hypnotic modality. Although certain techniques bring an almost instantaneous, sometimes deep, immersion in hypnosis, in most cases time is required for the individual to adjust to the hypnotic mode of perception and behavior. Hypnotizability tests, which elicit hypnotic responses, merge into an induction process with no demarcating line, except one we have arbitrarily defined. Induction techniques, when prolonged, tend to carry the individual even further into the trance state to perhaps, but not necessarily, to the maximum level measured by the scale. Accordingly, we can conceptualize that state as one of degree. A person is not either in or out of a hypnotic state; one is in such a state lightly, significantly, or deeply. Thus the hypnotizability tests, described in chapter 4, appear to measure not only the ability of an individual to be hypnotized but also the depth to which it is possible to hypnotize that person. The point, lost on a number of even well-known hypnosis researchers and clinicians, is that depth adequate to achieve the suggested response is not automatically manifested the moment a person is exposed to a hypnotic induction or self-hypnotic experience (Kahn & Fromm, 1992).

Another misconception among lay people and many professionals is that unless the individual is deeply involved he or she has not truly been hypnotized. Therapists often hear a new patient react to the first hypnotic induction with a statement such as, "But doctor, I wasn't hypnotized. I could hear you all the time." To many, being hypnotized seems to mean being in an unconscious condition, one in which the voice of the therapist is not heard and his or her suggestions not remembered upon awakening. There is further the implicit misconception that unless such a state was achieved, hypnotic suggestions will be ineffective and hypnotherapy contraindicated.

The Therapeutic Value of Light and Medium States

Certain phenomena, such as regression and posthypnotic hallucinations, require a rather deep state to be elicited. Such phenomena represent the more striking aspects of hypnosis and tend to establish the conviction of its reality to the observer. It is also true that hypnotic suggestions planted in the deeper trance states have an increased probability of being carried out and of lasting longer. Because we know that less than one quarter of unselected individuals are usually capable of reaching deep hypnotic levels, practitioners tend to be discouraged on the grounds that they could hope for effective results only with a minority of their patients.

Fortunately, the picture is not that discouraging. Not only do many hypnotherapeutic suggestions hold when implanted during light and medium states of hypnotic involvement but also some practitioners have argued that in certain types of therapy the condition of light hypnosis is to be preferred (Conn, 1959). For example, if our goal, as in the analytic therapies, is to lift into consciousness material of which the patient has previously been aware and also to ensure that this new awareness has been consciously assimilated and integrated to the fullest degree, then material that has been discovered while the patient has been only lightly hypnotized may bring about greater therapeutic change. Deeply repressed material can, as maintained by Anna Freud (1946), come temporarily to consciousness,[1] but in bypassing ego integration can be soon forgotten and rerepressed. Nothing happens and the patient does not change. E. Hilgard and Tart (1966) emphasized the need to obtain patient self-assessments of depth on a numeric scale during hypnotic experiments because of normal fluctuations in depth. Kahn and Fromm (1992, p. 394) pointed out that "just as depth fluctuates during trance, so too do the relative amounts of the self versus the other that are involved." A permissive therapist can use silence during trance to enhance the patient's private thoughts, fantasies, and self-suggestions. However, the directive or authoritarian model therapist who continually provides hypnotic suggestions moves the patient's experience almost entirely from the other therapist-initiated end of the self-versus-other continuum

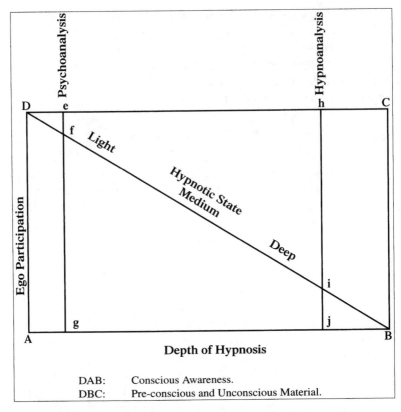

Fig. 7.1 The relationship of trance depth to various therapies, psychoanalytic and hypnoanalytic.

The Relationship Between Depth of Hypnosis and Ego Participation

To elucidate further, we formulate the relation of trance depth to various therapies, psychoanalytic and hypnoanalytic, in Figure 7.1.

In the rectangle in Figure 7.1, the dimension AB represents the depth of trance, extending from A, a completely alert condition, to B, the deepest possible hypnosis. This might represent what Erickson (1952) termed a "plenary trance." At right angles might be designated the degree of ego participation, correlated at least, if not theoretically identical, with the factor of conscious awareness. As the state of hypnosis (represented by the area DBQ) increases, the condition of conscious, egotized experience (represented by the area DBA) lessens. At the AD position, an individual is completely alert, fully in contact with his or her outer world, and retaining all critical faculties. As one moves along the diagonal line DB through induction and deepening procedures, one's behavior and experiencing increasingly take on the characteristics typical of hypnosis. Contact with the external world (except that with the therapist) is gradually withdrawn. Criticality is lowered as the individual regresses into more primary behavior and thought. First preconscious then unconscious and primary process ideation become more evident. Theoretically, at point B, the ego ceases participation, and the patient would lapse into a comalike state, which if it were ever completely reached would result even in breaking off contact with the therapist. We opine that under such a circumstance we would have to wait for natural forces within the patient to change, during a period of several seconds to perhaps 10 to 20 minutes, which would reestablish contact with reality.

Characteristics of Very Deep Hypnosis

In a remarkable Stanford University PhD dissertation, Sherman (1971) studied participants who had been placed in very deep hypnotic states, much more profound than are secured in most therapeutic hypnosis. They described their experiences as "being everything, feeling oneness with everything, loss of knowledge of individual identity"; "no self"; "absolute mental quiet, no thoughts or images." According to Sherman, these participants had "passed beyond" all those cognitive patterns that define one as a specific person and separate from other people and the environment. What is left is undifferentiated awareness — the awareness of purely "being" through which the person is identical to everything in the universe. Such a state seems to be similar to the condition of "satori," the goal of Zen meditation (Watts, 1957). Satori aims at a loss of individual identity and a complete merging with the universe. It seems likely that Buddist monks who sequester themselves to long-term solitary meditation in caves or similar environments may, as evidenced by their varied writings, obtain similar states perhaps with meditation facilitating the kind of focused attention involved in the deepest hypnotic states. This, of course, is entirely speculative until controlled research is conducted. Nonetheless it is a fascinating hypothesis worthy of study by the enterprising researcher who is willing to go beyond mundane experimentation.

Men exposed to the winter in Antarctica have frequently reported fuguelike states and have shown significant increases in hypnotizability (A. Barabasz, 1980a). Experimentally controlled research (A. Barabasz, 1982; M. Barabasz, A. Barabasz, Darakjy, and Warner, 2001) on the effects of 6 hours of sensory restriction in a sound- and light-free chamber has also shown increases in *Stanford Hypnotic Susceptibility Scale* scores. Participants were also able to use their increases in hypnotizability to produce pain relief.

We also speculate that this is the condition of experiencing reached by participants at point B on our scale in Figure 7.1. However, the achievement of such levels of depth is extremely rare and accomplished with only a few individuals after protracted and skillful induction. We simply do not see such states in the general practices of clinical hypnosis. At no time in our experience has any patient ever passed completely beyond the limits of communication.

Handling the Individual Who Resists Coming out of Hypnosis

We need have no fear that our participant will go into hypnosis so deeply that we cannot bring him or her back to the normal waking condition. Occasionally a participant will so much enjoy the tranquility of the hypnotic state that he or she will be somewhat slow to emerge. For example, suppose we have explained that alertness will be achieved upon counting backward from 10 to 1, but the individual's eyes do not open or only do so slowly. We have counted to 5, and he or she has either not opened the eyes or does so slowly. All that is necessary is to suggest to the individual something like the following:

> It really is enjoyable to relax in this comfortable state and I wish it was possible to stay in this position. Unfortunately, I have someone coming whom I must see this next hour. However, I promise you that we can repeat this experience if you wish at your next session. Why don't you bring yourself out of hypnosis in your own way and at your own speed. By simply permitting yourself to continue to feel very good and counting down from 10 to 1, at 5 you can let your eyes open and become fully awake and alert upon reaching 1, yet you can retain the pleasure of the present moment. I will be quiet while you do this.

We have never found a patient who did not respond to such an approach. There is no cause for alarm or fright simply because a patient is somewhat slow in responding to suggestions for terminating hypnosis.

Before learning this technique, I (A.F.B.) was faced with an interesting dilemma. A panicked person phoned my office to explain about a "hypnosis experiment gone wrong." A high school drama teacher had hypnotized one of his students and "couldn't bring her out." Upon my arrival, the student in trance was receiving considerable attention as she sat motionless in an armchair. People were blowing in her closed eyes, clapping their hands, and saying, "Please wake up … please, please come out of it." She just seemed to go deeper and deeper into hypnosis. I merely cleared the room of the onlookers but remained within her range of hearing. I carefully explained to her drama coach, "Everyone knows its impossible to stay in a hypnotic trance on your own, without the therapist present to give hypnotic suggestions." She would simply come out of it naturally. The well-intentioned people that were trying to awaken her were in fact helping to take her more deeply into hypnosis. Her eyes opened slowly and she apologized by saying, "I must have fallen asleep." I learned a month later that this 18-year-old senior was dating the drama coach. They had some sort of disagreement, just hours before her hypnosis with him, and she was still angry with him. Obviously, she paid him back by controlling him by her deepening rather then awakening from hypnosis.

Returning to our consideration of Figure 7.1, note that line EFG is drawn at the left-hand side of the figure to represent the condition typical of psychoanalysis where the patient is reclining on the couch, hence probably in a light hypnoidal state. He or she is told to be preoccupied with inner associations and that it will be easy to concentrate inside, ignoring external stimuli. This moves the patient inward from the AD axis and permits the release (line segment EF) of preconscious material and unconscious derivatives as described by Freud (1900-1953). There is still a large part of the "self" egotized, as represented by line segment FG.

In the deeper states of hypnosis, such as are sometimes employed in hypnoanalysis, the reverse is true. A great deal of unconscious and possibly primary process material becomes accessible as represented by line segment HI. However, there is present at that time only minimal conscious ego participation in the process as measured by the short line segment ij. Without wishing at this point to proceed too far along hypothetical lines, we might ask whether the greatest therapeutic movement in an analytic treatment would occur at stage EFG or at level HIJ. Would the greatest production occur where there is a small amount of raw material (EF) and a large processing factory (FG) or where there is a large quantity of raw material (HI) and a relative small factory to integrate and process it (IJ). From such speculation we might arrive at the position that either in an alternation of hypnotic depth or in the intermediate trance states are found the optimal conditions for lifting repressions and integrating newly discovered insights into a significant personality change. From such a viewpoint, neither the state in which traditional psychoanalysis is conducted nor deep hypnoanalysis would represent the most efficient condition for therapeutic movement. But let us leave further speculation along these lines to our book on hypnoanalytic techniques and return to a consideration of procedures for measuring and altering hypnotic depth.

Measuring Trance Depth

The depth of the state can be inferred by testing the individual's ability to execute various phenomena (using, for example, J. Watkins's scale, 1949); this involves interrupting the deepening procedure. A more subjective approach can be tried using an informal number scale whose coordinates have been set by the therapist. This can be especially valuable when a patient has been once hypnotized and we want to know whether he or she is as deeply involved as during the previous session, is less deeply so, or has achieved an even deeper state. The individual may be instructed as follows:

> Let us use the number 0 to represent your state of mind when you are unhypnotized, completely alert and not hypnotically involved at all. Levels 1 and 2 indicate a light hypnotic relaxation. Let 10 represent the deepest stage you have ever achieved in hypnosis. Now tell me, what number would represent your present level of involvement?

Perhaps the individual says "7." One can then continue the deepening procedure if desired to get the patient at least to the same depth as he or she was previously. As one works further with that patient, he or she might sink into new levels of depth and report that he or she is now at levels 12, 15, and so on. Such a scale, of course, is not validated; it is subjective, and it varies with every individual. However, it does provide a useful yardstick to the therapist in estimating just where his or her patient is during the induction-deepening procedure. It seems to have an internal validity to the patient.

Deepening Techniques

Hypnotic movement often deepens the state. By that we mean that each hypnotic suggestion that is carried through intensifies the individual's involvement in the process, which is a good rationale for putting the negative visual hallucination test item of the SHSS:C at the end of a number of progressivly more difficult items. On the other hand, hypnotic suggestions that are administered but not executed by the patient may have the effect of lightening or, in rare instances, terminating trance. It is important, therefore, that suggestions be timed and proceed in a systematic way from the simple to the more complex. One does not suggest a posthypnotic hallucination before one has achieved such easier responses as eye closure or arm drop. As in many other life situations, nothing succeeds like success. When one moves through a hierarchy of suggestions ranging from simple movements to complex alterations of perception and thought, the state of hypnosis progressively deepens. Each suggestion successfully executed makes easier the accomplishment of the next one. Weitzenhoffer (1953) termed this phenomenon "homoaction." Therefore, as long as we continue to administer suggestions, especially of a difficulty and complexity that increase by small degrees, we will be deepening the state.

Fractionation

The principle of deepening through hypnotic movement was termed "fractionation" more than 100 years ago (Vogt, 1896). In its simplest form, the individual is hypnotized, awakened, rehypnotized, reawakened, and so on. As the movement in and out of trance is continued, the individual tends to sink deeper and deeper into involvement in the hypnotic state.

A more systematic use of this principle that can be used after an initial induction is as follows:

> When I say an odd number, such as 1, let yourself relax more deeply. Go down into a more profound state. However, when I say an even number, such as 2, alert yourself slightly. Let yourself come up a little. But then as soon as I say the next odd number, 3, go down even deeper than before. Go down and down and continue to relax more profoundly until I say the next even number, 4. [Continue this way.] Go down on 5. Then up a bit on 6. Down again further on 7. And up, 8. Down, 9. Up, 10.

At this point, emphasize the word "down" strongly and wait a few seconds after each "down" suggestion. Speak "Up, 10" much more lightly and go almost immediately to "Down, 11." Now continue as follows: "12-13," "14-15," "16-17," "18-19," and so on. The even number is spoken lightly and rapidly, and the odd number is articulated almost immediately afterward, drawled out, and there is a pause after speaking it before going to the next pair, "20-21." This procedure can be continued as long as it is felt desirable to deepen the state further. The technique can function by engaging and distracting conscious processes, thus effectively preventing conscious interference with the establishment of trance.

The Summer Day (A Freedom From Distraction Scene)

Inducing the participant to visualize a very pleasant, relaxing scene is often effective in achieving greater hypnotic depth. The following is one typical example of this approach:

> Just imagine that it is a warm summer afternoon and you are lying on a green, grassy slope on a hillside miles away from where any-

body or anything could disturb you. It is extremely peaceful. The grass is very soft and thick. There are a few trees in the distance but the landscape is like a meadow, covered with thick, green grass and a few wildflowers. It is quiet and the sky overhead is a deep, rich blue with only a few soft, fluffy clouds floating in it. The sun is beating down, and you feel so peaceful, so relaxed, so safe, and so comfortable that you are allowing yourself to drowse more and more. It is as if the only thought you have is one that goes 'round and 'round in your head and says, "deeper relax, deeper relax, deeper relax."

The therapist may continue to describe this scene as the patient becomes increasingly involved in the pleasurable fantasy.

Progressive Warm, Heavy Feeling Procedure

Another deepening technique can be added to this summer scene if the therapist wishes, as follows:

There is a warm, numb feeling beginning to form in your forehead just above the eyes. Now it starts to spread over the top of your head, into your face, and all through your head. Your head feels warm and heavy. This is like a numb wave of warmness that is sweeping down through your body. It brings the most pleasant sensation of heaviness and relaxation. Now it moves down through your neck, and your neck becomes heavy. You make it heavy. Heavy, heavy, heavy. This warm, numb, heavy feeling now goes through your shoulders and down into your arms and hands. They feel like the limbs on the trunk of a tree. And now this warm, heavy feeling moves into the trunk of your body, down through your chest and your abdomen, and the trunk of your body feels warm and heavy. This feeling now drifts down into your legs, your thighs, the calves of your legs and into your feet, and they, too, feel warm and numb and heavy.

This pattern may be repeated several times. Some therapists prefer to have the warm, numb, heavy feeling or a relaxed feeling start in the patient's feet and move up the body. The patient's report of the way that causes him or her to respond best should be the one of choice after it has been tried.

Descending-Stairs Technique

This procedure combines visualization with implicit motor movement. It also brings in tactile and kinesthetic imagination and the concept of going "down," and it is open ended in the sense that it can be continued as long as necessary. The verbalization might go somewhat as follows:

> Imagine that you and I are standing at the top of a staircase looking down. The steps are covered with a soft, plush carpet of your favorite color. [Note opportunity for choice by the patient.] As you look farther down, the stairs seem to fade out into a soft, warm darkness. We will walk down these stairs as you slide your hand along the smooth, hardwood bannister. I will walk with you and count steps. Each count is another step down the soft, plush, carpeted stairs. Here we go, stepping down, 1, 2, 3, 4, 5, 6, 7, 8, 9, 10. Warm, heavy feelings spread over your entire body as your feet sink into the soft carpet, and the gentle darkness floats around you more and more with each step. Let us walk down more stairs together, plush, carpeted stairs as you slide your hand along the smooth bannister, 11, 12, 13, 14, 15, 16, 17, 18, 19, 20.

This deepening process is open ended, and the therapist can continue to count the descending stairs with a reinforcing repetition of the image of the plush carpet, the smooth hardwood banister, and the dimming of the light about every 10 steps.

Descending-Escalator Technique With or Without Timed Breathing

This version of the technique is from A. Barabasz (1977, pp. 168–169). The procedure is intended to reduce the implicit motor movement of the previous procedure in favor of kinesthetic imagination, where the concept of going down becomes involuntary or automatic. For some patients it is perceived as easier and safer, as footing security is not an issue. This technique may involve the timed-breathing technique described in the next induction.

The wording is as follows:

> Simply let yourself relax to the very best of your ability, easing up all over now [pause]. Relaxing further and further all the time, I want you to take note of your breathing, listening only to the sound of my voice now, just notice that as you exhale, you become more comfortably relaxed [pause]. Each time you exhale, your whole body can become more and more deeply relaxed, calm, and serene. Easing up and relaxing, appreciating the deeper and deeper waves of relaxation [pause]. Relaxing more and more comfortably heavy, comfortably warm and heavy. A good relaxed feeling as your whole body eases up all over [pause].

Now, to help you go even deeper into relaxation, even further, I want you to picture yourself standing at the top of a long, long escalator, just watching the steps move down slowly in front of you [pause]. While you watch the steps move downward, notice that each time you breathe out, each time you exhale, you become automatically more relaxed. More and more deeply relaxed. Relaxing now as you watch the escalator stairs go down, down, down [pause]. As you watch the stairs go down, you go down deeper and deeper into relaxation, further and further. Now, imagine yourself grasping the handrails of the escalator safely and securely, you step on the first stair [pause], and now you actually go down the escalator. As you go down the escalator, it becomes easier and easier to go more deeply into relaxation. Going deeper and deeper all the time now, as you continue to ride the escalator down further and further and further [pause]. A good calm serene feeling as you go still further [pause] to deeper and deeper levels of relaxation automatically. Going with the relaxation freely and gently, just easing up all over more and more [pause], deeper and deeper levels of calm as you continue to ride the escalator down.

Now, while you continue to picture yourself riding down the escalator, safely and securely, I am going to help you achieve an even deeper calm, a deeper level of relaxation [pause]. Becoming more and more relaxed each time you breathe out, I am going to count from 1 to 3 and on the count of 3 I want you to simply let your muscles switch off completely, thereby doubling your present state of relaxation [pause]. One [pause], 2 [pause], and 3. [The following should be stated more firmly and confidently, but a warm empathic nonauthoritarian tone should be maintained.] Doubly down now, doubly relaxed down even further now and further [pause]. It's easier and easier to become more and more fully relaxed, calm and serene, more and more totally at ease. A good, comfortable heavy feeling as you go all the way down now, all the way, a good, comfortably warm, relaxed feeling.

Notice the many factors involved in this fantasy that facilitate the deepening process. First, there is a relationship between the therapist and participant ("you and I" standing and walking down together). Next, there is the soft plush carpet that permits the participant to choose his or her favorite color. The motor concept of "stepping down" by analogy suggests "going down" into a deeper hypnotic state. The increasing darkness also implies a progressive reduction of external stimuli. Repetition and monotony add to the deepening effect.

Variations of these approaches involve having the individual go down an elevator in a large building or down a mineshaft as the light above fades out. Sometimes an individual shows fear or resistance to going down stairs. Perhaps at a tender age, he or she fell down the cellar steps. In one case I (A.F.B.) was preparing the patient for hypnotically assisted systematic desensitization and had her instrumented with skin conductance, heart rate, and pulse transducers (refer to them as "sensors" when in the presence of the patient) on my polygraph. As the escalator instructions continued the patient appeared outwardly calm. Then the polygraph pens nearly came off the graph paper, indicating a severe arousal of anxiety. Yet the patient continued to appear outwardly calm. I inquired, "Part of you seems distressed?" and then paused. She explained about once getting her high-heeled shoe caught in an escalator stair, which precipitated a broken leg. She said nothing during the induction because she "wanted to cooperate" and felt "I knew best." The point is, when you have doubts about a patient's reactions, simply ask the patient in an open-ended manner. In such cases the same deepening effect can be secured by having him or her walk up stairs into an increasing light until "floating on a cloud."

Timed-Breathing Technique

This technique can be employed in the initial phase of the descending-escalator technique or used on its own. Observe the normal breathing of the patient and say, "With each breath you will be more calm, deeper and deeper." Then repeat "Deeper calm, Deeper calm, Deeper calm" over and over, timing it with every exhalation. This can be continued for several minutes. It is essential to emphasize normal rather than deep breathing. Continued deep breathing blows off too much carbon dioxide and can produce hyperventilation. Hyperventilation can rapidly produce numbness of the fingers, loss of control over breathing volition, and epileptiform seizures in persons susceptible to seizures.

The Metronome

The same timing method can be employed using a metronome, obtainable at stores specializing in the sale of musical instruments. Set its speed at about 60 beats to the minute and then say to the participant, "As you hear this ticking [or beeping] sound you will relax deeper and deeper. It is as if the ticking were saying to you 'Deeper relax. Deeper calm. Deeper relax. Deeper calm.'" Time your remarks so that "deeper" and "relax" or "calm" each coincide with a tick. Repeat your "deeper relax" 10 or more times in synchronization with the metronome. Then inform the patient to continue to think "deeper relax" or "deeper calm" with each tick in order to sink into a deeper and deeper state. No more need be said. The patient can be left, preferably relaxing on a couch, listening to the metronome for up to 30 minutes or more at a time.

The ticking of some metronomes may be quite loud and act as a distraction to deep relaxation. In this case, place the metronome as far away from the patient as needed within the confines of the office. On occasion, we have found that the patient regresses into a normal sleep instead of a hypnotic state after listening to the metronome for a long time. Although suggestions can sometimes be given during normal sleep to turn it into hypnosis, it is preferable to awaken the patient and begin the induction again.

Floating in a Cloud

Ask the patient to imagine that he or she is floating in a soft, fluffy cloud. Feeling the soft cloud, wrapped all around like a fleecy blanket, often deepens the state by encouraging a regression to infantile fantasies.

Revolving in the Cloud

An extension of the floating in a cloud technique can sometimes be used. This technique involves manipulation of the kinesthetic and vestibular sensations. It might go as follows:

> You are now floating in this soft cloud miles above the earth. You can see the tiny houses and people way below you, and you feel a great sense of strength and peace. It seems now as if you are revolving around and around in that cloud so that first you see the earth below you. Then you are rotating backward so that it is now behind you. Now you are turning so that it is above you. Now, it is in front of you. And you continue floating over backward, around and around. And the earth continues to change as it is below you, behind you, above you, in front of you. Below. Behind. Above. In front. Around and around.

This narration can be kept up for some time as individuals feels themselves rotating around and around as oriented by the place of the earth far below.

Revolving-Wheels Fantasy

A number of patients react to this induction by entering a most profound state, as follows:

You are in the country lying on a grassy slope. You notice in front of you a large old-fashioned wagon wheel. It is so close and so large that it almost fills your field of vision. As you stare at it, you are very aware of the huge hub, the thick oak spokes, and the iron rim around the outside edge. If you look closely at this iron rim, you will notice that there are points of light imbedded in it as if they were tiny light bulbs. In fact, there are seven such points of light evenly spaced around the rim of the wheel. Look at each one of them. The first. The second. The third. The fourth. The fifth. The sixth. And the seventh. Now focus your eyes on that seventh tiny point of light on the rim of the wheel. As you stare at it, the wheel begins slowly to revolve. It is turning very slowly around and around and you are continuing to focus your eyes on that seventh point of light as it goes with the wheel around and around and around. It seems as if there is a voice also coming from the wheel that keeps saying over and over again, "deeper, deeper, deeper." And as the wheel turns and you follow that seventh point of light with your eyes, it goes around and around and around, and the voice keeps saying "deeper, deeper, deeper." Around and around and around. Deeper, deeper, deeper.

Now you begin to notice that the revolution of the wheel is gradually becoming more rapid. It is going around, and around and around, and the voice keeps saying "deeper, deeper, deeper." It is getting harder and harder to keep focusing on the seventh light on that spinning wheel that is going around and around and around with the voice saying "deeper, deeper, deeper!"

And now the spokes begin to blur because the wheel is spinning so fast around and around and around. And you can hardly keep focusing on the seventh point of light. In fact, it is now going so fast that all seven lights blend into a fiery ring of light around the outside rim of the wagon wheel that is spinning around and around and around. And the voice with it is saying "deeper, deeper, deeper."

And now it seems as if you are slowly retreating back from the wheel, or as if it were moving back and away from you, and you can see a second spinning wheel coming into the field of view. Now there are two spinning wheels with fiery rings of light around their rims, going around and around and around. And two voices saying, "deeper, deeper, deeper."

And the wheels are now getting smaller as they move away from you so that a third spinning wheel surrounded by a fiery ring of light comes into your field of view. There are now three spinning wheels going around and around and around and three voices saying, "deeper, deeper, deeper."

And still they move away from you so that a fourth, then a fifth, and then a sixth wheel comes into view. Six spinning wheels going around and around and around and a half dozen voices softly saying, "deeper, deeper, deeper."

As they move away from you even more wheels come into view, 7, 8, 9, 10, 11, 12 spinning fiery rings and a dozen voices very softly saying, "deeper, deeper, deeper."

And now they are moving so far away into space that it seems like a hundred tiny spinning wheels of light are going around and around and around, miles and miles from you and hundreds of tiny voices are softly whispering, "deeper, deeper, deeper, deeper, deeper."

And the tiny rings of light are slowly fading away, and the whispering voices are getting so soft you can hardly hear them as they say, "deeper, deeper, deeper, deeper." And finally, all the light is gone and all the voices are gone, and there is nothing left but a great soft warm darkness that fills the entire world, and you feel deeply at peace with the whole universe.

As this narration is being given to the patient, the voice of the therapist gradually changes. At first, while describing the wheel as it begins to turn, the therapist's voice is strong but slow. As more wheels appear, the rate of the therapist's speech and words per minute should gradually increase, "around and around and around." Then the therapist's voice softens, until at the end saying "deeper, deeper, deeper, deeper" very rapidly but very softly. Finally, the fantasy ends in a "soft warm darkness" much like the origins of our life in the womb. These techniques can often carry the patient into a profound hypnotic regression.

It should be noted that some individuals cannot respond at all to this fantasy. Others report that they were annoyed by the slow development of the fantasy. As always, check the patient's reactions to it after alerting is complete. A small but significant number of patients enter a state so deep that after about the third wheel they become completely amnesic to the later developments.

Miscellaneous Deepening Procedures

As you begin to resonate with your patient over many sessions, many other fantasies can come to light and can become more useful to the facilitation of deeper levels of hypnosis. Communicate comfortably and confidently with your patient. Simple scripted protocols are merely a doorway to deeper levels of hypnotic responding. Some patients are carried into a deep state by simply listening to their favorite music in hallucination. Others are affected by reading beautiful poetry in imagination or looking at great hallucinated paintings. Individuals tend to respond when the modality that is most natural to them — visual, auditory, kinesthetic, or motor — is tapped. The therapist learns to adapt the descriptions to the needs of each individual or patient. In general, hypnotic suggestions tend to build on one another. This is called "homoaction." The participant becomes increasingly involved in the hypnotic fantasy and gradually severs his or her perceptions from external reality or other internal preoccupations. The imagined becomes the real, and existence for the moment is within that strange state of consciousness that we call a hypnotic trance.[2]

Notes

1. Material discovered and brought to consciousness can represent happenings of an actual event. Hypnosis is not a truth serum.
2. It is almost impossible to establish a standardized set of induction and deepening techniques to be read by a research assistant (or from a recording) to each participant in a research group. Most experimentalists do not even try, which is why most experimental research in hypnosis does not involve deep hypnotic levels.

Chapter 8
Placebo, Hypnotic Suggestion, and the Hypnotherapist

Every good salesperson knows how to use suggestion. Members of the healing professions call it "placebo." Salespeople and therapists have much in common as both are trying to influence human behavior. In fact, suggestion or placebo may be the most frequent form of therapy ever used, if we consider its employment throughout all the ages of history, in every culture, civilized and primitive. As Kirsch (2002) noted, placebos are usually physically inert substances or medical procedures that are identical in appearance to an active pharmacological or medical procedure being tested. Placebos are used to determine the psychological effects of administering a particular treatment for a disorder. Placebo effects are the effects attributed to placebos.[1] Placebo effects operate within every type of therapeutic intervention. Even in psychoanalysis, the suggestive-placebo factor is operating concurrently with interpretations and insight. People often change their behavior, feelings, attitudes, and symptoms when told to by someone who holds a position of prestige and respect. Kirsch (2002) reminded us that it is difficult to extend placebo effects tests to psychotherapy because all of the effects of psychotherapy are due to the psychological properties of the the treatment, therefore "there is nothing to control for." At this point it is important to remember that hypnosis is not psychotherapy but rather a physiological state that can be induced or spontaneously experienced. Therefore, those effects that can be accounted for by placebo rather than hypnosis can, and should, be accounted for.

One of the major hurdles faced by drug companies in the quest to attain approval of a new medication by the Federal Drug Administation is to show, by experimentally controlled research, that the supposed effects of the drug are, in fact, greater than that of suggestion or placebo. Curiously, the majority of those in the healing profession, and even a substantial number of our colleagues involved in hypnosis research and practice, seem unaware that hypnosis has been subjected to stringent tests similar to those required of drug companies. Indeed, a substantial minority of our esteemed colleagues seem to go on merrily equating hypnosis with placebo. Like a drug meeting Federal Drug Administration approval, hypnosis has shown it can produce effects significanly greater than placebo.

Hypnosis and Hypnotic Suggestion Versus Suggestion or Placebo

The late Campbell Perry (2004) explained that response to placebo is probably the best index of suggestibility that can be found because any response to a pharmacologically inert substance must stem from its suggestive properties and the prestige or credibility of the person who prescribes it. Obviously, testing hypnosis against a placebo pill for responses to experimentally induced pain would be a stringent test for hypnosis effects indeed. Although dramatic demonstrations of the use of hypnosis as a substitute for anesthesia during major surgery without pain for the patient include thousands of cases over a long span of history (see, e.g., Esdaile, 1957; Marmer, 1959; Meares, 1961). In the foreword to Lillian Fredericks's (2001) book on hypnosis on surgery and anesthesiology, Dabney Ewin, MD, Tulane University professor of surgery and psychiatry highlighted Magaw's (1906) review of more than 14,000 consecutive anestheias at the Mayo Clinic using hypnosis in major surgery. However, controlled experimental research was yet to be done.

McGlashan, Evans, and Orne (1969) contrasted hypnotic analgesia in high- and low-hypnotizable individuals in both hypnosis and suggestion-placebo conditions. Only the high-hypnotizable individuals in deep hypnosis obtained significant pain relief. Furthermore, the high-hypnotizable individuals showed a small pain increase in the placebo condition. The point is, as Perry (2004) stated, "This study demonstrates, unequivocally, that hypnosis is something other than suggestibility; otherwise the high hypnotizables would have obtained pain relief from the placebo comparable to what they experienced in hypnosis."

This finding, apparently overlooked by those who still hold the unfounded belief that hypnosis can be equated with suggestion or placebo, was replicated by the social influence (sociocognitivist) proponent Nick

Spanos (Spanos, Perlini, & Robertson, 1989) even though the same hypothesis was tested in a very different manner.

The McGlashan et al. (1969) study remains unchallanged to this day. It is a classic example of stringent research design and participant selection using the *Stanford Hypnotic Susceptibility Scale*, Forms A and C (SHSS:A, SHSS:C, respectively), and two clinical ratings. Exhaustively careful controls were employed to ensure that the low-hypnotizable participants were provided with every legitimate and deceptive bases to expect hypnosis to relieve pain and persuasive social influence to ensure that the high- and low-hypnotizable participants expected that the placebo drug to be even more powerful than hypnosis. For example, as part of the social influence ruse to convince participants that the placebo was a strong drug, a physical examination was conducted and participants were not released from the drug condition until "free from all side effects." The placebo analgesia condition included providing participants with information about the phamacology of analgesia and the particular drug being used. Its virtues were extolled as superior to hypnotic analgesia. It was explained that the powerful drug was being used as a standard to measure the efficacy of hypnosis because it was much more stable, reproducible, and uniformly more effective than hypnosis in producing pain relief. Participants were told that the drug was a powerful new experimental analgesic still packed in Darvon capsules for convenience because it was not yet commercially available. The assistant who randomly scheduled the partipants to "Darvon" or "Placebo" conditions did not know that both sets of capsules contained placebo.

The hypnosis condition had to be equally plausible to the low-hypnotizable participants who had also met the study's criterion hypnotizability scores that rated at the very bottom of the *Stanford Hypnotic Susceptibility Scale*. Perry (2004) discussed his role in the preparation of the low-hypnotizable participants. Perry was given the task of persuading the non-hypnotizable participants to firmly believe that they could achieve pain relief with hypnosis. Cleverly, he administered an electric shock to their hands, and explained that it was the level of shock they would get after analgesic hypnosis. To persuade the low-hypnotizable participants to believe they could respond to hypnosis, Perry administered the shock, which was 50% less intense than the earlier shock, after the participants were exposed to deep relaxation hypnotic instructions. Much to Perry's dismay and wonderment, all but one of the low-hypnotizable participants (nonhypnotizable participants who had not the slightest movement of the arm in an arm-levitation test and who had low *Stanford Hypnotic Susceptibility Scale* scores) were thoroughly convinced they had finally been able to experience hypnosis.

The low-hypnotizable participants were socially influenced and highly motivated into expecting the hypnosis to achieve analgesia. There were many other very carefully implemented controls. Finally, participants were ready for the experiment, which showed unequivocally that hypnosis effects can only be wrought from hypnotizable people and that the effects are far greater than those obtainable with suggestion or placebo. The finding was tested again by Spanos et al. (1989) and fully supported.

When Suggestive Hypnotherapy Is Appropriate

In some psychological treatment approaches great efforts are made to eliminate or minimize the effect of suggestion. However, if our main goal is constructive change of our patient, therapeutic suggestion, within or outside the condition of hypnosis, is an appropriate tactic, providing it

1. eliminates symptoms or improves the patient's condition,
2. is successful in maintaining the therapeutic gains, and
3. is accomplished without the precipitation of some other equivalent or equally severe symptomatic substitution.

In many cases, it may be the treatment of choice because of its simplicity and rapidity, even though the same result could have been accomplished by other more complex psychological techniques.

Criticisms of Suggestive Hypnotherapy

There is a tendency, especially in psychoanalytic circles, to belittle the effect of hypnotic suggestion as superficial, accomplishing only temporary results and perhaps even harmful ones, and to maintain that anxiety or the formation of substitute symptoms can be expected as a consequence. These practitioners usually argue that only a resolution of the basic conflicts underlying a psychogenic disorder will achieve permanent and complete symptomatic relief. This position was stated by Sigmund Freud (1935) and his daughter Anna Freud (1946). The potential of suggestion to alter physical and psychological functioning is so strongly established that research on the efficacy of new therapeutic procedures—pharmacological or other—requires very sophisticated designs to rule out the suggestive factor as a significant ingredient.

There is little controversy regarding the direct effect of hypnotic suggestion on physiological functioning, except the disbelief held by many medical skeptics who believe that a purely psychological approach can influence such conditions as real pain, that pain is organically "caused" by a known lesion, or that physiological processes can be significantly altered by psychological intervention. The literature today showing the effect of psychological variables on physiological functioning is simply too tremendous to argue at this point. However, study is needed to determine those organic processes that are most responsive and those that are resistant to psychological intervention. What is most surprising is the tremendous lack of knowledge among nonpsychiatric physicians concerning the significant contribution to the therapeutics of organic medical problems that hypnotic suggestion can make.

The Personality of the Hypnotherapist

Hypnosis is an intensive doctor-patient relationship and an altered state of consciousness. The therapist's qualifications, experience, confidence, and prestige can help provide the patient with the security and trust required to enter the hypnotic state at a depth sufficient for psychotherapuetic change.

We have already discussed the comparative ease with which hypnosis can be induced in some individuals by hypnotherapists who have attained the experience leading to status in the field as compared with the results achieved by others who are not so respected. Unless the patient believes that the "doctor"[2] has knowledge and power, he or she will probably show little symptomatic change in response to the hypnotic suggestions, even though a significant degree of trance had been attained. Prestige, of course, may depend on many factors. Some practitioners feel that it is acquired by having a lavishly furnished waiting room or many diplomas on the walls, by a great reputation in the community, or by charging high fees. All these undoubtedly influence the patient's expectations of success and, hence, the probability of a positive therapeutic outcome.

Many years ago I (J.G.W.) received a call from a woman in a neighboring city stating that she had read my book on *Hypnotherapy of War Neuroses* (J. Watkins, 1949) and that she would be traveling to my community. She requested, in fact insisted on, an immediate appointment. Because I was engaged then only in part-time private practice, I was able to see her the next day.

She stormed into my consultation room and proceeded at once to describe a condition that she felt would be relieved by hypnotic suggestion. At the end of our session she whipped out her checkbook and demanded, "How much do I owe you?" Being relatively unsure of the efficacy of my treatment, but somewhat impressed by her obvious means, I mentioned a sum slightly larger than the usual fee but that was still relatively modest. She wrote out the check, handed it to me with utter disdain, and said, "Huh! I make more than that in 5 minutes." I seriously doubt that the suggestions I had given her had any significant benefit. Overcharging can impair a therapeutic relationship, just as undercharging can mar one's professional image.

Although such factors as fees, office furnishing, diplomas, and so forth do add to the image of the hypnotic practitioner, even more significant is an ability to resonate with the needs of the patient and empathically administer suggestions with an understanding of the patient's motivations. Expensive clothes, high fees, and a prestigious office location cannot take the place of sensitivity, psychological sophistication, and experience.

One of the most significant factors tending to increase the probability that hypnotic suggestions will be carried out is the confidence displayed by the doctor. The therapist who is hesitant and administers suggestions in a weak or vacillating voice will transmit this uncertainty to the patient. If the therapist does not believe in hypnotic procedures, he or she will probably instill doubt in the patients. The successful practitioner of hypnotherapy not only is convinced of the efficacy of clinical hypnosis but is also certain that he or she can succeed in inducing the hypnotic state and the hypnotic suggestions (or at least most of them) will be appropriately responded to by the patient.

At first, it is best to work with patients with substantial levels of hypnotic ability and accepting attitudes toward the modality. Obviously, the therapist must know that he or she is able to hypnotize. This does not mean the therapist does not recognize that with some individuals there will be failure, but it does imply that the therapist must not have an "I'm not sure I can do it" attitude. This belief in therapists is fatal to their success. One becomes a negative therapist on oneself, and by such a conviction covertly suggests failure. Hypnotic patients are especially sensitive at picking up the covert beliefs and attitudes of their doctors. Therefore, the trouble that beginning workers in the field often have is not one of failing to learn technique but one involving their own self-assurance. therapists who are skeptical of hypnosis as a true phenomenon will also be handicapped in their work. The therapist's underlying skeptical attribute is covertly (unconsciously in many cases) transmitted to the patient. Thus the therapist will have great difficulty inducing a true hypnotic state.

During a period when I (J.G.W.) was working in analysis, I had great difficulty in hypnotizing patients referred to me. My analytic "father" did not approve of hypnosis, and despite the excellent insights he helped me to work through and his skill as one of the recognized old masters of the field, he transmitted in subtle ways his disapproval of hypnosis—one that he had received when he was personally trained by Freud. As a result, during those years I found myself unable to treat successfully by hypnotherapy many of the referrals sent to me, even though at that time I had already written one book and a number of papers and had achieved some recognition in the area. Later, my interest in developing the field of hypnoanalysis by integrating analytic insights with my hypnotic experience enabled me to overcome this temporary inhibition and resume effective practice with hypnotherapy. All this is only to emphasize that if you find difficulty in your initial work with hypnotherapy the problem might lie in inadequate successful experience, which can be corrected by working with good patients under the supervision of an experienced hypnotherapist or by working to resolve such unconscious blocks that might be acting as countermotivation.

Not all practitioners find themselves suited to the practice of hypnotherapy. Occasionally we meet former students who tell us that they never felt adequate using hypnosis and that they did not now use it. However, they generally indicated that their training in the field increased their understanding of psychosomatic conditions, their respect for the doctor-patient relationship, and their recognition of the importance of unconscious processes in determining behavior and symptoms.

Sometimes further study in the area can correct earlier blocks. A psychiatrist who had taken one of my (J.G.W.) hypnotherapy workshops at her medical school came back to take a more extensive course I was offering at a different university some 12 years later. She reported that she seldom employed hypnosis after her initial contact with it, but after the later course, she began to use hypnotherapy frequently and successfully in her practice.

Similarly, a board-certified internist took one of my (A.F.B.) workshops in hypnosis and both of my graduate-level classes in hypnosis and therapy but still did not begin to enjoy the confidence she needed to incorporate it in her practice until she retook both classes. She now reports using hypnosis in her practice almost daily, but she still seems amazed about how well her patients respond.

The belief that hypnosis can in many cases be effective and permanent is essential for the practitioner who wants to employ the technique successfully. Freud stated that he gave up the use of hypnosis because he despaired of securing permanent cures through it. However, there is considerable evidence (Kline, 1958) that the real reason was that he was a poor therapist and that he did not relish the close interpersonal relationship between the good hypnotherapist and the patient. In fact, he stated that he put his patients on the couch because he did not like to face them and look them in the eye.

Psychoanalytic Objections to Hypnosis

The objections to hypnosis voiced by psychoanalysts include primarily the following:

1. The results are temporary.
2. The ego is bypassed. Hypnotic suggestions and insights received through hypnotic suggestion are not egotized and integrated.
3. The underlying dynamic causes of external symptoms (and of course here we are talking about psychogenically, not organically, caused symptoms) are not resolved. Soon the underlying conflicts initiate a return of the symptoms or of equivalent ones (Meldman, 1960).

Even though researchers have shown these objections to be invalid, the prestige of the early founder of psychoanalysis is such that analytic writers (Blanck & Blanck, 1974) continue to echo the same criticisms, apparently with no awareness of the research and literature to the contrary.

Psychodynamic Reasons That Hypnosis Treatment Can Be Permanently Successful

When dealing with the impact of direct suggestions on physical conditions, we need not be concerned with this controversy, but for the benefit of dynamically oriented psychiatrists and psychologists we must point out several analytically sound rationales about why symptom relief by hypnosis often is permanent, though not necessarily always so.

First, many psychogenically caused symptoms continue to plague individuals after the original conflict that initiated the problem is no longer present. This is because of their maintenance by secondary gain (reinforcements). Consider the case of a man who developed a hysterical limp because of repressed anger at his mother-in-law, whom he had to keep in his home. The offending person died, but the symptom continued because his sympathetic wife had been pampering him for many years: "I know you've had a hard day's work at the office, darling, and your leg's been giving you trouble. Just you sit down here in the easy chair and let me make your favorite drink." No wonder the limp continued. But the real psychological conflict that marked its inception was no longer present, and the power for its continuation was not very strong. His resentment at his mother-in-law had long ago dissipated. Accordingly, such patients can respond quite well to a session or two of hypnotherapy in which they sees that they no longer need to endure the symptom's inconvenience. For example, this man's realization of this will strengthen if, following his relinquishment, the affectionate concern of his wife for his welfare does not diminish. Undoubtedly, many patients have hysterically caused symptoms long after the psychodynamic justification for their existence is gone, simply because of the secondary reinforcements they receive. Hypnosis is the treatment of choice for such conditions.

Second, psychogenic symptoms, which still have some dynamic motivation for their maintenance, can be temporarily eliminated through hypnosis. They do not necessarily return, because the change brought about in the individual's life by the cessation of the symptoms initiates a new motivational system that keeps them suppressed. The world now reinforces the person's loss of the symptom.

Consider the case of the obese woman who developed an overeating habit because of her resentment at being neglected by her husband. Perhaps he became so involved in his job that he spent all his spare time away from home engaging in business activities. As his wife lost her figure, he became even less interested in her. Thus, she and her husband are caught up in a mutually destructive relationship. The more he stays away from her, the more she eats and gains weight. The fatter she becomes, the less he is attracted to her.

Now enters a practitioner who suggests that the woman lose weight with hypnosis. Reluctantly she tries it and soon finds that she can get along with lowered food intake. As she begins to regain an attractive figure, her husband develops a new interest in her: "Hey honey, you're looking swell. Why don't we go out for dinner tonight, and dance a little afterward?" Then the neighbors flock around: "Mary, you're looking wonderful these days. That new dress is stunning on you."

Why should she go back to overeating? She is now receiving attention, the lack of which motivated her neurotic eating behavior. If sufficient reinforcements from her world continue, the symptom is gone, and it does not return. Through hypnotic suggestion, she achieved a permanent change in her life. No insight was required.

Symptom suppression can be much more than temporary when the entire reinforcement structure is changed as a result. In such cases deep, psychoanalytic therapy, with "working through" aimed at insight, is an unnecessary and wasteful approach.

Third, if hypnosis is an intensive interpersonal relationship experience, then the patient will often introject the voice of the therapist. How many times have we internalized the admonitions, suggestions, and praise of a parent or some other significant figure in our life? It is as if happy individuals travel through their existence hearing unconsciously the praises and positive reinforcements of an introjected parent saying "Good boy" or "Good girl," "See what you can do," "You are very capable," or "I am proud of you," and so on.

In intensive relationship therapy, with or without hypnosis, the good therapist is often introjected. If the therapeutic experience was a significant one, the teachings, interpretations, and suggestions offered by the

212 • Hypnotherapeutic Techniques

important healer become permanently internalized within the patient. They continue to be "said" by the therapist introject within the patient long after treatment sessions with the real doctor have terminated. The suggestions are repeated covertly, and the patient's following of them is reinforced and strengthened. Such an inner dynamic structure can account for many of the innumerable cases where hypnotic suggestion has removed a psychogenic symptom; permanently for all purposes —confounding traditional psychoanalytic theory.

It is not maintained here that these three conditions operate all of the time. There are many psychologically caused problems that do not respond to simple hypnotic suggestions. There are many others that, as maintained by the psychoanalyst, are temporarily alleviated but not cured, and a few in which the removal actually precipitates an even more severe problem. But the flat insistence that hypnotic suggestion can have only temporary results is simply not true. There are too many cases that prove the opposite. The experience of many hypnotherapists is filled with such examples, and these have been frequently reported in the literature.

On the other hand, we cannot side with our cognitive-behavioral-minded colleagues who claim that the symptoms are the illness, that it is never necessary to analyze underlying dynamic reasons for their existence. The most reasonable position might be that many organically caused conditions can be constructively influenced by hypnosis, and that some psychogenic symptoms will respond favorably and permanently to hypnotic suggestion. Others might require more intensive and deep treatment by hypnoanalytic techniques. We reject the claims of those who cry "never" and of those who insist "always" as to the indications for symptomatic treatment. The real problem for the practitioner is to discriminate those conditions that can be handled through hypnosis—either by simple hypnotic suggestions or by the more sophisticated approaches we describe in this chapter—from those that require some analytic therapy involving insight and personality reorganization. Here, too, hypnosis can contribute, but through more complex methods than direct hypnotic suggestion.

Perhaps we can think of hypnosis as an intervention in the psychological equilibrium of an individual. Sometimes this can tip the scales in favor of constructive forces and initiate a benevolent cycle of favorable motivations and reinforcements. For many patients this can be sufficient.

Levels of Hypnotic Suggestion

Intervention can be approached at different levels. This is somewhat comparable to the situation in organic treatment where a symptom or harmful process is interrupted at different points. Thus, in the treatment of a

disorder the therapist might intervene with a variety of alternative therapeutic strategies.

Direct Attack on Symptoms

In hypnotherapy we can attack the symptom directly, aiming for its elimination or initially only for its partial alleviation. We can attempt to secure
an immediate (one session) response, or we can plant hypnotic suggestions aimed at a more gradual effect.

For example, during World War II, I (J.G.W.) treated a soldier who had
developed a hysterical limp. It was important to him to gradually relinquish this symptom, because to do so rapidly would imply that he had
never really been wounded. A damaged limb is supposed to take time to
heal. Accordingly, he was told, under hypnosis that his leg would improve
gradually, that he would note its improvement each day, and that within a
few weeks he would be fully recovered. In about 3 weeks, he relinquished
his cane, and by the time of his discharge, only the slightest impairment of
function could be noticed. He could return home and save face. He would
not be charged with malingering; he had suffered a real disability.

In this case a pseudorationale was employed, but to the patient it was
logical and made sense. An attempt to take the symptom away from him
immediately might have provoked severe resistance, resentment, perhaps
a refusal to come for further treatment, and even a relapse into a greater
disability.

At times, the potency of a psychological treatment like hypnosis can be
demonstrated by temporarily increasing instead of diminishing the severity of a symptom. A patient suffering from severe tension headaches complained, "My headache is real; just talking won't do any good." I (J.G.W.)
hypnotized him and give the suggestion that when he emerged from the
hypnotic state his headache would be twice as severe and would remain so
until I touched him on the shoulder. At that time the patient would return
to his normal level of discomfort. He emerged from trance and accusingly
said, "Your treatment has made me worse; my head hurts more than when
I came here." I replied, "Of course. I made it that way; see, now I will bring
it back to the condition it was in when you came into the office." I touched
his shoulder and he immediately noted the difference. I then told him,
"You see, this treatment is strong enough to influence your symptom. If it
is strong enough to make it worse, it can be strong enough to make it better." The patient was convinced of the potency of a talking therapy and
immediately became more responsive to hypnotic suggestions aimed at
alleviating his distress.

Indirect Effects Through Nonspecific Suggestions

Rather than working directly on a symptom, a therapist can direct the suggestions toward the general strength and well-being of the patient:

> You are beginning to feel much better. As you do, a sense of confidence starts to go all through you. You realize that your body is mobilizing to correct this condition. Each day you feel more confident that you will succeed in regaining your health.

Here the hypnotic suggestions are aimed at simply inducing patients to mobilize their own resources. Indirectly the therapist may be stimulating the patient's immunological systems and thus helping to increase antibody development, T cells, B cells, and helper and suppressor cells (Ruzyla-Smith, Barabasz, Barabasz, Warner, 1995) and to stimulate those physiological processes that operate to distinguish between patients with low morale and those who fight to overcome their illness or disability.

Ego Strengthening

Hypnosis can be employed to strengthen the ego. If individuals have strong egos they are either capable of repressing discordant elements in their personalities and maintaining the repression, or strong enough to confront them and resolve them through insight therapy. Either way, a strengthening of the ego can be beneficial. Accordingly, a therapist might tell patients in hypnosis, "You are developing a sense of inner vitality. Each day you realize that you are building a stronger and stronger personality. You notice how much more frequently you are successful in achieving your goals and what a feeling of adequacy you are beginning to develop. You are more and more convinced that you can reach your goals," and so on.

The Cumulative Effect of Hypnotic Suggestions

Hypnotic suggestions can have a cumulative effect, a principle frequently used in television commercials. As the public is well aware, commercials are repeated over and over again. It is through repetition that the public is taught to think exactly what the manufacturer wishes it to think. Thus, many might be able to recall, even today, what brand is related to "You've come a long way, baby" (a Virginia Slims slogan).

Another example of this type of repetition happened a few years ago with the musical jingle "What'll You Have?" Millions of people learned to respond with "Pabst Blue Ribbon." The thought of a particular brand was tied to the question that most bartenders ask a new customer. Similar suggestions can be tied together with great effect when using hypnosis.

Authoritative Versus Persuasive or Permissive Hypnotic Suggestions

The patient's confidence in the hypnotherapist is an essential ingredient in any approach. After the hypnotic state has been induced, the therapist can choose to use a very direct, authoritative manner: "When I place my hand on your shoulder the pain in your back will leave immediately, and when I count to 5 you will become alert and feel just fine."

On the other hand, the doctor may elect for a more persuasive or permissive approach, such as, "When I place my hand on your shoulder, the muscles in your back will [or can] begin to relax. You will [or can] feel a sense of warmth in them as you recognize that the blood circulation there is improving. This is because you can [you have the power to] release the tension that is causing the pain."

Suggestions Administered under Hypnosis and Posthypnotically

Sometimes it is desirable to remove a symptom while the patient is under hypnosis but defer its relinquishment for a while after the patient has returned to the normal state. This can be done to test whether the symptom can be influenced under hypnosis—a great deal, slightly, or not at all—and is especially indicated when the symptom may be psychogenic and serving some dynamic function. It is often surprising to note that when the therapist has removed the symptom by hypnosis but reinstated (by hypnotic suggestion) it before bringing the patient out of the trance state, the patient may give it up spontaneously within a comparatively short time. It seems that by demonstrating to the patient at a covert (subconscious) level that the symptom is no longer needed, he or she can arrive at this conclusion on a more conscious level. The patient then voluntarily eliminates the symptom and does not feel pressured prematurely by the doctor into doing so.

For many conditions, especially organically caused pain, therapists can choose to keep the symptom removed or alleviated after patients have emerged from the hypnotic state. Accordingly, if the symptom has been removed by hypnosis, therapists can tell patients before alerting them from the trance that "the change will continue after awakening." The subsequent length of time during which the symptom is gone (an hour, a day, a week, a month, etc.) tells us something about the severity of a patient's condition, and in the case of a neurotic disorder, it tells of the strength of underlying motivations for developing and maintaining the symptom.

Symptom Substitution

A technique that a therapist sometimes uses in treating neurotic disorders is to replace the patient's presenting complaint with a less disabling symptom. A concert pianist who has developed an occupational neurosis involving stiffening of the fingers may accept a transfer of this stiffness from the hand to the foot. The musician can still be administering self-punishment, if that is the dynamic reason for the condition, but the condition no longer prevents the pianist from earning a living. Although there are reports of the successful use of this technique, we much prefer to use approaches aimed at the resolution of the symptoms rather than their transfer or substitution.

Tying Suggestions Together for Smoking Cessation and Obesity

Perhaps the most elegant example of the tying-together technique is the H. Spiegel and D. Spiegel (1978–1987, pp. 210–219) intervention for smoking cessation. The technique ties together the obvious truths that smoking is a poison and that, to the extent smokers want to live, they cannot continue to poison their bodies. After the hypnotic state is induced, patients are told to concentrate on three critical points:

1. "For your body, smoking is a poison. You are composed of a number of components, the most important of which is your body. Smoking is not so much a poison for you as it is for your body specifically."
2. "You cannot live without your body. Your body is a precious physical plant through which you experience life."
3. "To the extent that you want to live, you owe your body respect and protection. This is your way of acknowledging the fragile, precious nature of your body and, at the same time, your way of seeing yourself as your body's keeper. You are, in truth, your body's keeper. When you make this commitment to respect your body, you have within you the power to have smoked your last cigarette."

The Spiegel and Spiegel procedure ties together the incompatibility of continued smoking with protecting one's body. It is clearly impossible for people to be protective of their bodies while smoking. The hypnotic suggestions tie together their purpose (protecting the precious physical plant that they need to live) with the recognition that smoking is a poison (destruction of the physical plant they need to live). As the Spiegels noted, the emphasis is on what the patients are *for* rather than what they are against.

In a study completed at the Harvard Medical School and Massachusetts General Hospital, researchers (A. Barabasz, Baer, Sheehan, & Barabasz,

1986) tested the Spiegels' approach with 307 clients who had failed to quit smoking with nonhypnotic procedures. All patients had lifelong smoking histories. Clinicians' experience level, contact time, and procedural thoroughness varied in six interventions of one to five sessions, and an additional intervention combined hypnosis with restricted environmental stimulation (REST). Hypnotizability was assessed using the *Stanford Hypnotic Clinical Scale*. The major results suggest positive treatment outcomes to be related to greater hypnotizability, greater ability to become absorbed, greater therapist experience level, greater procedural thoroughness, and longer client-therapist contact time. Consistent with our earlier discussions about experience with hypnosis, the least effective intervention (4% abstinence at 4-month follow-up) involved psychology and PhD interns using a single-session approach. Group and individual hypnosis using two to five sessions and highly experienced hypnosis psychologists and psychiatrists respectively yielded 36% abstinence at 10 months and 30% abstinence at 17 months. Using three to five sessions with the addition of 60 to 90 minutes of REST (reclining in a sound-attenuated, light-free chamber with low-level white noise) plus hypnosis and administration of the Spiegels' smoking cessation instructions yielded 47% abstinence at 19 months. The abstinence rate resulting from REST and the Spiegel hypnosis approach of three to five sessions was comparable to H. Watkins's (1976) five-session treatment that used hypnosis to tie together the urge to smoke with relaxation and coping with anger.

The Spiegel method also has successfully treated patients with obesity. A controlled experimental study (M. Barabasz & Spiegel, 1989) tested the effects of hypnosis for weight control. Researchers assessed hypnotizability by administering the SHSS:C. Forty-five participants who were 28% to 74% above optimum weight completed the study with therapists who were blind to the hypnotizability scores. Participants were exposed to a simple cognitive-behavioral self-management technique and to the H. Spiegel and D. Spiegel (1978–1987) hypnosis intervention, modified to include specific food aversion for each patient's declared problem food. For example, "Oreos are a poison to your body just as overeating is poison to your precious body." These participants lost significantly more weight at a 3-month follow-up than did participants exposed only to the self-management treatment. A significant correlation between weight loss and the *Stanford Hypnotic Susceptibility Scale* scores for the same group supported the specificity of hypnosis in the program. Participant attrition was about equal across all treatment groups, suggesting all treatments were perceived as active. The findings from this study were the most efficacious of the 20 experiments included in the Kirsch, Montgomery, and Sapirstein (1995) meta-analysis of hypnosis as an adjunct to cognitive-behavioral psychotherapy. Even by the most conservative estimate, Kirsch et al. explained that clients receiving the addition of hypnotherapy benefited more than at least 70% of clients receiving the same treatment without hypnosis. Given such findings in a widely cited award-winning meta-analysis, we raise the question as to whether it is even ethical practice to employ cognitive-behavioral therapy alone when hypnosis makes such a demonstrably dramatic positive difference.

Hypnosis as a Tactic within Insight Therapy

Although generally we prefer to aim at a personality reorganization of our patients by analytical treatment, hypnosis can often be useful in helping the individual through, for example, a period of sleeplessness. Or suggestion can be used as a tactic within a hypnoanalytic therapy. For example, a blocking of drinking or smoking behavior, which dams a patient's impulses, may temporarily increase drive for movement and process in the insight treatment. Resistances can be mobilized and thus brought to the fore where, through analysis, they can be resolved. We do not always resolve the symptom, but, by the hypnotic suggestions, we have activated the conflict that underlies it.

Finally, we should note that hypnotic suggestions can be directed against not only symptoms and behaviors but also attitudes, feelings, motivations, prejudices, or even relationships. The possibilities for their use are infinite and limited only by practitioners' conception of the structure and scope of the disorder with which they are confronted, plus their own ingenuity and skill in applying this potent tool. In the next chapters, we consider specific conditions that can be treated with hypnotic suggestion, and case examples that illustrate hypnotherapeutic technique.

Notes

1. Placebo response has long been considered a direct manifestation of an individual's suggestibility (Barber, 1969; Gliedman, Nash, Imber, Stone, & Frank, 1958; Kirsch & Lynn, 1999; Shapiro & Morris , 1978).
2. By "doctor" we refer to all qualified healing arts practitioners who employ hypnosis therapeutically whether or not they are physicians.

Chapter 9
Relieving Pain With Hypnosis

To see the smiling tranquil face of a patient after undergoing major surgery or other excruciatingly painful medical procedure with no anesthetic except the words of the hypnotherapist is an unforgettable experience. Then to witness a 6-year-old cancer patient, who had been taught self-hypnosis by her counselor, reassure her mother with the words "Mommy it's OK, I'm going off to play with Cleo [an imaginary friend]. I'll come home when the doctor's gone," is even more remarkable as the bone marrow aspiration procedure is then completed amidst the child's giggles of playfulness. These are but two awe-inspiring immersions into the domain of hypnotic trance phenomena (A. Barabasz, 2003a, 2003b).

The Experience of Pain

The Christian Bible teaches that because of Eve's transgression in eating the forbidden fruit, women shall bring forth children in pain. The acceptance of pain as a necessary burden may be the one common thread among most religions. For centuries, pain was regarded as an inescapable accompaniment to disease or damage to the body. Pain is an almost universal experience, one that people seek to avoid.

Two specific components of pain appear to have been identified; namely, sensory pain and suffering. Sensory pain provides needed information to the individual that something is wrong that requires treatment. More often than not, the pain indicates the site of the disturbance. All pain experiences include both of these components even though an individual may not discriminate between them unless questioned. Sensory pain provides the key cues as to the specific location and descriptors of the pain, such as *hot, burning, cold, aching, intermittent,* or *continuous.* It serves a protective purpose to the organism and should not be eliminated. People have been known to die because of the failure of their bodies to provide the warning of sensory pain.

Suffering is the affective component of pain; it describes how disturbing or bothersome the pain is to the patient. This component describes the overall impact and interpretation of suffering. The normal muscle soreness suffered by an individual after an intense resistance training workout such as weight lifting (caused by the production of hydroxypromoline and micro muscle tears) certainly hurts, but the lifter is not bothered by it in the same way as a similar pain produced by accidental injury. Similarly, the pain of childbirth of a welcome child produces hurt in the mother, but it frequently is without suffering. By contrast, competitive weight lifters who experience a macro tear of a muscle can experience enormous suffering because they will be substantially set back in their training efforts or may be put out of competition for an entire season, or both. Alternatively, the pain of cancer may not be intense but the suffering can be overwhelmingly frightening; it is the suffering, the affective component of pain, that leads to what can become immobilizing depression.

Dissociated Control, Covert Pain, and the Hidden Observer

The Hilgards (E. Hilgard & J. Hilgard, 1983) discovered that while direct suffering is related to overt, consciously experienced pain, there is also a component of pain that is covert. This pain is registered at unconscious levels. Thus, the experience of pain can be hypnotically suppressed in laboratory participants who have a hand placed in ice water. They reported feeling only numbness and held the hand in the solution long after they ordinarily would have removed it. However, their reactions to the following query are interesting: "Although you are hypnotically insensitive to pain, perhaps there is some part of you that is experiencing it. If there is, lift the index finger on your other hand." In many cases, the participant lifts the finger and communicates at hypnotic levels that he or she is "unconsciously" suffering. Ernest Hilgard termed this phenomenon the "hidden observer" and described it as a dissociated cognitive structural system. Accordingly, we must reckon with the fact that pain can be overt and covert. For specific analgesic purposes, we are concerned primarily with overt pain, and we judge our therapeutic efforts successful if we can alleviate it. However, it seems that the repression of some part of the pain into covert levels must involve effort and can have an effect indirectly on other functioning, even as unconscious motivations are known to play a significant role in the formation of neurotic symptoms.

The suppression of any stimulating source such as covert pain has its advantages and potentialities for influencing psychological equilibrium. Therefore, we consider it wise to inquire about possible disturbing thoughts and dreams through which suppressed or repressed stimuli can be manifested. Cheek (1962) suggested that information about the meaning of a pain can be obtained through the use of an unconscious finger-signal technique. Patients are asked questions about when and where the pain first became important to them. The questions are answered "yes," "no," "maybe," or "I don't wish to answer." These replies are transmitted in hypnosis back to the therapist by the patient's lifting of different fingers that have been conditioned to such responses. The finger-signal technique can also be employed to find out the patients' underlying reaction to various procedures or their predictions of possible outcomes. The technique has become known as ideomotor signaling and is frequently referred to in the literature and workshops on hypnosis training as such (Ewin, 2003).

Research summarized by the Hilgards (E. Hilgard & J. Hilgard, 1983) shows that the trance state seems to have little effect on the perception of pain. It is the suggestion administered in the hypnotic modality that determines that result. Therefore, the induction of hypnosis should be considered as only a preliminary and preparatory procedure to the skillful use of suggestive hypnotherapy. However, bear in mind that hypnotic response through hypnotic suggestion goes far beyond those responses that can be wrought by mere waking suggestibility.

On the other side of the question, Spanos and Chaves (1989) and Kirsch and Lynn (1995) believe that the operative variables in hypnotic pain relief are due to contextual cues in the social environment, expectancies, demand characteristics of the setting, or role-playing on the part of the participant or patient. However, these perceptions are based primarily on laboratory studies with healthy university students as participants and have not yet been shown to have applicability in anesthesiology or the outpatient treatment of pain.

Carefully controlled studies using participants (Orne, 1974) who are simulating hypnosis have clearly demonstrated that highly hypnotizable individuals were able to eliminate pain completely whereas participants who were asked to simulate or fake hypnosis with highly motivating instructions were not able to do so. Hypnotic suggestion also seems to be different from the placebo effect common in the administration of drugs.

In their classic experiment in the field, McGlashan, Evans, and Orne (1969) showed that those individuals high in hypnotizability show analgesia in response to hypnosis but not to placebo, and low-hypnotizable individuals show the same minimal response to hypnosis as they do to a placebo. Perry (2004) noted that this finding showed that participants obtained pain relief in the placebo suggestion condition that was comparable to what they experienced in hypnosis. The sociocognitivists completely replicated the study (Spanos, Perlini, & Robertson, 1989) even though the later investigation tested the hypothesis in a very different manner. In fact, the Hilgards (E. Hilgard & J. Hilgard, 1975, 1983) found that highly hypnotizable participants responded less well to placebos than did unhypnotizable participants, thus lending early support to the trance theories about hypnosis as an altered state of consciousness that are now widely accepted.

Although the reality of hypnotic analgesia seems quite firmly established among informed workers, one controversy on this point was, for several years, quite interesting. Sutcliffe (1961) demonstrated that the galvanic skin response (GSR) (an inaccurate measure of psychophysiological arousal; see A. Barabasz, 1977, pp. 130–131), which tends to decrease when people are experiencing pain, also decreased in hypnotized participants who were given suggestions of analgesia. An electrical shock stimulation involving a combined buzzer and shock was used. Even though the hypnotized participants denied that they felt pain, they showed an equal or greater change in GSR as did control participants who heard the buzzer but were given no shock. Sutcliffe argued that the analgesic participants were either misperceiving or misrepresenting their true feelings, because if the hypnotic analgesia truly relieved them from pain they should have shown less change of the GSR than the control participants. However, this apparent blow to hypnotic control of pain was disproved by Bowers and Van der Meulen (1972). They evaluated GSR responses and heart rate in a group of 7 dental patients whose caries were treated under hypnoanalgesia and compared them with a control group of 7 patients whose caries were treated under chemoanalgesia. The GSR changes produced by the hypnosis group were the same as those produced by the patients receiving chemoanalgesia.

More recently, the brain's reaction to hypnoanalgesia has at last been revealed by the work of David Spiegel and his associates. As in the studies from our lab (A. Barabasz, 2000; A. Barabasz et al., 1999), Spiegel showed that EEG event-related potentials in response to hypnosis to attenuate the pain stimulus clearly produces an attenuated brain response to the painful stimuli. Once again we have direct physiological evidence of the trance state of hypnosis (see Figure 9.1 and Figure 9.2).

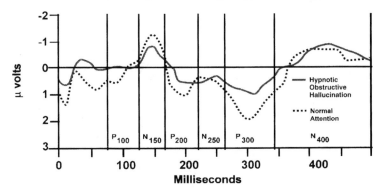

Fig. 9.1 This figure shows suppression of EEG event-related potentials in patients' responses to pain for a hypnotic obstructive hallucination compared with normal attention. From "Hypnotic Alteration of Somatosensory Perception," by D. Spiegel, P. Bierre, and J. Rootenberg, 1989, *American Journal of Psychiatry, 146*, pp. 749–754. With permission.

The point to remember is simply that pain is not interpreted as a danger to our overall health and well-being that does not cause suffering. The existential point of view interprets pain as what it means to sufferers in terms of their interaction with the outside world and believes this is what counts most (Frankl, 1963, p. 159).

The more pain has been investigated, the more complex the phenomenon appears. Melzack (1974) reviewed studies that have attempted to differentiate the qualitative and component aspects of pain and discovered 102 terms necessary to describe the different aspects of pain. They categorized these descriptive terms under three headings: sensory pain, which included such adjectives as *throbbing, pounding, pinching, cramping,* and so forth; affective, which included *fearful* and *terrifying;* and evaluative, which included *annoying, miserable,* and *unbearable.*

As an inner experience, pain can no longer be viewed as a simple reaction to a stress, disease, or tissue damage. Not only are there tremendous differences between individuals in their perception and tolerance of pain but the discomfort from a specific lesion can vary greatly from time to time depending on the interplay of various psychological factors. Motivation, attention, distraction, learned habits, perception, and interpersonal relationships all play roles that influence the perception of pain and its suffering.

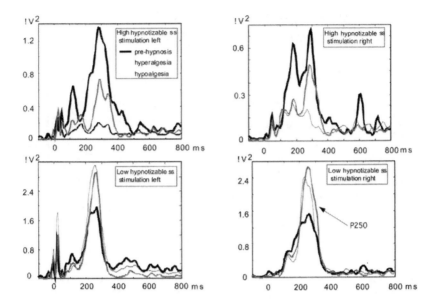

Fig. 9.2 These figures show the grand mean global power of event-related potentials under pre-hypnosis, hyperanalgesia, and hypnoanalgesia obtained at 129 electrode sites. Left panels show event-related potentials obtained with stimulation of the left hands; right panels pertain to the right hands; top panels show results of high-hypnotizable individuals; and bottom panels show results of low-hypnotizable individuals. From "Temporal Aspects of Hypnotic Processes," by W. Ray and V. De Pascalis, 2003, *International Journal of Clinical and Experimental Hypnosis, 51*, p. 159. With permission.

Morphine,[1] for example, does not knock out the sensory pain but considerably influences its suffering. However, it is the realm of suffering that shows the greatest variability, the least constructive value to humans, and the greatest opportunity for therapeutic intervention.

Useful Theories of Pain

The decision to use hypnosis in controlling a pain involves examining a number of considerations prior to applying any of the hypnotic techniques. Because pain can be referred from an originating site to another where it is apparently experienced, application of a specific hypnotic analgesia at the point where it hurts can result simply in its referral to another area. A more generalized approach may be required. This is especially true if the pain is serving a psychodynamic function; for example, the individual's need to be punished for some transgression, real or imagined. In such cases hypnosis directed at the pain site is not likely to solve the problem, except perhaps temporarily. The patient may require a more intensive and insightful kind of treatment that uses approaches we describe in our Volume II, *Hypnotherapeutic Techniques* and that is practiced by clinicians who are trained in hypnoanalytic psychotherapy or ego-state hypnotherapy, or both (Emmerson, 2003; J. Watkins & Watkins, 1997).

Consistent with the issues we discussed previously, but contrary to widespread belief, hypnosis is significantly more effective in relieving organically caused pains than those stemming from hysterical or other psychogenic sources that involve underlying needs in the patient.[2] Referral sources need to be educated in this regard. More important, the individual suffering from a severe organic pain is usually highly motivated to accept any promising treatment and consequently is often more amenable to hypnotherapy. Such patients are also much more compliant with the hypnotic protocol and have a far better record of mastery of self-hypnotic techniques for pain control.

At this point, however, we are concerned with procedures for alleviating pain by hypnotic suggestion rather than through some complex hypnoanalytic resolution of unconscious conflicts. If the patient is found to have such neurotic mechanisms such as underlying guilt, masochistic needs, and so forth, these psychological conditions may require treatment first before hypnotic suggestion can be effective. Our Volume II will describe techniques useful in this latter objective that can be employed by the more experienced psychotherapeutically sophisticated practitioner. Hypnosis for pain relief is, of course, contraindicated for psychotics with hallucinated pains.

Gate control theory. Although many theories have been proposed to account for pain, the widely accepted gate control theory proposed by Melzack and Wall (1965) accounts for the various aspects of pain, which makes it particularly useful as a guide to the use of hypnosis. According to this theory, pain stimuli are transmitted to the higher brain centers through two different sets of pathways called the sensory-discriminative system and the motivational-affective system. The first system is concerned with the location and severity of the pain. The second system transmits those impulses that involve suffering. These two systems appear to be anatomically verified. It is hypothesized that pain stimuli in the large and small fibers ascending the spinal cord pass through a gate control system. At this point, the impulses interact and serve to modulate stimuli transmitted to the motivational-affective and sensory-discriminative systems by certain transmission cells. It is thus possible through surgical, chemical, and psychological intervention at this point to interfere with stimulation of the sensory-discriminative system while permitting normal passage of the impulses through the motivational-affective system.

We are interested precisely in such an intervention. Thus either through chemo- or hypnoanalgesia we can alleviate suffering without impairing functioning or eliminating nature's protective signals. This is our hypnotherapeutic goal. Because we are concerned primarily with hypnotic techniques that can achieve that objective, we will not proceed further into the complexities and theories of pain. For the reader who wishes to learn more about theories of pain, we recommend reading books by Ernest Hilgard and Josephine Hilgard (1975) and Joseph Barber (1996), which represent thorough treatises on this topic as related to the use of hypnosis. The chapter devoted to pain in the classic H. Spiegel and D. Spiegel (1978–1987, pp. 251–262) book is also of great value.

Displacement of pain. As shown in Figures 9.1 and 9.2, considerable experimentally controlled data are now available to show that pain relief with hypnosis typically involves a gating of perceptions so that the pain stimuli are not recorded at the cerebral level with little more than a recognition of the stimulus. However, this does not mean that there may also be alternative pathways to explain the control of pain. J. Watkins and Watkins (1990) explained that multiple personality patients (dissociative identity disorder) can eliminate the pain in the overt personality by displacing it to underlying alters. Curiously, this phenomenon may first have been observed by Ernest Hilgard (E. Hilgard & J. Hilgard, 1983) in the discovery of a patient's ability to dissociate pain into a covert cognitive-structural system called a hidden observer. J. Watkins and Watkins conceptualized the hidden observer as the same phenomenon as ego states. Ego-state theory (J. Watkins & H. Watkins, 1997) assumes that human personality develops through integration and differentiation. At one end of the continuum, differentiation is adaptive. Ego states process relatively permeable boundaries as in normal moods. At the other end of the continuum, ego-state boundaries become less permeable or hardened. Normal differentiation becomes maladaptive dissociation, and multiple personalities (dissociative identity) disorders may therefore be created. In the intermediate range of the differentiation-dissociation continuum, covert ego states can be found in most normal individuals. Normal individuals, such as multiples and hidden observer participants, can displace (dissociate) pain into covert ego states. In such cases, the pain is not actually eliminated. It is simply displaced to another ego state, as would be the case with a dissociative identity disordered individual. As we know, dissociative identity disordered cases are characterized by high hypnotizability (Kluft, 1987), and, in fact, the disorder has been labeled as an instance of "spontaneous hypnosis" (Bliss, 1986).

Beahrs (1986) viewed the dissociative process in dissociative identity disordered personalities as a form of self-hypnosis intended to protect the patient from the pain and abuse he or she received as a child. In other words, when confronted by more pain, guilt, and rage then they can tolerate, abused children may dissociate this mental hazardous waste into personality alters created for the purpose of providing internal garbage cans. The notion is that the original and primary personality then no longer feels the misery. The mechanisms, when initially employed, were probably adaptive and helped the child cope with an overwhelmingly hostile social environment, but as dissociation in this more severe form developed, it became maladaptive and symptom causing. As observed in numerous clinical cases of those with dissociative identity disorder, the skill of dissociating pain, learned as a child, can easily continue to be practiced as an adult. For example, J. Watkins and H. Watkins (1990) described the case of Diana. The predominant alter in a dissociative identity disordered personality, which normally did not experience much pain, complained at a therapy session that she had a severe headache. John Watkins told her simply, "You know how to eliminate the pain, don't you? You have practiced this for many years." The patient responded, "Of course I do." Watkins said, "Well why don't you just go do that right now." Diana closed her eyes and in a few moments looked up and brightly volunteered, "OK, it doesn't hurt anymore now." Watkins then asked, "Is there anybody who knows about Diana's pain?" Mary, a misery-ridden child-personality alter, emerged shouting, "Damn you, my head just started to hurt." Watkins pointed out that for years, Mary had been receiving the pain and rage that Diana, the jolly primary state, did not want to experience. Session after session of therapy went by where Diana, with her easygoing smile and friendly manner, reported the good events of the day; if the events were bad, she never seemed to suffer from them. And then how many times later in the same session would Mary appear, often spontaneously — as is the case with dissociative identity disordered patients — enraged, crying, and suffering from these very same incidents. Since childhood, Diana had learned to dissociate her pain and anger by displacing them into other personality alters, primarily Mary. Mary was suicidal and homicidal, and John Watkins spent many worrisome days and nights concerned about whether she might emerge and kill her own (Diana's) children or herself.

It is my (A.F.B.) position that removing pain with hypnosis is normally a process of gating the pain perception as reflected by the EEG graphs appearing in Figures 9.1 and 9.2. Nonetheless, the work by J. Watkins and H. Watkins clearly shows us that the wise clinician should be aware of alternative pain-reducing mechanisms where the use of hypnosis may not mean the patient is getting away from the pain but is merely displacing it into underlying ego states. There it is stored, and the possibility of noxious sequelae can later return in some other undesirable form. Obviously, the clinician who is treating a patient in pain who might be dissociative identity disordered or borderline dissociative identity disordered should be extremely cautious. Clinicians should also be aware that normal individuals can at times displace pains to ego states. Furthermore, as J. Watkins and H. Watkins pointed out, the same questions about possible displacement must be raised when pain and suffering is seemingly alleviated by medications.

Dissociated-control theory. The late Ken Bowers (1992) advanced a dissociated-control theory of hypnosis that complements and extends the work of the Hilgards. Whereas Ernest Hilgard (1977) conceptualized dissociation as a way of repressing or suppressing cognitive processes from consciousness though perhaps amnesia, Bowers maintained that the brain's subsystems can be activated directly through the executive-control system. Contrary to sociocognitive role-playing explanations, carefully controlled research (Eastwood, Gaskovski, & Bowers, 1998; Hargadon, Bowers, & Woody, 1995) showed that consciously evoked pain strategies were not needed to produce a reduction in pain by hypnosis and that any strategies that might have been evoked were evoked effortlessly and automatically. As Patterson and Jensen (2003) discussed, these findings are entirely consistent with A. Barabasz (1982); A. Barabasz and Barabasz (1989); Freeman, Barabasz, Barabasz, and Warner (2000); Miller, Barabasz, and Barabasz (1991); and J. Smith, Barabasz, and Barabasz (1996).

Our focus here is the mind-body interaction with hypnosis as the facilitator. The patient learns hypnotic techniques to self-control pain. To ensure the pain relief effects are the greatest, the patient must recognize that he or she need not use hypnosis in all situations. Fredericks (2001, p. 51) said the patient should feel comfortable about deciding when it is appropriate to use such mastery over pain techniques. The patient should be allowed choice as to when to control pain, particularly pain associated with "exposure to psychological threat," and the removal of pain as a defensive reaction. The therapist should emphasize to the patient simply that he or she is capable of pain relief, control of the related psychological, and emotional concomitants. Fredericks also pointed out that the doctor should endeavor to remain disinvolved with the ethical and moral issues the patient might be concerned with as to when to use such powerful hypnotic techniques. Essentially the tactic is to use the behavioral technique of contracting with the patient to allow the patient to manipulate pain when he or she feels it is psychologically appropriate. This deepens the therapeutic alliance and can preclude the immediate need to resolve psychic conflicts.

Pain Relief: Simple Distraction or Dissociation

As discussed by J. Smith et al. (1996) in the *Journal of Counseling Psychology*, E. Hilgard's (1977, 1984, 1992) neodissociation theory explains that dissociation occurs when attention is focused. Activities are dissociated when "one of them goes on automatically, with little conscious effort, as the other is carried out with attention focused on it" (J. Hilgard & LeBaron, 1984, p. 4). The "executive ego" is the managing director of the attentional system, which simply means that it can time the system to meet environmental demands. Thus, the dissociation that occurs in hypnosis is partial and functional. The importance of imaginative involvement (A. Barabasz, 1982) in producing reality separate from, but in some sense concordant with typical reality orientation, is encompassed by the neodissociation conceptualization of hypnosis (J. Hilgard, 1974). Neodissociation theory (also see chapter 3) assumes total involvement of the person within an imaginative adventure; that is to say, the hypnotic state makes it possible for the person to let go of reality and to experience fantasy. It is important to understand that the reality-oriented ego is not disowned but downplayed to benefit from fantasy (E. Hilgard, 1977). The hypnotized individuals remain in control of the entire pain-control situation, able to leave hypnosis, reject any hypnotic suggestion, or substitute their own hypnotic self-suggestion.

Alternatively, Spanos and his colleagues conjectured that hypnosis, for pain control, is nothing more than simple distraction (Spanos, 1982; Spanos, Gwynn, Dellamalva & Bertrand, 1988). Spanos believed that anyone, hypnotizable or not, can reduce pain through simple distraction by doing anything with much effort by engaging in unrelated tasks (Spanos, 1982; Spanos et al., 1988).

Unfortunately, even the most sophisticated reviews of hypnosis for pain management frequently combine distraction and dissociation in treatment, making it impossible to ascertain which intervention accounts for the observed results. For example, Kohen and Olness (1993, p. 375) referred to the "distraction value" of certain hypnotic suggestions but noted that "a direct permission to ignore" the pain is dissociative. J. Hilgard and LeBaron (1984, p. 111) noted, "Distraction that compels attention away from the pain may be non-hypnotic or hypnotic," depending on the degree of fantasy involved.

Two experimentally controlled studies have been conducted to differentiate the effects of distraction compared with the effects produced by actual hypnosis. J. Smith et al. (1996) focused on pain control in an ethnically diverse sample of severely ill children just 3 to 8 years of age. The 36 children suffered blood disorders or cancers such as leukemia and solid tumors.

Acute invasive pain-producing medical procedures included, for example, bone marrow aspirations (physical restraint of the child can involve as many as six people to hold the child down as the skin is swabbed with alcohol and a large needle inserted through the bone). Children's parents were trained to use distraction and hypnosis to reduce pain and anxiety. (For details of both procedures, see chapter 10, titled "Hypnosis in Anesthesia and Surgery.") Several measures to reduce pain and anxiety were obtained from the children and their parents. Independent raters and nurses also judged the children's videotaped distress responses. Data were collected during painful medical procedures for baseline, distraction, and hypnosis conditions. The findings showed dissociation to be responsible for the greatest pain relief. Hypnotizable children (the majority of participants) showed dramatically lower pain, anxiety, and distress scores (frequently no distress reaction at all) in response to hypnosis in contrast to the low-hypnotizable children. Distraction, the method taught to hospital staff as the technique "that works," did produce significant positive effects for observer-rated distress but not for self-reported distress scores for the low-hypnotizable children.

Freeman et al. (2002) tested the effects of hypnosis versus distraction on pain control for adults in a very different manner than J. Smith et al. (1996). As recommended by A. Barabasz and M. Barabasz (1992), participants were exposed to rapport building, education about hypnosis, and repeated inductions. Ten high-hypnotizable participants and 10 low-hypnotizable participants were exposed to cold pressor pain (the arm and hand are immersed in circulating ice water while standardized pain reports are obtained) during balanced experimental conditions of waking relaxation, distraction, and hypnosis. To better discriminate between hypnosis and distraction, the researchers developed a new distraction procedure that involved the memorization of a sequence of colored lights. High-hypnotizable participants showed significantly greater pain relief in the hypnosis condition compared with both the control and distraction conditions. High-hypnotizable participants also demonstrated greater pain relief than the low-hypnotizable participants in response to hypnosis. Furthermore, quantitative EEG findings showed significantly greater high theta (5.5 Hz) activity for high-hypnotizable participants as compared with low-hypnotizable participants.

Both of these carefully controlled, yet very different studies, clearly failed to support the sociocognitive position exposing the false notion that pain control by distraction is the same as that produced by hypnotizable individuals in a deep hypnosis condition. Furthermore, both studies provided additional evidence suggesting that the mechanism of action for pain control with hypnosis is dissociative in nature.

Why Use Hypnosis for Pain?

Nobody wants to hurt, and pain interferes with healing, so it is no wonder that one of the most rewarding uses of hypnosis is its ability to influence the perception of pain. Hypnosis can make a substantial contribution to the disciplines of surgery and anesthesiology, because the control of pain remains one of man's most pressing problems. It engages much of the time and efforts of physicians, counselors, and psychologists who are treating patients for conditions in which pain is prominent. If only the pain problem of a patient could be quickly and easily solved, the effective application of many other procedures to the treatment of disease or disability would be greatly facilitated. Moreover, hypnosis can contribute to the management of many other aspects of surgical procedures, preoperatively, during the operation, and in the postoperative recovery period. Central to all of these benefits, however, is the ability of hypnosis to alleviate or eliminate pain. However, hypnosis should be thought of not as competing with chemical analgesics but rather as complementing their use when they are ill advised for the patient's treatment.

The use of various drugs, including alcoholic beverages, for the alleviation of pain had been practiced long before Morton discovered ether in 1846. This was about the time that the Scottish physician Esdaile (1957) reported on 345 major surgical procedures employing hypnosis as the sole anesthetic in India. E. Hilgard and J. Hilgard (1983) listed 15 different types of surgeries, discussed by numerous researchers, for which hypnosis was used as the sole anesthetic to completely ameliorate pain for procedures such as appendectomies, gastrostomies, tumor excisions, and hysterectomies. Rausch (1980) used self-hypnosis for a full cholecystectomy and then walked back to his room immediately without the slightest experience of pain. Patterson, Questad, and Boltwood (1987); Gilboa et al. (1990); and Finer and Nylen (1961) reported at length about the use of hypnosis as the sole anesthetic for patients with repeated extensive burn surgeries.

Numerous studies have described patients with a wide variety of problems who have responded to hypnosis, including those patients with pain associated with dental work (J. Barber, 1977; J. Barber & Mayer, 1977; Hartland, 1971), cancer (J. Hilgard & LeBaron, 1984; Sacerdote, 1972; D. Spiegel, 1997; D. Spiegel & Bloom, 1983), reflex sympathetic dystrophy (Gainer, 1992), acquired amputation (Chaves, 1986), childbirth (Haanen et al., 1991; McCarthy, 2001), spinal cord injury (Jensen & Barber, 2000), intractable pain (Lea, Ware, & Monroe, 1960), sickle cell anemia (Dinges et al., 1997), arthritis (Appel, 1992; Crasilneck, 1995), temporomandibular joint disorder (Crasilneck, 1995; Simon & Lewis, 2000), multiple sclerosis

(Dane, 1996; Sutcher, 1997), causalgias (Finer, 1982), lupus erythematosus (S. Smith & Balaban, 1983), postsurgical pain (Mauer, Burnett, Ouellette, Ironson, & Dandes, 1999), unanesthetized fracture reduction (Iserson, 1999), and mixed chronic pain (Evans, 1989; Jack, 1999). Other types of pain problems reported to respond to hypnotic analgesia include low back pain (Crasilneck, 1995), and headaches (Crasilneck, 1995; Spinhoven 1988). Even this long list of pain etiologies is by no means exhaustive. In short, hypnosis has been reported to be useful for nearly every clinical pain problem imaginable. It must be generally concluded that hypnosis is an effective analgesic in many types of cases and should be an integral part in any program of pain control. That goal, at least, is being achieved. Hypnosis is now the pain-control method of choice for interventional radiological procedures at Harvard Medical School's Beth Israel Deaconess Medical Center in Boston (Lang et al., 2000; Lang & Berbaum, 1997). Recoveries are faster, patients are more satisfied, and the hospital saves considerable sums of money while reducing risk exposure. Other hospitals are sure to follow the lead of the Harvard teaching hospital and the achievements of David Spiegel's group at Stanford Medical School.

Hypnotic Techniques for the Control of Pain

Hypnotic procedures used in alleviating pain can be classed under three major headings: direct hypnotic suggestion, altering the experience of pain, and directing attention away from pain.

Direct Hypnotic Suggestion

The first and simplest approach is for therapists to inform hypnotized individuals that they will no longer feel the pain. Here the authority of the doctors and their relationship with the patients is pitted against the pressure of the pain stimuli in an effort at suppression. At times, this is effective (Shepard, 2001), especially with highly hypnotizable people who have great faith in their doctors. In fact, by placing all their prestige against the pain, doctors are using a powerful interpersonal relationship tool, but this can also be a double-edged sword.

If the hypnotizability of the patient is weak or if the impact of the pain stimuli becomes overwhelming, not only can the pain return in force but also the credibility of the doctor is likely irrevocably jeopardized. Sometimes, when commanded to give up their symptoms, the patients give up the doctor instead. This is especially easy to do if the patient resents what appears to be an attempt at domination. A rebellious "child within" the patient is mobilized. The patient comes back to report (sometimes with ill-concealed pleasure), "Doctor, your treatment didn't work." This demanding, authoritative approach (which Sandor Ferenczi termed "father" hypnosis) can be indicated when there is a genuine emergency and temporary pain relief is a vital necessity (Shepard, 2001). This is also the time when this procedure is most likely to be successful. A patient in trauma might be near a state of spontaneous hypnotic trance or at least especially receptive to a rapid induction of hypnosis. Nonetheless, to succeed the therapist must be experienced enough to be absolutely confident in the execution of the induction.

It seems amazing how easy it often is for a therapist to successfully hypnotize and administer hypnotherapeutic suggestions to a patient whom the therapist has considerable respect or sometimes even affection for. The point is that the prerequisite rapport has been established. The same patient might have been relatively unhypnotizable by another less experienced practitioner, or at best achieved only a light trance or merely had some minor responsiveness to suggestion without having entered hypnosis. Although some patients appear to resist hypnosis, regardless of who attempts the induction, the situation can often be improved if the therapist follows the injunction — which is good in almost any type of therapy — "When in doubt work on the relationship." Rapport is the key element in any hypnotic intervention; resonance is even better.

If, as is so often the case, the pain is one that requires relief every few hours, we recommend two approaches. First, the therapist should make an audio recording of the entire induction and the hypnotic suggestions of pain alleviation, including the termination of the hypnosis at the end, which might involve counting backward from 10 to 1. As a guard against misuse of the recording by someone other than the patient for whom it is intended, the therapist should (a) placard the recording medium accordingly, and (b) use the patient's first name as appropriate throughout the recording. Then whenever the patient feels the need for relief from the pain, he or she simply plays the tape. Because the tape has been made by the therapist specifically for the patient, and the suggestions are timed to fit the patient's speed of response, the effect is to repeat the hypnotic experience with the doctor and to emerge with the same result, one that generally holds about the same length of time as the original.

Because part of the patients' experience of clinical hypnosis is their close interpersonal relationship with the doctor, it is possible that the effects of the unreinforced tape can wear off after a while. The effects can usually be renewed either by another face-to-face session with the therapist or by playing the tape in the therapist's presence. This effort reestablishes the relationship and potentiates the effectiveness of the hypnotic suggestions.

Self-Hypnosis

The second approach, which can be used when it is not possible for the therapist to come personally and administer another hypnosuggestive treatment, is to teach the patient auto- or self-hypnosis. (See the technique of self-hypnosis proposed by H. Watkins in chapter 6.) If an auto-hypnotic procedure is indicated, the doctor should use a similar approach during the initial induction of the patient. Thus, the technique of focusing the patient's eyes on the uplifted hand and suggesting that its heaviness will cause it to lower can be adapted equally well to an induction by the doctor and later as an auto-hypnotic technique. This technique simply teaches patients to say to themselves the same suggestions that the therapist would. One individual indicated that it was more effective for her if she visualized the doctor speaking the suggestions (induction, deepening, and therapeutic) to her and imagining herself as listening to them. This visualization seemed to reestablish the close interpersonal relationship she felt with him even when he was not present.

Visualization or imagining is a very effective method of presenting suggestions. That which can be pictured in the mind has more power than words do to affect behavior and experience for most people. After all, words are supposed to be stimulus cues to behavior, but if they do not have genuine meanings, they will probably have little effect. For example, Harding (1967) described a successful approach to the pain of migraine headaches. He used suggestions of visualization, such as "Migraine headaches are caused by the blood vessels in the head becoming excessively swollen. Now, picture the blood vessels in the head. See them large and swollen. Now picture them growing smaller and smaller, returning to normal, carrying the normal amount of blood to the brain." Images such as these seem to have more effect on autonomic processes than simple commands or instructions do.

Migraine headaches are considered to be caused by an excess of blood in the cranial blood vessels and their resulting distension. Another way (A. Barabasz, 1977) a therapist can use hypnosis to rapidly eliminate migraine headaches is to induce hypnosis and ask the patient to visualize ways of warming the extremities that appeal to the patient. This action redirects the patient's blood flow and creates peripheral vasodilatation. In so doing, the patient's blood volume is reduced in the head and the migraine is alleviated (also see A. Barabasz & McGeorge, 1978). This form of hypnosis is usually much more effective than merely telling the patients that their heads will not hurt. Certain patients, particularly those from British heritage might be more kinesthetic minded than visually oriented. If they are unable to visualize a vascular bed or a single blood vessel, they might get a better reaction from suggestions that stress feelings of warmth, comfort, tingling, relaxation, and so on. When the therapist is uncertain as to what sensory modality is most significant to a patient (visual, auditory, kinesthetic, gustatory, olfactory, or touch), suggestions that incorporate vivid impressions from several or all of these senses can be employed. Thus, when relaxing individuals, the therapist might ask them to picture a peaceful scene, see the clouds and the blue sky, hear the gentle murmur of a stream, feel the warm air on the skin, and smell the delicious scent of the wildflowers. The more vivid the suggestions and the more significant sensory modalities the patients employ, the more genuine they become to them and the more the patients can throw themselves into a meaningful, realistic experience.

Changing the Suffering and Meaning of Pain

The essential impact of hypnosis is to alter the suffering component of pain, not its presence; the patient's pain experience can be modified and made to feel different. We can tell the hypnotized patient that the discomfort in the arm will be sensed as a mild pressure. He or she will know it is there, but will not suffer from it. The patient can be informed that the dull ache in the back will be felt as a slight sensation of warmth. Such suggestions, given an adequate hypnotic trance state, probably disrupt normal physiological pain processes less than attempts to eliminate them do, as we can see from the research on recent brain response to hypnosis as shown in Figures 9.1 and 9.2. The brain's response shows an attenuation of response rather than obliteration of the sensation entirely. So far, the controlled experimental evidence shows us how the brain responds to hypnosis for pain relief, so at long last we now have a scientific method available to assess the relative effectiveness of different approaches while still not knowing precisely how hypnosis gets the brain to do this. One might reason that the complete suppression of pain impulses traveling through the nervous system requires a greater counterforce than allowing their expression in ways that are more acceptable. Furthermore, if there is an underlying dynamic reason why a patient needs to have pain, such as for self-punishment, the fact of its creation, and presence, might meet this need. For example, the body often turns unacceptable emotions into pain. Thus, the individual who cannot express rage at a spouse might instead experience some anginal (chest) pain. As soon as he or she can express the anger, the pain subsides. The suppressed rage on one hand initiates heart spasms, and on the other hand it is displaced into the consequent suffering. The patient does not experience anger; he or she feels pain. The displacement of its suffering component into a more benign form significantly reduces the patient's disability. By such procedures, we help individuals to live with their discomfort even though we may not be able to eliminate it.

Another method is to teach the patient to ignore the pain. Thus, we told a 50-year-old woman with breast cancer, "You need not pay attention to any uncomfortable feelings coming from below your shoulders. You will ignore them because you are so busy and interested in listening to good music, enjoying television, reading books, and conversing with friends." In this case, we were using distraction as a technique to lead the patient to dissociate the pain. However, as we know (Freeman et al., 2000; J. Smith et al., 1996) distraction by itself is a poor alternative to pain relief with actual hypnosis. The hypnotic evocation of dissociation is what makes it truly possible for the patient to not pay attention to the pain. When we dissociate a body part, to make it no longer a part of ourselves, we do not pay further attention to it and it no longer bothers us. Numbness can be hypnotically suggested in one area and then transferred ("permitted," or "requested" to "travel") to other areas where it is needed but that are less accessible. It is also best "imaged" when the hypnotic suggestions are tied to memories, such as "You can remember when the dentist injected Novocain into your tooth. Reexperience it now in relation to [the afflicted area]," that the patient desires to render insensitive. The numbness can often be made more effective if it is established as the opposite of the pain. Hence, the therapist tells the patient, "When you have numbness you feel nothing but numbness there."

Dissociative Interventions

Hypnotic dissociation is an extremely complex process that we do not entirely understand. In its extreme forms, it is seen in the multiple personality (dissociative identity disorder) cases where one part of the self may not even know of the existence of another part. We prefer to consider these part-person entities as "ego states," and they will be discussed in considerably more detail in Volume II (see also J. Watkins & Watkins, 1997). Amnesia represents another example of dissociation. Individuals do not remember experiences and behaviors that happened to them at another time. Perhaps normal forgetting is a dissociative process. However, when people are found in a strange city unable to recall their names, homes, or families, we recognize it as an abnormality and consider it a mental illness.

The hysterical paralysis of a part of the body so that it no longer functions within the individual's "body ego" is comparable to the dissociation of a part of one's experiential life so it is no longer a part of the "mental ego." The separation of some part of one's physical or psychological functioning so that it is no longer felt as within one's self — as "me" — is a fascinating study that can be initiated or undone effectively by the use of hypnosis. We consider its theoretical and technical manifestations at length later. However, for the moment let us accept the fact that dissociation of bodily and mental processes does exist, that it is possible to manipulate this phenomenon by hypnosis, and that, accordingly, we can effectively employ it for the treatment of various conditions, both psychological and physiological.

In a sense, we had already begun to use it when we told our patient to "ignore" unpleasant sensations coming from some part of the body. It is necessary to extend these hypnotic suggestions further. We might say to the patient,

> Your right arm is no longer a part of you. Your self stops here at your shoulder. The arm has no feeling or movement. You cannot move it, because it is no longer connected to you. You feel that there is a space between the end of your shoulder and the beginning of that arm. Therefore, there is no connection between it and yourself. Because it is no longer within your own being, it no longer has the power to send you painful impulses. It is dead and attached like a board to your shoulders. You experience no sensations coming from it.

We have temporarily dissociated the patient's arm from the rest of the body. Accordingly, any impulses coming from it will be ignored. Patients do not respond to them; they have no feeling in that arm and experience no pain there. Notice that during the hypnotic suggestions that were given (except for the initial reference) the arm was described as an "it," "that" arm, and so on, not "your" arm. We were attempting to make this limb an object, to remove it from subject, from self.

Not only can a part of the body be dissociated but the entire body can also be dissociated. Suggestions of dissociation can be as follows: "You are now standing by the door in your room looking at that body that looks like yours over there in the bed. It may be suffering in pain, but you are not because at the present time you and it are not the same." In chapter 11, we describe the use of this procedure for childbirth. The dissociative technique is one of the most dramatic procedures within the armamentarium of the hypnotherapist, and it usually requires a patient who is above average in hypnotizability. If this technique is to be maintained for some time, the therapist generally must give the suggestions for its initiation as the patient is quite deeply hypnotized. Dissociation in its pure sense is difficult for the individual who can enter only a very light trance.

Ego Strengthening and Pain Reduction

If one thinks of the human ego as a kind of mental muscle, an organ developed to aid them in adjusting to reality, then this ability to cope with distress is related to its strength. Individuals who become emotionally devastated at minor frustrations are considered psychologically to have a weak ego. Coping with pain is much like adjusting to any other of life's adversities. The strong individual can carry a greater load. If people are physically strong, they can lift a greater weight; if psychologically strong, they can lift a greater life burden. Accordingly, if we can strengthen a weak ego in pain-ridden patients, we can better teach them how to ignore the pain, dissociate it, suppress it, or endure it without suffering.

The use of hypnosis with suggestions specifically aimed at building the patient's ego began nearly 40 years ago with Hartland (1966). The procedure can be useful for a number of therapeutic goals, including the relief of pain. He suggested repetitively that the individual will feel more alert, more energetic, and physically stronger and fitter each day and will tire less easily. The therapist tells patients that they will become deeply interested in whatever they are doing, that the mind will become calmer, and that they can think more clearly. The therapist suggests to patients that they will be less easily disturbed, more relaxed, and imbued with greater confidence and that each day they will feel more optimistic.

Of course, the number of such positive hypnotic suggestions could be extended indefinitely. There is some question as to whether the ego is strengthened most by much repetition of a few suggestions or by a wide variety of suggestions. However, there is no doubt that many individuals respond quite favorably to such an approach and develop an improved outlook on life and increased motivation to cope with their problems. Hartland's approach to using hypnosis is not unlike Coue's (1923) approach: "Every day in every way I am getting better and better."

Summary

Hypnosis is widely recognized as a treatment for patients with conditions in which pain is prominent. Although hypnosis contributes to the management of many surgical procedures to alleviate or eliminate pain, hypnosis is best thought of as complementing rather than competing with chemical analgesics. Direct hypnotic suggestion procedures can be extremely effective in emergency procedures. Patients with long-term acute and chronic conditions can be taught self-hypnosis. Self-hypnotic procedures are most likely to be successful for pain relief if they are not used to shift the responsibility for the pain relief entirely to the patient. Recent brain activity research shows that hypnosis has direct effects at the sensory level, which attenuate pain perception. However, hypnosis has long demonstrated its value in altering the suffering and meaning of pain. Dissociative interventions can be extremely complex and are not entirely understood, but these techniques can be enormously effective in either alleviating or modifying a patient's pain. At the psychotherapeutic level, pain tolerance can also be substantially increased by ego-strengthening procedures.

Notes

1. Hypnoanalgesia appears to fade in effect at about the same rate as chemoanalgesia. A patient once treated by John G. Watkins was alternated between hypnoanalgesia and pain medication. In each case, she would remain pain free for about 3 hours.
2. In a recent experiment involving the hypnotic suppression of pain, a participant's hand was hypnotically anesthetized and then thrust into ice water, thus creating what is called "cold-pressor" pain. The participant was unmoved and reported having no feeling in his hand, but about a minute later he developed a violent stomachache.

Chapter 10
Hypnosis in Anesthesia and Surgery

A century ago, Dr. Alice Magaw used hypnosis for more than 14,000 painless surgeries, at the then not-so-famous Mayo Clinic, without a single anesthesia-related death. At the time, the death rate was 1 in 400 from the use of ether, even at the nation's best hospitals (Magaw, 1906).

Patient Orientation and Indications for Hypnosis

When patients first enter a hospital for major surgery, they are rapidly bereft of their defenses. They are interviewed by impersonal hospital personnel and then must sign consent forms and releases, which appear, even to the most casual observer, to allow the hospital personnel do almost anything without recourse from the now helpless patients. Then blood tests, venipunctures, enemas, x-rays, and other tests are frequently performed. No wonder that even the hardiest individual begins to feel a sense of insecurity, which can turn into fear, and in some patients, outright terror.

Anesthesiologists who are willing at this time to visit patients, introduce themselves, and give reassurance can have a significant effect on the equanimity with which patients face surgery and their post-surgical course. Mention of the recovery room will alert patients to the fact that when awakened, they will be in a different room from the one in which they departed from consciousness, and perhaps will be surrounded by other patients. This helps to prevent them from being startled by the new surroundings. The more details concerning the operative procedure that can be shared, the more likely the patients will be to cope with them. We can usually handle much better that which we understand.

The classic major indications for the use of hypnosis in anesthesiology were noted by Marmer (1959), an outstanding early authority in this area. These include (a) the ability to overcome anxiety and fear, (b) the provision of a more comfortable reaction from anesthesia and postoperative recovery, (c) the capacity to raise the pain threshold, and (d) the ability to induce anesthesia or analgesia.

New applications of hypnosis for surgery were developed and tested by Henry Bennett (1993), including (a) to reduce the amount of chemoanesthesia needed or to replace it entirely, (b) to reduce the amount of blood loss during surgery, (c) to return blood circulation to the surgically targeted area during the healing process, and (d) to increase speed of healing and recovery after surgery.

After induction of hypnosis, Bennett said to the patient, "We would like your help. It will be better for you and better for us. I would like to speak with you about becoming a more active participant in your anesthesia and your surgical repair." Of course, while under anesthesia, the patient is not expected to do anything consciously. He or she is asked to let the body respond involuntarily, "such as the way blood flows to your face and makes you blush when you're embarrassed." For example, spinal surgery patients, in hypnosis are simply told, "To make sure you will have very little blood loss in your surgery, it is important that the blood move away from the area of the spine and out to other parts of your body during the operation. Therefore, the blood will move away from your back during the operation. Then, after the operation, it will return to that area to bring nutrients and to heal your body quickly and completely." Hypnosis is simple to administer, even to those who are only moderately hypnotizable.

But does it work? To date, more than 100 such spinal-surgery patients at the University of California (Davis) Medical Center have gone though this hypnosis procedure. The patients using hypnosis lost an average of just 500 cubic centimeters of blood while the average loss by the control patients undergoing the standard medical procedure and the group taught deep relaxation techniques both lost the usual 900-plus cubic centimeters of blood. The patients exposed to the hypnosis protocol are happier and the providers save money.

The trauma of stress often makes a patient more hypnotizable. There is less of an attitude of criticality, which normally needs to be suspended for best results. Accordingly, hypnotic suggestions for relaxation, freedom from fear, and ability to sleep the night before the operation may be much more effective in helping patients to be at their best the morning of the surgery than a simple prescription of sedative medication. The less patients need to be medicated prior to surgery, the more likely that their postoperative recovery will be rapid. Furthermore, suggestions to the effect that patients will remain calm in the operating room and will feel comfortable there can do much to remove both initial fear and post-traumatization. Surgical patients have occasionally been so traumatized by their experience that a long-lasting anxiety, neurosis, or a phobia has been initiated, requiring an extended period of psychotherapy. The more relaxed and comfortable the surgical patient, the less likely that we will have a psychiatric patient later. The principle of mastery over a very significant experience determines whether it terminates in mature growth or leaves a frightened and ego-weakened individual. Both Marmer (1959) and Crasilneck and Hall (1985), who have had much experience with hypnoanesthesia, stressed this relationship factor in the reduction of presurgical tension.

Major surgical procedures can be performed with hypnoanesthesia alone. Many have been done, but unless the hypnotic treatment is supplemented with chemoanesthesia, the patient needs to be an excellent participant, capable of a deep trance, and one who has had adequate training before the surgery begins. Only about 10% of patients meet these criteria. The greatest value for hypnoanesthesia appears to be its integration with chemical anesthetics so that less medication than usual needs to be administered. When considered from this viewpoint, hypnosis is prepared to make a significant contribution to the majority of surgical procedures.

Hypnosis is, perhaps, the treatment of choice when the patient has a phobia of anesthesia, perhaps a carryover from a previous operation. In some cases, the patient is allergic to sedation medication and hypnosis is indicated. There are also poor surgical risks in which the chemoanesthesia alone poses a genuine hazard. In such cases hypnosis, more often than not, is the anesthesia of choice. Fredericks (2001, p. 94) noted that hypnosis is particularly effective and specifically indicated when inadequate spinal or epidural anesthesia is encountered where the patient is suffering a good deal of pain, or the area where the surgery has to be performed is exceedingly large and the amount of local anesthetic required would be too great and possibly toxic. Schultz-Stubner (1996) routinely used hypnosis instead of cerebral sedatives, especially for high-risk patients, because of the safety of hypnosis.

Patients should never be pressured into accepting hypnosis. However, if they prove to be highly hypnotizable they may well consent, providing they are assured that other anesthetic agents are available for immediate use should they feel the need for reinforcement of the hypnoanesthesia.

Wise anesthesiologists, even when working with highly hypnotizable patients, are prepared for any unforeseen eventuality that may require their full repertoire of procedures.

Medical Procedures Appropriate for Hypnosis

The range of medical procedures, which now have a history of success with hypnoanesthesia as the sole or principal anesthetic, is indeed broad (Gauld, 1988). Kelsey and Barrow (1958) reported using hypnosis successfully to maintain a pedicle graft when it was important for the patient to be "locked" in a fixed and immovable position for a long period of time. Marmer (1959) described specific cases involving laminectomy, thyroidectomy, vein ligation and stripping, rectovaginal repair, urinary bladder cystectomy, cholecystectomy, hernia repair, hemorrhoidectomy, hysterectomy, pneumonectomy, mitral commissurotomy, and cardiac poudrage, to mention but a few. In each of these cases, he indicated either that hypnoanesthesia was used alone, or, if in combination with drugs, the amounts and types of chemoanesthesia employed were dramatically lessened. He also described the specific surgical techniques and the postoperative courses involved. Elvira Lang's (Lang, Joyce, Spiegel, Hamilton, & Lee, 1996) unit at Harvard's Beth Israel Deaconess Medical Center uses hypnosis as the standard anesthetic for a wide range of painful invasive procedures.

In cases requiring only local anesthesia, the therapist can make hypnotic suggestions specific by touching or stroking the areas indicated. Thus, a therapist might say to the patient, "As I touch this area on your hand, it will become numb. It will feel as if covered by a leather glove. There will be no sensation of pain in it. You can ignore this hand while I work on it." Suggestions of this kind can by pyramided, that is, the patient can be told, "Each time I touch the hand, the feeling of numbness will increase."

A useful variation is to suggest that a piece of ice is being held on the area to be anesthetized. The feeling of coldness is built up through repeated and vivid picturizations. It can then be experienced by the patient as a hypnotic hallucination.

During the period of hypnotic induction, including the suggestions of anesthesia or analgesia undertaken by the anesthesiologist or by a clinical or counseling psychologist prior to the actual operation, the effectiveness of the hypnoanesthesia can be checked by clamps. My (A.F.B.) preference is to use a rubber-protected hemostat to demonstrate to the patient and the physician performing the procedure that pain has indeed been controlled with hypnosis. Tests of this type should be administered prior to the actual surgery, assuming that there has been adequate time for orientation of the patient beforehand.

In the treatment of burn patients (Ewin, 1986a, 1986b) two problems often arise for which hypnosis can provide a solution, including debridement of dead tissue and the changing of dressings. Both can be very painful, and it is not normally possible to spray the afflicted area with a chemical analgesic, because it is under the old dressing. Although sedation medication may be of help, a general anesthesia would be contraindicated. In such cases, patients can be taught to develop a glove anesthesia on one hand and then instructed to transfer this anesthesia to the afflicted area by pressing their anesthetized hand lightly over the area covered by the dressing. The anesthesia is transferred, and the dressing can be removed with minimal discomfort or none at all (Gilboa, Borenstein, Seidman, & Tsur, 1990; Patterson, Questad, & Boltwood, 1987).

Another common problem in the management of burn cases is that of anorexia. Here hypnosis is used to stimulate feelings of hunger and appetite. Images of delectable foods pictured by the hypnotized patient, combined with suggestions of desire to eat, can often work wonders with such cases. Of course, the same kind of hypnotic suggestions can be used in treating anorexia stemming from other reasons (M. Barabasz, 1996), so long as the hypnosis is carefully used as an adjunct to a comprehensive psychotherapeutic approach.

Milton Erickson (1967) described an approach for the management of pain in which patients are instructed in hypnosis to "compress" their pain experience into a very short and intense period. Thus, by suffering intensely for a minute or two, patients can then be pain-free for many hours. This approach appears to be promising, but no objective data as yet have been reported as to its efficacy in comparison with other techniques of altering pain. Obviously, this would make an excellent Ph.D. dissertation, series of laboratory experiments, or set of clinical trials.

John Watkins (1978) described a cancer case that initially was resistant to hypnosis. He was successful the next day in inducing a trance and relieving the pain after analyzing two of his own dreams, which were experienced on the night following the failure. These dreams pointed to his personal investment in being successful with this case, as a demonstration of the potency of hypnosis, in order to impress skeptical medical colleagues. Resolution of his own dreamed "ugliness" enabled him to establish a more resonant relationship with his patient the next day; a relationship she sensed as committed to her welfare for its own sake rather than an attempt at a "therapeutic trophy." This case illustrates the importance of a sound doctor-patient relationship as a prerequisite to success in hypnotherapy. As Kluft (2003) pointed out, the wise doctor treats the patient rather than the disease. Encounters with patients that tap unknown parts of their minds can be misperceived as a threat to their identity, function, stability, or even safety.

One of the greatest drawbacks for the use of hypnosis in surgery is the amount of time sometimes required to induce a deep enough level of trance. Esdaile often spent many hours with each patient before operating. Today, the amount of surgery being done, and the many demands upon the time of the anesthesiologist and surgeon, often precludes the expenditures of many hours in conditioning a patient, which may extend over a number of days. Patients frequently arrive in the hospital the evening before the surgery is scheduled, or even the morning of the surgery. There is time at best for brief visits from their doctors, and so much needs to be accomplished in so short a time. Furthermore, if the doctors involved must charge relative to the amount of time they spend with each case, the cost to the patient who will be given hypnoanesthesia can be prohibitive. Because so many good chemoanesthesias are now available, and the technical aspects of using them well-known to anesthesiologists, the more time-consuming psychological approaches to pain control, such as hypnosis, tend to be ignored. As is being demonstrated in the interventional radiology unit at Harvard Medical School, we are beginning to rethink the way we have been doing this in the past and finally developing ways of involving less costly adjunct medical and psychological staff to assist under supervision.

Despite the drawbacks, hypnosis makes a substantial contribution to surgery and anesthesiology in many cases, and in some, there are special indications, which prove it to be the anesthesia of choice, such as a danger of cardiac or respiratory decompensation. Knowledge of uses of hypnosis and its limitations should be part of the training of every surgeon and anesthesiologist. Personnel skilled in its application, typically a licensed clinical or counseling psychologist, should be available when needed. Hypnosis is not always the most convenient and effective anesthesia; it is definitely the safest and certainly one of the best ways to ensure involvement of the patient in his or her own treatment.

Hypnosis in Surgery: Psychological Factors

Surgery is an intervention into the physical body, which can alter its functioning in extremely complex ways. Less attention has been focused on the fact that it is also a psychologically traumatic experience. Normal mental and emotional functioning may be highly disturbed as a result of surgery or before it in anticipation of the feared event. If we view the human individual as a physiological-psychological-social system of equilibrium that functions as a whole, then tissue insult can precipitate a drastic reorganization of psychological functioning.

That patients often get depressed as a result of surgery is a well-observed fact. That the process can also operate in reverse is not nearly as well accepted and understood by physicians. Put succinctly, we are more cognizant that tissue insult can cause psychological disturbance than we are that psychological disturbance can initiate tissue damage. Recently, the role of emotional factors in the maintenance (and even initiation) of malignant processes has been rather clearly demonstrated through controlled research studies (see Achterberg, Simonton, & Simonton, 1976). Consequently, the effects on behavior and sensation of such procedures as lobotomies and neural blocks can be equally matched by the consequence of tension, stress, and emotional conflicts on bodily functions.

From this holistic viewpoint, the physical technique of performing a surgical operation plus the postoperative management represent only a part (albeit the most significant part) of the total impact on an individual. The wise surgeon and anesthesiologist will give much attention to the psychological factors within their patients, which can heavily influence the outcome of the procedure. If understood and mobilized, the patients' chances of a successful recovery are greatly enhanced. If ignored and badly handled, their postoperative course may be a rocky one. In some cases, these psychological factors will determine the difference between recovery and death.

We are concerned with the total psychological function of the patients — emotionally, perceptually and cognitively — as they approach the operation, during it, and in the postoperative reaction to it. Hypnosis is only one of many psychological interventions. However, it is a specific technique that can be employed for specific purposes before, during, and subsequent to surgery to facilitate management and can become an extremely potent therapeutic procedure to supplement and facilitate the surgical intervention. It is common for the physician who thinks primarily in physiological terms to underestimate the value of hypnosis.

Every surgeon has been confronted by the anxious, tense, fear-ridden patient who may relapse into an attitude of fatalistic resignation, become paralyzed with terror, or even refuse sound medical advice. Such a patient avoids a needed surgical procedure, sometimes at the cost of his or her life.

Preoperative apprehension is often a significant complication to postsurgical adjustment. Contrary to popular belief, the individual who manifests complete calm is not always the one who shows the best recovery. Many people achieve this apparent placidity by an excess of control and become postsurgically prone to the development of phobias and obsessions. More than 40 years ago, Janis (1958) discovered that there is an optimal level of anxiety. Individuals who exceeded it and those who were below it showed a less satisfactory postoperative adjustment. However, patients who had been informed about the anticipated experiences related to their operations were less likely to become angry or emotionally upset during the period of convalescence.

As an adjunct to providing such information and reassurance, the therapist can produce a tape that uses basic hypnotic relaxation accompanied by instructions given to the patient at hypnotic levels. A patient who listens to the recording during the preoperative period will be less tense on the day of the operation and usually demonstrate a more rapid recovery. There is much evidence to verify the fact that patients who approach their operations fear-ridden and with negative attitudes are poorer surgical risks than those who can relax, understand the nature of the surgery, and prepare for maximum cooperation. This initial fear can be significantly reduced if both the surgeon and anesthesiologist will give adequate reassurance to the patient prior to the operation. However, if hypnosis is to be used to assist in a surgical procedure on a patient who is undergoing psychotherapy, especially if it is intensive or analytic therapy, it would be wise to consult the treating psychotherapist. In some cases, hypnosis may be contraindicated for psychological reasons.

Fear-Ameliorating Techniques

Consider the initial contact of the patient on arriving at the hospital. He or she is often questioned in a nonempathic way about his or her residence, religion, ability to pay, and so forth, by an admissions interviewer. The patient begins to feel like an object, a "thing." The patient may be faced with the most fearful event of his or her life. Yet no one is considering the patient's emotional needs. At this stage, phobias about the surgical procedure and questions may well be brushed off by the contacting person, who more often than not is a representative of the business office rather than a member of the professional staff. The hapless patients find themselves in a strange, impersonal environment, surrounded by efficient people who nevertheless have little time to nurture. Friends and relatives may leave or be escorted out, and patients are free to believe the worst.

It is at this stage where a contact with the surgeon, however brief, can be of tremendous support. The surgeon who is not in too big a hurry to dismiss the patient's fears but is willing to allow them to be expressed will find that the anxiety level will lower, and the patient's preoccupation with them can be directed into constructive questions about the conduct of the forthcoming procedure. Our coping mechanisms can handle a known danger more effectively than an unknown one. Accordingly, the good surgeon will at this time, or at least before the operation, rehearse with the patient what will be done. Ideally, this should involve a step-by-step explanation of each stage of the procedure.

The patient is probably in a highly suggestible mood then. He or she will react with greater calm if the surgeon describes the procedures in a quiet but firm (confident) manner. This simultaneously informs the patient of what to expect and transmits the message that, "I know what I am doing. The operation will be conducted competently."

Wording can be very important. Thus, "discomfort" is not as alarming a term as "pain" or "hurt." "Separate" may not stimulate as much anxiety as "cut." While the surgeon is rehearsing the operation or thoughtfully explaining it in advance to the patient, he or she is also desensitizing the patient. The suggestions, which the surgeon implants in the patient at this time, may have a powerful effect, even without hypnosis.

This "rehearsal" of the surgical procedure can be accomplished better in hypnosis. The patient is hypnotized by one of the methods described in the previous chapters, and the various steps in the procedure reviewed. Hypnotic suggestions, using nontechnical language, can be given at this time. The hypnotic procedure is aimed not only at relaxing the patient and reducing tension but even more positively at minimizing bleeding, stimulating constructive attitudes, hope, and the will to recover. A wording of such hypnotic suggestions might go as follows after a reasonable level of hypnotic depth has been achieved:

> Now that you are deeply relaxed you find that you are calm and secure. You know your medical procedure will be skillfully conducted so you can make a rapid recovery. You understand what is to be done; there is no need for worry. The entire surgical staff is competent and prepared to handle every aspect of it. You know you are in good hands. You look forward to the correction of your medical problem and the improvement in your life. You are very strong inside and powerful. You can handle this situation well. You can let your surgeon, your anesthesiologist, and the entire surgical team perform their roles efficiently while you remain quiet and calm under the anesthesia. It is good to know that capable people are taking care of your welfare.

Such hypnotic suggestions can be administered by the surgeon, anesthesiologist, or by a consulting psychologist or psychiatrist skilled in hypnotic techniques. However, it is quite important that the patient meet his or her surgeon and the anesthesiologist face-to-face. The patient needs to know just who the significant people are, and in whose hands his or her body, and perhaps life, is now placed.

Reactions and questions voiced by the patient should be listened to carefully. The patient who states "I am afraid that I may die" is not being "neurotic." In fact, the concern is genuine. There is evidence that individuals who enter the operating room harboring such an attitude may indeed be far poorer surgical risks. Although it is not wise to argue with the patient, efforts should be made to change this belief. Whether this "belief" is a cause or an effect of inner destructive processes will be discussed in Volume II. It can operate like a self-suggestion. People who believe that they are going to die are indeed more likely to die. Incidentally, some practitioners (Cheek & LeCron, 1968) ask the patient in hypnosis what is the best time for his or her surgery. This is a question directed at the patient's unconscious processes. The reply may have substantial validity.

Individuals who have had their anxiety lowered by an explanation of the procedures to be done, reassurance, rehearsal, and positive suggestions aimed at improving attitudes (either in or out of hypnosis) will often require much less preoperative medication, thus enhancing the chances of recovery. There are times during surgery when it would be desirable to secure a response from the patient following some procedure, which under chemoanesthesia is seldom possible. It is almost always possible when hypnoanesthesia is the method employed.

Hypnotic Communication With the Patient

Ewin (2003) teaches the "ideomotor" method of communicating with patients to elicit replies from covert processes during surgery and other medical procedures. In hypnosis, it is suggested that when a question is asked, "the unconscious" will answer by lifting a finger on one hand to indicate its reply. Thus, a lifting of the forefinger might signify "yes," the middle finger "no," the little finger for "I am not certain," and the thumb for "I do not choose to answer." Ewin explained that it is possible to communicate in this way with a patient who can no longer verbalize. Cheek and LeCron (1968) reported that it has been used to secure responses from dying patients even after they appear to have slipped beyond the realm of communicating. Cheek and Ewin noted that through such a technique they have been able to elicit reactions from individuals regressed to preverbal levels in the earliest periods of their infancy. With this technique, the therapist can also ask the patient to "predict" his or her recovery date, which is often but not necessarily always true.

If the patient is hypnotized prior to surgery, suggestions can be given such as, "During the operation you will remain very quiet. It will not be necessary for you to move." This assists in providing the surgeon with a quiet field in which to work. Such suggestions also permit the patient to endure long and uncomfortable procedures in cases where a general anesthesia is contraindicated.

It has been assumed that under a general anesthesia, in which deep muscle relaxation is secured, the patient is also unable to hear and react to words spoken in his or her presence. However, researchers have found that patients who were subsequently hypnotized were often able to report much of what was said and done during their operation (Bennett, 1993, Cheek, 1964; Levinson, 1965; Pearson, 1961). Negative or unflattering remarks made by members of the surgical team were received and recorded at covert levels and had a decided impact on recovery (Ewin, 1990). Even though Trustman, Dubovsky, and Titley (1977) threw some doubt on these findings, doctors and nurses would be well advised to guard their tongues while operating. Remarks such as "I don't think this old tub of lard will make it" or "This one's sure circling the drain; probably won't last long no matter what we do today" can be devastating and have an effect similar to what might occur if the patient were hypnotized and then told, "We don't respect you very much and we expect you to die." In the high-surgical-risk case, such a remark could make the difference between recovery and death during the postoperative period.

If patients under anesthesia can react to negative suggestions, they can also be constructively influenced if the surgeon, anesthesiologist, or other professional take advantage of this period to make remarks emphasizing successful completion of the various stages of the operation and instilling suggestions aimed at enhancing postoperative recovery. This has clearly demonstrated its value when minor surgical procedures are performed with regional anesthesia complemented by the use of intravenous anesthesia or sedation combined with narcotics. Fredericks (2001) noted that "because of convenience and ease of administration, most surgeons use this technique almost routinely" (p. 94). Rather than "hypnosis," this technique is usually referred to as MAC (Monitored Anesthesia Care). Wolfe and Millet (1960) demonstrated the value of this procedure for surgery with full general anesthetics. Suggestions might go as follows:

> There, that's been taken care of. It should not bother you any more. When you wake up you will feel comfortable, just fine. You will be able to sleep soundly, pass water, breathe well, and cough if necessary. You need not feel nauseous.

Of course, the entire surgical team should be aware of the importance such suggestions may have when the patient is apparently completely anesthetized and be sympathetic to the possibilities of constructive psychological intervention at this time. Otherwise, these remarks will be received with derision by those doctors or nurses who are ignorant of the findings regarding their significance.

There should be no hesitation in suggesting such aspects of cooperation and recovery as is desired. Among the most useful suggestions that can be given to improve the course of a patient's postoperative recovery are (a) freedom from retching, (b) the ability to cough without pain, (c) increased fluid intake and appetite for food, (d) the need for lesser amounts of narcotics and sedation, and (e) control of vomiting and hiccoughing. Ideally, these are implanted prior to surgery with hypnosis, but they can also be given or reinforced while the patient is still on the operating table.

The Personal Relationship During Surgery

Helen Watkins (1976) reported a case in which a middle-aged woman, whom she had been psychotherapeutically treating for alcoholism, decided to secure a face-lift, hoping to erase the lines that marked the years of neglect to her health, body, and appearance. Because hypnosis had been an integral part of the psychotherapy, the patient asked her physician if it could be used to assist her through the operation. Upon discussing this situation with the surgeon, the psychotherapist asked him in what ways she might help the patient to undergo the operation. He mentioned first of all the reduction of tension and pain, and then remarked, "Of course, I wish her bleeding could be restricted."

The therapist made no promises, but when next the patient was hypnotized, after suggestions were administered regarding quiet, peace of mind, and freedom from pain, she was also told, "You don't need to bleed." The operation, performed under local anesthesia, was quite successful, and the patient emerged with a greatly improved face and morale. The surgeon noted that in contrast to other cases bleeding was minimal. However, the patient later reported to her therapist that during the operation she had a very strong impulse to bleed, almost as if some inner compulsion was saying to her, "Bleed! Bleed!" She would then answer back with another part of herself, "I won't bleed. Helen doesn't want me to bleed." By telling the patient, "You don't need to bleed," and repeating it, she was actually reinforcing the patient's "I won't bleed. Helen doesn't want me to bleed." Helen was throwing her own resonance and therapeutic relationship into the patient's unconscious battle with herself. During the earlier surgery, her ego state commanding her to "Bleed!" was obviously dominant, and prevailed. During the recent surgery, Helen's "resonance," which allied with the opposing "Don't bleed" ego state, prevailed. This inner struggle continued throughout the entire operation. Despite the inner battle of ego states, her apparent relaxation and quiet transmitted none of this to the surgeon. Only after the surgery was completed did the physician tell the therapist about the patient's medical record, noting that 2 years previously she had had a hysterectomy because of excessive bleeding, but that the pathology report had shown no evidence of tumor. The therapist and the patient during the course of the analytically oriented therapy disclosed many evidences and psychodynamic reasons for a self-punitive, masochistic tendency, which seemed related to her need to bleed. Bleeding, like many other physical functions, can in some patients have a strong psychogenic component and can therefore, be psychologically influenced by hypnotic suggestion.

This particular case illustrates a number of significant points regarding the use of clinical hypnosis. It should be noted that the intensive relationship with her psychotherapist, developed over many sessions, provided the motive to the patient to inhibit bleeding. The unconscious need to bleed stemming from masochistic impulses was pitted against the therapist's hypnotic suggestion not to bleed. Had the patient (who was obviously a bleeder) sought relief on a long-term basis from this symptom by hypnosis, we would anticipate that the inhibiting suggestion would have soon broken down.

Hypnotic suggestions aimed at suppressing symptoms, at least those that have a strong underlying psychogenic motivation, usually succeed only temporarily. Therefore, the hypnotic approach would probably be inadequate in a psychotherapeutic treatment of this condition. A deeper, more complex and dynamically oriented psychotherapy, perhaps using hypnosis adjunctively, would likely be required to eliminate it (see J. Watkins & H. Watkins, 1997). However, the simple hypnotic suggestion to suppress the bleeding symptom was successful in temporarily inhibiting this response during the period of the operation, thus demonstrating how direct hypnotic suggestion can be successfully used for time-limited effects during surgical operations without the necessity of psychodynamic resolution of underlying conflicts, providing it does not contradict the patient's psychodynamic motivational structure. Without Helen's resonant "therapeutic self" intervention, we (A.F.B. and J.G.W.) do not think the simple suggestion alone would have been adequate. The same wording given by a nonresonating inexperienced therapist would not have been successful. The contribution of this case is primarily to demonstrate how "direct hypnotic suggestions" can be successfully used. It was the meaning in the interpersonal situation, not the words that established sufficient security for the patient to withhold bleeding.

One finding, which was first noted in the 1840s by Esdaile (1850/1957), was the greatly lowered incidence of surgical shock in patients whose procedures were completed under hypnosis. This indicates that such shock may be as much a psychological reaction to the trauma as physiological. At least, it is a phenomenon that deserves to be much more carefully researched.

Many minor procedures in which a general anesthesia is not indicated can often be expeditiously performed using hypnosis; even a light hypnotic state can be very effective. In one example, involving catheterization of a frightened 7-year-old girl, David Spiegel explained (reported by Hebert, 1998, p. 2–3),

> We had to insert a catheter through the urethra to inject a dye into her bladder. We couldn't anesthetize the child because we needed her cooperation, but it's a terrible thing for a small girl to have done to her. The last time they did it, it took three nurses and her father holding her down, while she was screaming and struggling. This time, I used hypnosis, restructuring the stressor for her, getting her to focus on being in place where she'd rather be than in the procedure room. In her case, it was a Beanie Baby Store. She got though the procedure with a few tears and mild discomfort, but in far less time and with no struggling at all. Best of all, nobody had to hold her down.

In our study (J. Smith, Barabasz, & Barabasz, 1996) with 3- to 8-year-old children undergoing painful medical procedures, we compared hypnosis and distraction. Parents and their children were shown the video *No Tears, No Fears* (Kuttner, 1987), which presents a balanced approach to the use of distraction and hypnotic techniques to cope with pain and fear during actual medical procedures. Training in distraction and hypnosis took place in separate sessions. One volunteer parent for each child was trained first in one procedure and then the other by one of four trainers and was given the expectation of equality of potential effects for distraction and hypnotic procedures. However, all four trainers said that they had "greater faith" in the distraction technique because this was the method in use by the hospital. This was a great experimental advantage for "distraction" and probably why it was somewhat effective. Spanos and Coe (1992) were right: The "beliefs" of the therapist can prevail. They did not conclude, though, that the "beliefs" of the researcher (including their own) could affect the outcomes of an experimental study.

Training for the hypnosis condition involved developing a favorite place for hypnotic induction where the parent and child could go on an imaginary journey to a location the child selected. Once the location was selected, parents were taught how to help the child develop and elaborate the imagery. In training for the distraction condition, the parent was instructed to help the child by activating the toy, noting interesting aspects of the toy and how much fun it was. For both distraction and hypnosis, parents were taught equivalent three-step procedures including (a) introduction, (b) involvement, and (c) intervention. For the hypnosis condition, in the induction step the child was prepared to use hypnotic skills by choosing the location for a favorite place hypnotic induction. For the distraction condition, the first step involved the introduction and discussion of the prop (pop-up distraction toy with loud sounds) to be used during the procedure. The child selected a favorite pop-up toy from dozens provided by the trainer that were intended to have the capability to divert or redirect attention to it. The depth assessment phase was described as a "warm-up" exercise for the imagination. As in the Wall and Womack (1989) study, parents were asked to use the arm-lowering item (in which the child is requested to hold out an arm and then think about trying to hold something heavy) from the *Stanford Hypnotic Clinical Scale: Child* (1978–1987). It was used for both distraction and imaginative involvement conditions. A handout of the script was provided to each parent to help ensure adherence to the procedure should the parent become anxious during the painful medical procedure. The third step consisted of the actual intervention.

The hypnosis condition employed a story, and the distraction condition used the toys the child selected. Both interventions were infused with coping suggestions. Parents practiced interventions in a role-play training session with the trainers so that proper application of each intervention could be ensured.

As foreshadowed earlier in this chapter, Cooper and Erickson (1959) showed that the sense of time is capable of manipulation hypnotically. Thus, through hypnotic suggestion, a procedure that requires many hours can be made to appear experientially to the patient as if it lasted only a very short time. Likewise, long dreary hours in the recovery room can be "shortened" by hypnosis with the suggestion that the patient will experience each hour as if it had lasted only a few minutes.

Summary

Given improved safety and the applicability of chemoanesthesiology to a broader range of patients, hypnosis will probably never be used as extensively as the exclusive anesthetic in surgery as by Esdaile. However, as hospitals become more aware of the tangible benefits of hypnosis in terms of demonstrated reduced costs, fewer complications, and reduced recovery-room time, hypnosis will, no doubt, continue to experience a gradual but positive increase in its use. As physicians become increasingly cognizant of the significant impact psychological factors can have on their success, and as more of them become trained in hypnotic procedures, hypnosis will become increasingly accepted and used as an integral part of their specialties.

Chapter 11
Hypnosis for Childbirth Pain
and Trauma

A man can have sexual relations with a woman, and it is a biologically local performance. The sperm cells are secreted, and once that process has been completed — the manufacture of the sperm cells — the man's body has no longer any use for them. They serve no purpose to him. They are useful only when the man gets rid of them by depositing them into the vagina. And so, a man's sexual performance biologically is a purely local phenomenon and can be accomplished very quickly, in the space of seconds. It's just local, and once he has deposited the sperm cells he's all through with the sexual act. Biologically speaking, when a woman has intercourse, to complete that single act of intercourse biologically, she becomes pregnant, a condition that lasts for nine months. She lactates; that lasts another six months. And then she has the problem of caring for the child, teaching it, feeding it, looking after it, and enabling it to grow up. And for a woman, the single act of intercourse, in our culture, takes about eighteen years to complete. A man — eighteen seconds is all that is necessary. How is a woman's body built? Very few people stop to realize it — how completely a woman's body enters into the sexual relationship. When a woman starts having an active thoroughly well adjusted sexual life, the calcium of her skeleton changes. The calcium count increases. Her foot gets about a fourth of a size larger, her eyebrow ridges increase a little bit. The angle of jaw shifts, the chin is a little bit heavier, the nose a trifle longer, there's likely to be a change in her hair, her breasts change in either size or consistency or both. The shape of the spine alters a bit. And so physiologically and physically the girl becomes different in as short a time as two weeks of ardent lovemaking. Because biologically her body has to be prepared to take care of another creature for nine months inside, and then for months and years afterward, with all her body behavior centering on her offspring. And with each child, there's tendency for a woman's feet to get larger, the angle of her jaw to change. Every pregnancy brings about these tremendous physical and physiological changes. A man doesn't grow more whiskers because he is having intercourse, his calcium count doesn't alter any, his feet don't enlarge. He doesn't change center of gravity one bit. It is a local affair with him. But intercourse and pregnancy are a tremendous biological, physiological alteration for a woman. She has to enter it as a complete physical being. (Milton Erickson, as quoted by Haley, 1973)

Natural Childbirth and Lamaze Methods

In 1933, Grantly Dick-Read (1968) introduced a technique of delivery, termed "natural childbirth," which aimed at reducing pain by teaching the expectant mother to relax. Dick-Read held that it was tension that produced the pain, and that this tension was a consequence of the fear with which a woman approached labor and delivery. To reduce this fear, he would teach expectant mothers the facts about childbirth, because we are less prone to fear that which we understand. He followed this with exercises in breathing, relaxation, and the use of suggestion. At first, he insisted that his suggestions were in no way related to hypnosis. However, later he admitted that the combination of relaxation followed by suggestions was very similar to the procedure practiced by therapists

The "Lamaze" method (Lamaze, 1958) has become the most popular method in the United States. The expectant mother is taught many of the less fearful facts of pregnancy and delivery, respiratory exercises, neuromuscular control, and conditioning methods aimed at eliminating fear. It is theorized that an individual develops a recurrent and self-reinforcing cycle of fear-tension-pain, which in turn creates new and greater fear, and so on. By breaking this cycle through knowledge and relaxation, the mother approaches the delivery as something more natural, more like that of other species of mammals.

Both "natural childbirth" and "Lamaze" have documented reductions in pain for a substantial fraction of expectant mothers so trained, with about one fourth to one third of mothers requiring no chemical analgesic of anesthetic. Of those requiring such chemical interventions, prepared mothers used less than unprepared mothers (E. Hilgard & J. Hilgard, 1983).

All of these same elements enter into the tactics employed by the skilled hypnotherapist of today who is employed in the field of obstetrics, be he or she the obstetrician, an anesthesiologist, or another skilled professional trained in hypnosis (e.g., a counseling psychologist, clinical psychologist, or psychiatrist). The advantages of hypnosis, of course, lie in the range of pain control techniques available and the ability to induce trance with dissociation, giving the mother greater control. The effects of hypnosis to delivery can, therefore, go well beyond dependence on fear reduction, relaxation, or the occurrence of uncontrolled spontaneous trance.

Theorizing about Hypnosis and the Relief of Childbirth Pain

Just why women using hypnosis experience a less painful or painless delivery has been a matter of speculation by a number of workers in the field. Ernest Hilgard and Josephine Hilgard (1994) explained that hypnosis functions to control pain by dissociation reduced awareness of information that is transmitted to the higher brain centers. The EEG event-related potential research provides clear evidence supporting such reduced awareness, as shown in Figure 9.1 (D. Spiegel, Bierre, & Rootenberg, 1989). Essentially, childbirth-related pains registered by the woman's body are also thought to be recognized by covert awareness during hypnotic analgesia and anesthesia but masked from perception as painful by an amnestic barrier between dissociated levels of consciousness. Such awareness can be reached by evoking the "hidden observer" (see chapter 3). Most important, carefully controlled experimental research (Hilgard, Morgan, & MacDonald, 1975) has shown that hypnosis produced a significant reduction in overt pain reports compared with suggestion without hypnosis. Supporting the neodissociation explanation, covert reports through key pressing and automatic talking were unchanged. The point is that such reductions by dissociation were responsible for pain control. Perhaps the registering of sensory pain is blocked by the amnestic barrier (immediately forgotten) so that it does not enter conscious awareness.

Decades ago, Doctor Anslie Meares (1961), who conceptualized hypnosis as a form of atavistic regression, hypothesized that a hypnotized individual regresses or returns to a type of experiential existence that characterized humans during the stages of evolutionary development from an anthropoid animal into primitive man. This then reestablishes abilities of pain isolation and control that were characteristic of humans then, abilities that have been largely lost by civilized times. Meares also held that the conscious experience of a mother's love becomes possible when chemoanesthesias are not used and that this enables the mother to achieve a more total and realistic anesthesia through hypnosis. The conscious experience of delivery results in a closer mother-child bond than when it is blurred by a chemical anesthetic.

Earlier still, Otto Rank (1952) held that birth was traumatic to the child and the original source of neurotic anxiety because it involved separation from the mother. Whether or not this is correct, certainly the addition of chemoanesthesia, which drugs the child prior to separation, could only add to the hazard the infant faces in coming into this world. A birth that was traumatic to the mother may be equally traumatic to the child and may have strong unforeseen effects on its later emotional development.

Nevertheless, the birth experience is an extremely significant one to the mother. If it is accomplished without undue pain, attitudes toward the child may be more positive than if the baby's delivery was accompanied by much suffering. It is the beginning of the mother-child relationship. It should be started under the most favorable circumstances possible for the future well-being and emotional health of both.

Because hypnosis is not suited to all individuals, the judgment as to whether to use it as an anesthesia and analgesia in the case of a gravid (pregnant) patient should be made early and should consider many different factors. A last-minute decision to employ hypnosis (perhaps as the woman in labor is being wheeled into the delivery room) can result in failure and traumatization. However, excellent results in eliminating or at least reducing pain by hypnosis can be obtained with a minimum of training — in fact, far less training than required for less effective techniques such as Lamaze or the Dick-Read natural childbirth methods.

Effectiveness of Hypnosis for Childbirth

Scientific evidence that hypnosis should in most cases be the pain relief method of choice comes from numerous case reports and from controlled statistical studies. Unfortunately, most studies lack hypnotizability test data from standardized scales. However, the little systematic information now available regarding the use of hypnotizability tests to predict successful and unsuccessful outcomes is promising. Most research also fails to gather data indexing the amount or lack of pain felt, as was done in the J. Smith, Barabasz, and Barabasz (1996) study that we discussed in the previous chapter. Instead of using patients' pain reports, investigators have based their "objective" measures on the reduction in the amounts of chemoanalgesia or chemoanesthesia required. Such measures are based on the assumption that those suffering the greatest pain should demand more relief; however, such a correlation between the amount of pain felt and the amount of medication demanded is just as imperfect as the response to chemical analgesics.

Katchan and Belozerski (1940) obtained pain report data from 501 cases. Despite the authors' failure to predict outcomes in more than 60% of the cases (apparently their expectations for success made no difference), they were able to conclude that 29% of the cases obtained complete analgesia, 38% obtained partial analgesia, 21% resulted in failure, and 12% showed questionable responses. Thus, nearly 70% of the cases had at least partial and helpful analgesia or complete analgesia using hypnosis as the sole pain-relieving agent.

The first more carefully controlled study involved 210 women. Davidson (1962) randomly divided them into three equal groups. The control group received no training; the hypnosis group received 1.5 hours of training in self-hypnosis; and the third group was taught the Dick-Read natural childbirth relaxation procedure. Patients reported pain on a scale of 0 (*no pain*), 1 (*slight pain*), 2 (*moderate pain*), and 3 (*severe pain*). The Dick-Read relaxation method average score was 1.68, well below the 1.95 reported by the control group. The hypnosis group achieved dramatically lower pain with an average score of just 0.83 — a remarkable achievement for only a single hypnosis session.

Brann and Guzvica's 1987 study permitted participants to self-select either hypnosis or relaxation training, with 48 volunteers in each group. The research showed that the time involved in the first stage of labor (onset of labor to dilation of the cervix) was significantly lower for those in the hypnosis group compared with the relaxation training group. First-time mothers (primigavidas) benefited most. Perhaps more important, those in the hypnosis group reported significantly greater satisfaction with the labor process, greater ease of going to sleep when desired, and much less anxiety about the entire birthing process. The hypnosis patients also felt more self-control and were more satisfied than the relaxation-trained patients.

No doubt inspired by the work of Brann and Guzvica in England, Jenkins and Pritchard (1993) conducted the largest controlled study to date in Wales. A total of 862 participants were studied, with half consisting of primigravidas and the other half of second-time mothers (secundgravidas). Each group was split between those receiving hypnosis and age-matched controls. Each of the hypnosis participants underwent six sessions of individualized hypnosis. As in the Brann and Guzvica study, primigravidas in the hypnosis group showed dramatic lower duration of first stage labor (3 hours less than the controls). The second stage (dilation of cervix to delivery) was also significantly less than the controls. The secundgravidas also spent less time in the first stage of labor than the controls. Perhaps because of asymptote, the effects of hypnosis on their second stage of time and labor was not significant. Overall, volunteers in the hypnosis condition required significantly less need (or no need) for analgesic chemicals in contrast to the controls.

Harmon, Hynan, and Tyre (1990) conducted the most elegantly controlled study extant as should be expected of the research from the United States conducted in that era. Hypnotizability was addressed, as was patient perceived pain. Sixty primigravidas, who were recruited rather than volunteered, were tested and then divided into high- and low-hypnotizability groups before random assignment to hypnosis or nonhypnosis conditions. In other words, half of the high-hypnotizable participants and half of the low-hypnotizable participants received hypnosis, whereas the other half received the standard relaxation training treatment, which included breathing exercises similar to the Dick-Read natural childbirth method. The hypnosis groups used significantly less analgesic chemicals, had more spontaneous deliveries, and had shorter first stages of labor than those receiving relaxation suggestions and breathing exercises.

As in the A. Barabasz and M. Barabasz (1989) study of chronic pain patients, Harmon and his colleagues also administered a measure of pain tolerance using ischemic pain to test the effects of hypnosis period. While in antenatal training, a blood pressure cuff (sphygmomanometer) was placed on the patients' arms and inflated to produce pain by cutting off arterial blood flow to the lower arm. The high-hypnotizable participants receiving hypnosis training produced the most significant reduction in pain. Obviously, obtaining a pain-reduction measure using experimentally induced pain at a far removed site from the birthing channel is less than ideal, but it is a step in the right direction.

Benefits of Hypnosis in the Practice of Obstetrics

The research to date shows a number of minimum benefits we can expect from the use of hypnosis in obstetrics. These benefits include at least the following: (a) reduction in the duration of the first stage of labor (averaging about 3 hours less); (b) chemoanalgesia and anesthesia; (c) reduction or elimination of pain; (d) decreased shock and more rapid recovery; (e) better patient cooperation; (f) lowered incidence of operative delivery; (g) facilitation of anesthesia of the perineum, delivery, episiotomy, and suturing; (h) reduction or elimination of many undesirable postoperative effects; (i) much less required training than natural childbirth and Lamaze methods; (j) unlike chemoanesthetics, hypnoanesthesia cannot harm either mother or child; (k) most mothers find childbirth using hypnosis an extremely gratifying and satisfying experience and (l) in certain emergencies, such as abruption placenta, the use of hypnosis can be life-saving.

Posttraumatic Stress and High Hypnotizability

"I could see everything in the mirror; the forceps, the episiotomy, my whole body being laid open. Somehow, I just wasn't there. I seemed to be floating around on the ceiling. It just really wasn't happening to me" (Reynolds, 1997, p. 831). The ability to be highly hypnotizable is a remarkable talent, but in obstetrics, as in certain other situations, it can be a problematic avenue to trauma. High hypnotizability is usually a great advantage in hypnotherapy, but as we have discussed in the earlier chapters, those talented individuals with high hypnotizability typically have an extraordinary capacity for both imaginative involvement and fantasy proneness (Rhue & Lynn, 1989; Rhue, Lynn, Bukh, & Henry, 1991).

Two features of childbirth make it potentially traumatizing: extreme pain and a sense of loss of control. The deleterious long-term sequelae are only beginning to be recognized. A post-delivery stress clinic has been opened in England to address this frequently ignored variant of posttraumatic stress disorder (PTSD). To begin with, PTSD, once thought to be a combat-related syndrome of men, is much more prevalent among women (Resnick, Kilpatrick, Dansky, Saunders, & Best, 1993). Indeed, the rate is more than 2.3 times that of men according to Helzer, Robins, and McEvoy (1987).

Little more than a decade ago, Malzack (1993) used labor pain as a "model for acute pain," reporting that 60% of first-time mothers and 45% of those bearing additional children described labor that made them feel either severe or extremely severe pain, with most noting it was the most intense pain they had ever felt. Such a painful experience is an ideal environment to precipitate PTSD in women with high hypnotizability who undergo childbirth, either with chemoanalgesia or natural childbirth but without training in pain management with hypnosis. Without hypnotic management, they can be left with long-term, detrimental effects and prolonged suffering. They exhibit avoidance of behaviors such as demands for cesarean sections for subsequent births. They become hypervigilant in an effort to try to ensure the traumatic event will not be repeated. Childbirth-related PTSD can precipitate long-lasting postpartum depression. In some cases, childbirth PTSD manifests itself by neglect or even physical abuse of the child, because he or she reminds the mother of the trauma experience.

Highly hypnotizable women, whether previously traumatized by child-birth or not, can learn to manage their talent to reduce labor time and have a pain-free or reduced-pain delivery. Alternatively, without knowledge about their talent and training in hypnosis, they will be prone to childbirth PTSD. Their talent for fantasy proneness and intense created imaginative experiences can distort perception of time and create the impression that labor has been going on forever. Resting periods seem attenuated, and contractions seem prolonged. Natural dissociative capacity can turn into a sense of loss of control, and as they imagine the worst, such as a deformed or retarded baby, these women become more and more anxious. The result is muscle tension, which slows dilation of the cervix and anxious overbreathing (i.e., hyperventilation) and increases catecholamine, which further inhibits uterine muscle function. The cycle worsens and worsens, and if these women do not begin with PTSD they will certainly be on the way to developing the syndrome.

Of course, all of the negative sequelae can be avoided given appropriate training in hypnosis from a resonant therapist. In addition, we recommend that when a therapist's clinical intuition suggests the patient might fit the above descriptions, he or she should take a complete history, including information on (a) possible rape or sexual abuse, (b) a history of nightmares, (c) a history of other events that were traumatic for the patinet, and (d) a history of trouble trusting authority figures. If the patient has been extremely detailed in her birthing plans, the therapist should recognize that this likely indicates a strong need for control and severe anxiety about childbirth. Excellent rapport is essential to a successful outcome for these patients. Such an outcome with hypnotizability working for, rather than against the patient, can completely reverse the effects of a previous birthing trauma.

Changing Attitudes About Labor and Delivery

Almost universally, women from industrialized cultures begin their pregnancy burdened by doubts and fears which have been implanted in them by their mothers and neighbors. Those who have been regaled as children with the horrors of childbirth are the patients who are most likely to develop complications that require special psychological attention. If these individuals are hypnotizable and given hypnotic suggestions that may have a long-lasting effect, one should consider how these same people may have received unconstructive and harmful suggestions earlier in their lives, suggestions about the pains of childbirth that now are creating great overt or covert anxiety in them. Kroger and other practitioners recognized decades ago that these women were in a sense hypnotized (perhaps at times of spontaneous trance) and exposed to antitherapeutic suggestions as children. In these cases, the use of hypnosis is indicated to correct prior negativity by cognitively reframing the harmful suggestions that they already have received. As Albert Ellis, the father of rational-emotive cognitive behavior therapy has exclaimed, it is not what happens to us but the attitudes we develop at an early age that determine our reactions to events (Albert Ellis, personal communication to A.F.B., 1980). From our perspective, attitudes of fear can be offset by continuous hypnotic suggestions of confidence, calmness, and peace of mind as pregnancy progresses. Nonhypnotic suggestions tying together childbirth and pain have often been repeated to the patient over many years. No wonder they are built-in, constantly recalled at both conscious and unconscious levels and difficult to eradicate. Furthermore, even when not voiced, these fears afflict many women who have been taught that it is not appropriate to express fear. Today, because so many anesthetics are available, expression of fear tends to be suppressed. Wise doctors will not attempt to stifle the genuine fears their patients have of the coming ordeal with hasty reassurance. Through Rogersian acceptance, the strength of such anxieties tends to decline and hypnosis can play the key facilitative adjunctive role. Reassurance and positive hypnotic suggestions about the birthing process are usually effective only after the patient has had a full opportunity to reveal her true attitudes about childbirth and to voice her misgivings. Such critical revelations may most efficiently be obtained using ego-state hypnosis (J. Watkins & H. Watkins, 1997).

Some practitioners have advocated that hypnotic suggestions should be given to the pregnant women that her child will be a joy to her so as to build up her positive expectations. Indeed, she has been hearing the same song from friends and relatives whose lives she has seen changed by pregnancy and the raising of children in both positive and sometimes disastrous ways. This technique might be a help to some women. To others, especially those who are more angry than pleased about being pregnant, such a procedure is contraindicated. If the child does not meet her expectations, she will likely feel cheated and can take it out by a rejection of the neonate.

During the period of pregnancy, much can be done to counter harmful beliefs and attitudes that have been suggested to patients when they were children. Hypnosis should be employed to modify such attitudes, and this may be of equal value to training in the production of anesthesia. As the attitudes improve, so also are pain thresholds raised. Likewise, as the gravid woman learns to produce anesthesia, such as in her hand, her confidence improves and her attitudes of fear will lessen. The psychological approach is a holistic one, involving her entire being. It is not an isolated set of piecemeal tactics that try to deal singly with each symptom. A holistic approach results in a general strengthening of the ego, thus making a woman better able to cope with pain and many of the other frustrations and discomforts associated with pregnancy, labor, and delivery.

Not only is it important to reframe unconstructive attitudes in the pregnant woman, it is equally important to develop favorable attitudes about clinical hypnosis and its benefits. Unsympathetic, naive, or misinformed nurses can, by their remarks, nullify weeks of careful work with the patient. Attitudes of skepticism and comments to the effect that they do not believe in it or that they are not "suggestible" (thus falsely implying that to have hypnotic talent is for the gullible) can have a profound negative impact when made by health personnel, thus undermining the effectiveness of the hypnotic intervention. Accordingly, when hypnosis is to be used, the nursing staff and health personnel who will be caring for the patient should have instruction in the modality, including its principles, possibilities, and limitations. They should also be instructed of the necessity that they give approval and support to the patient with whom hypnosis is to be employed. Their support will help greatly in bringing the patient to delivery with a strong conviction of its effectiveness.

Nurses who become aware of the suggestive import of their words will show this in many ways when hypnosis is not being used. Doctors can suggest doubt and dismay merely by a remark like, "If this doesn't work we'll try…" Instead of asking the patient, "How are your pains?" it is far better to say, "Are you feeling contractions?" There is an entire language that is associated with pain that can be avoided by the sensitive healing arts person, doctor, nurse, technician, or other health care personnel.

Who Does the Hypnosis During Obstetrical Delivery

The best individual to administer the hypnosis during an obstetrical delivery is the obstetrician, the doctor who has had the most contact with the patient. The doctor is the one whom the patient trusts to see her safely through this experience, the one who can be counted on to be present at the time of delivery, and the one who knows what medical complications might occur in her case. The obstetrician bears the final responsibility from the first consultation with the patient, presumably early in pregnancy, through labor and delivery. The doctor's relationship with the gravid woman has been a long one, established over a number of months. Accordingly, one might anticipate that, because clinical hypnosis is an intensive interpersonal relationship experience and an altered state of consciousness, the obstetrician will be the one to whom the patient would most likely make a positive hypnotic response. Furthermore, the obstetrician is generally endowed with the characteristics of a nurturing parent figure in a natural transference reaction established by the patient at this time. The obstetrician's influence should be most potent during the induction of hypnosis and the administration of the therapeutic suggestions.

However, hypnosis should be done only by experienced therapists who have established a very close interpersonal relationship with their patient and presupposes that the obstetrician has been trained in hypnotic procedures. Because many doctors have had little or no training in hypnosis or find that the practice of clinical hypnosis is not to their interest, once the decision to use it has been made, it is necessary to find or select a well-trained professional in this area to carry out the procedures. Recognizing that hypnosis can be a time-consuming technique, many ob-gyn doctors find themselves simply too busy and handling too many patients to use this approach, even though they know its value.

An anesthesiologist, trained in hypnosis, makes a second-best choice. Although this doctor probably does not have the long and continuing relationship with the patient, he or she is skilled in all the other procedures of anesthesia and can best handle an emergency such as the last-minute failure of the hypnoanesthesia to be effective. The labor, of course, may require many hours, and the professional who will act as the therapist should be able to spend considerable time with the patient throughout this period, as well as be present at the time of delivery.

Should the obstetrician be untrained in hypnotic techniques, and an anesthesiologist so trained also be unavailable, then a psychologist, psychiatrist, or other psychotherapist who is skilled in these procedures is the most suitable practitioner. These applied behavioral scientists are accustomed to communicating over long periods of time with patients, and, if they are competent, have developed many interpersonal relationship skills that can make them invaluable in dealing with the frightened or disturbed gravid woman. If the patient has been in psychotherapy, and her therapist is skilled in hypnotherapy (especially if this technique has been used in her psychological treatment), such an individual would be ideal to work with the obstetrician.

Some obstetricians maintain a continuous colleague relationship with this professional and arrange for this person to be involved in the early education and conditioning of their patients throughout the period of pregnancy. He or she then becomes most naturally a part of the "obstetrical team," and no new element or person is introduced to the patient at the last moment with whom she has to cope. Such an arrangement promotes a general feeling of security. If the doctor has not been personally acquainted with such a professional and does not have full knowledge of the training, experience, and skill that the therapist has to offer, then a few suggestions can be offered here that should help any physician to select a well-trained specialist in this field.

Most legitimate, ethical, and well-trained workers in the field of hypnosis belong to one or both of the two major hypnosis societies — the Society for Clinical and Experimental Hypnosis and the American Society of Clinical Hypnosis. Many qualified psychologists are associated with Division 30 (Society of Psychological Hypnosis) of the American Psychological Association. A few highly experienced practitioners are also diplomates of one of the subboards of the American Board of Clinical Hypnosis. These are the American Board of Medical Hypnosis, the American Board of Psychological Hypnosis, and the American Board of Hypnosis in Dentistry. Practitioners' affiliation with any of these organizations does not guarantee a successful hypnotic experience for their patients. However, it does ensure that the individuals have had qualifying courses in the field and are recognized by the respective membership committees or boards as being trained to use hypnosis.

Members of these groups are all qualified people in their recognized professions: medicine, psychology, dentistry, and so on. They are not simply therapists. They have full training, usually doctoral, in their major fields and have learned hypnotic techniques in addition. Accordingly, they have worked with many other patients and are bound by the same health care licensing procedures, principles of ethics, and responsibilities that inhere in the practice of medicine. Although there are occasionally other individuals who have had specialized training in hypnosis, the obstetrician or other physician who seeks their services should exercise extreme caution in using them, because there are currently a number of "therapists" attempting to offer their services to physicians who have neither the medical nor psychological background to be entrusted with this delicate and sophisticated psychological procedure. To hypnotize can be easily learned; to apply hypnosis skillfully and with appropriate precautions during clinical practice is an entirely different matter. Even a simpleton can cut open a belly with a scalpel; this does not make one a surgeon. Psychological sophistication does not come from a course in how to induce a trance, and the practice of clinical hypnosis or hypnotherapy is a job for a licensed clinician or counseling psychologist, not a technician.

Hypnosis for Delivery

It was previously thought that training in hypnosis should start early, preferably by at least the third or fourth month of pregnancy (J. Watkins, 1987, p. 229). However, new procedures we review next are brief and effective, and can be taught to women very near the projected time of delivery.

Training can occur individually or in groups. Certainly, the Harmon et al. (1990) study showed that group training can be effective. Certainly, it seems logical to save both time and costs by using a group procedure, because each pregnant woman will be experiencing the giving of birth. However, we wish to emphasize that although the event is technically the same that does not mean the experience can be expected to be the same. Each woman is quite unique. Each woman will bring her special hypnotic capacities, cultural issues, fears, and apprehensions to her training in hypnosis. As we know from previous research, (A. Barabasz et al., 2003), not only is clinician experience and resonance with the patient important for maximal results from hypnosis but also inductions tailored to the patient are more effective than scripted protocols when a significant degree of hypnotic depth is needed (Barabasz & Christensen, in press). So then, although the patient is female and pregnant, let the expectations of gender experience end there. Above all, treat the patient as she deserves to be treated — as a unique individual who brings special talents and unique issues to the hypnotic birthing experience. The techniques of induction and deepening can be adapted to her individual needs. The doctor-patient relationship may be closer at this time. By observing her unique responses to the induction procedure, one is better prepared to take maximum advantage of these during the period of labor and delivery.

Some believe that these advantages can frequently be offset by certain plusses that inhere in a group-training situation. In the group, an esprit de corps rapidly develops that involves both social motivation and competition. To win approval from the doctor, patients may vie with each other in trying to reach deeper levels of hypnotic response. The amount of time that is spent for induction practice can be considerably increased without tremendous cost if patients are trained in groups.

As each woman, new to the group, observes more experienced participants demonstrate hypnosis, her own confidence may be increased. Two-hour meetings, held about twice a month, are the norm. The value of the procedure in the eyes of the trainees is further increased as those who "graduate" return with their babies to relate their experiences to the group. Group motivation and support are powerful facilitators of the training process.

Whether done individually or in groups, the training steps are the same. They involve first answering questions about hypnosis and desensitizing the patient. Emphasis is placed on it as a "natural" procedure. Anxieties are resolved that might have occurred as a result of viewing horror films, listening to old-wives' tales, and countering the resistance that often is engendered by friends, family members, and too frequently even by doctors and nurses who are committed to the old traditional method using chemoanesthesias that still remains the predominant experience for many women. However, those that have had experience with delivery with hypnosis instead almost universally and unquestionably remark that it is the best way to go, an experience that brings together the mother and child and, more frequently, the father as well if he is present during the delivery.

Hypnosis in the Management of Pregnancy

A number of problems that occur during pregnancy may be substantially lessened once the patient has been conditioned to make hypnotic responses. These problems include nausea and vomiting, difficulty in voiding or problems with urinary and bowel control, insomnia, and excessive salivation. Skillfully planted suggestions can alter these processes in constructive ways, which may obviate the necessity of frequent drug prescriptions. Other problems that will often respond favorably to hypnotic suggestion are backaches, fatigue, cramps, and regulation of appetite where the gravid patient loses appetite and consumes an inadequate food intake for herself and the unborn child, or overeats and makes an excessive weight gain.

Nausea and vomiting are special situations that deserve psychodynamic consideration. If it appears that they represent a symbolic rejection of the child, hence an unconscious desire to expel it through the mouth, then hypnotic suggestion alone may not only be inadequate, but, because it is directed at an underlying motivation, hypnosis can precipitate other difficulties, possibly hemorrhage or abortion. Direct evidence is lacking on this point. Furthermore, the entire problem of symptom substitution is still controversial. However, psychological prudence dictates that when a symptom seems to be related to some unconscious need, attempts to remove it should suggestively be conservative and undertaken with precaution and with the recognition that the patient may require a more dynamic and insightful therapy.

Urinary and bowel control might be attacked more directly, perhaps combining hypnosis with behavior therapy techniques. Excessive fatigue can often be alleviated by short periods of hypnotic relaxation, during which suggestions aimed at instilling a feeling of rest are administered (e.g., "You will wake up feeling as if you have had a good night's sleep).

One of the most serious problems facing the obstetrician is persistent vaginal bleeding, with the continuous danger of spontaneous abortion. A number of case reports have been published that describe the effective use of hypnotic suggestion to reduce bleeding time in various conditions (Edel, 1959; Stolzenberg, 1955). Crasilneck and Fogelman (1957) reported a controlled study on the effect hypnosis had on such factors as clotting and bleeding time between the waking control state and hypnosis. Their results were negative. However, it must be constantly reiterated that hypnosis with volunteer experimental individuals is not the same as hypnosis in the clinical situation with patients who have a close relationship with their doctor.

During the period of pregnancy, not only does the woman's body shape change but also frequently there are significant alterations in self-concept, in the attitude toward the unborn child, and in the relationship with the child's father. In some cases, these should receive some kind of psychological treatment, which might include support, ventilation, and suggestion, with or without hypnosis. Because this is a time of stress for the patient, a psychological approach to the entire problem of pregnancy, labor, and delivery should be given significant weight. The obstetrical case cannot be considered as having been well handled if, as a result of neglect of these factors, the mother is traumatized, a pattern of rejecting her child is established, or long-lasting emotional maladjustments are set off, even though the delivery was accomplished without physical harm to either mother or child. In a program of psychological conditioning for expectant mothers, hypnosis can play an important role for many of them.

In cases of possible abortion, Cheek recommended use of his finger-response technique (see Cheek & LeCron, 1968, pp. 131–133) as a way of communicating with unconscious attitudes within the patient. Underlying motives might be uncovered that will throw valuable light on such questions as whether the expectant mother wants the child. Decisions as to the best types of psychological treatment to be initiated can be more wisely made, and at times even questions of whether the child should be put up for adoption might rest on such communications.

A high percentage of the hemorrhages that occur during the first trimester do so while the patient is asleep. These may be accompanied by frightening dreams related to labor. Such emotional disturbances should receive early psychotherapeutic treatment, either hypnotic or otherwise. Kroger (1963) suggested that prolonged sleep under hypnosis is one of the best methods to ward off a threatened spontaneous abortion.

Preparation for Labor

At the beginning of labor or just prior to its anticipated onset, a most important session will be held by the patient with her doctor. This is designed to get her psychologically ready for the birth experience. The session aims to focus and review all that the patient has learned prior to this time about constructive attitudes, freedom from fear, and her ability to induce anesthesia. As Kroger and Freed (1951) put it, good obstetric practice should be concerned "with preparation of the woman's mind and less with the administration of noxious drugs."

If the patient has previously been conditioned to establish a hypnotic anesthesia, care should be taken that it not be so continuous and automatic that she does not get the warning of the first uterine contractions, which warn that it is time to contact her physician and perhaps go to the hospital. If necessary, hypnosis can be induced in the already conditioned patient over the phone, and suggestions of pain relief can also be given.

This is the time for a new dose of reassurance. The patient should never feel that she has made an irrevocable commitment to the sole use of hypnoanesthesia. She can be told, "If it is necessary, we will supplement with a small amount of chemoanesthesia," or "We may need only a little anesthetic." The patient should be encouraged to ask for some anesthetic if she feels she needs it. The situation should never become structured as a test of her courage.

At this time the entire hypnotic procedure should be rehearsed, including a considerable amount of time spent in deepening. If the patient indicates fear that she will not be able to follow her hypnosis training should the doctor not be present, the therapist should ask her to carry through the procedure and step out of the room while she is doing so. Especially significant will be the patient's ability at this time to self-induce a glove anesthesia. The therapist should request that the patient do so and test with pinprick or clamp.

Management of Labor

Screaming patients in a nearby room may so distract the hypnotically trained patient as to weaken her conviction about her ability to achieve and maintain a hypnoanesthesia. Wolfe (1961) recommended that the patient be warned in advance somewhat as follows: "You may hear patients in labor in the next room who do not know how to take advantage of hypnosis and are, therefore, making a great deal of noise. Do not let the noise or conversation of these people, or the use of the word *pain*, interfere in any way with what you know and have proved you can do." It is sometimes valuable to make suggestions aimed at eliminating painful memories associated with delivery. In this case, it is recommended that a more permissive wording be used such as, "It is not necessary that you remember," rather than "You will not remember."

Erickson, Hershman, and Secter (1961) suggested a feedback technique to maximize confidence and cooperation in the patient when she is in labor. In this procedure the patient is asked, both in and out of hypnosis, just what she would like to feel during the birth experience. Perhaps she prefers to be awake and alert at the moment the baby appears. Perhaps she wishes to feel the uterine contractions but does not want to endure severe suffering. Maybe she wants to hear the baby's first cry and then go to sleep. The experience of giving birth will be one of the most significant ones in her life. She should feel herself a participant in planning and directing it, not a helpless victim of forces, pains, and numbing over which she has no control. This moment can be one of triumph for her, or it can be a severe psychological trauma with lifelong crippling effects.

If she has given birth before, and her previous experience, using either hypnoanesthesia or chemoanesthesia, was a particularly satisfying one, then suggestions to her that she will remember the exact feelings she had before and fuse them with her present ones may help to secure a replay of the previous favorable labor and delivery.

In making suggestions related to the uterine contractions and approaching delivery, instead of trying to completely suppress all feelings of pain, the doctor might suggest instead that the patient does not need to experience any more difficulty than she is willing to accept.

In general, we do not use glove anesthesia for childbirth because of the potential for paralysis of functions. We want to eliminate or reduce pain perception, not muscular ability to induce contractions. However, if a glove anesthesia is to be used and then transferred to the abdomen during labor and to the perineum during delivery, then it should be carefully checked beforehand. It is usually first induced in the hand, which is tested with a pinprick. Then the patient is instructed to transfer this anesthetic feeling, by stroking the hand, to some other area of her body. At this time some site is selected that is not experiencing any pain. This secondary area is then tested for anesthesia by a pinprick or clamp. If no signs of flinching occur, and the patient reports feeling no pain, she should be ready to accomplish the same effect during the labor and delivery. Some obstetricians prefer to suggest a numbing sensation over the entire lower half of the body rather than induce glove anesthesia and simply transfer it to the desired areas. Although a fairly deep degree of hypnotic involvement is necessary to secure a complete anesthesia or analgesia, even a light trance may be helpful in that it lowers the amount of chemoanesthesia needed to secure the desired result. A posthypnotic suggestion can be given that this numbness will reappear immediately following a signal to be given by the doctor.

In view of the findings of the Hilgards (E. Hilgard & J. Hilgard, 1994) on overt versus covert pain, it is probably wise to suggest that the patient will "feel" no pain rather than she will "have" none. Their studies have shown that pain has two components: sensory pain, which indicates the location and intensity of the pain stimulus, and suffering, a reaction that follows the first. It is this second reaction that we wish to suppress hypnotically.

A sophisticated and advanced method that can be effectively employed with the patient who can achieve deep hypnotic levels is that of general dissociation. It can be induced as follows:

> You are having the feeling of floating out of your body. The body remains here on the delivery table and you are walking over to that side of the room and sitting in the chair, where you can watch that woman lying on the table over there. She looks just like you. She is your size and has the same hair as you do. Her face resembles that which you see when you look in a mirror. She is going to have a baby. The doctors and nurses are there, and you are most interested in observing what happens. She does not appear to have much discomfort, and as you watch her she seems to be looking forward eagerly to her experience of giving birth. You will observe every part of her delivery from the chair in which you are seated across the room.

There is a possible psychological objection to this procedure, which may or may not have significance. No research data seems to be available on this matter at present. If the woman over there gives birth to the baby, will the observer across the room feel it is her own baby? Or will she feel an estrangement toward the infant, which affects her relationship with it? If this were true, it might also be true that anytime a baby is delivered under such heavy sedation that the mother is not aware of the birth, she would have a similar reaction. This potential problem deserves experimental study.

There are a number of advantages that accrue with the use of hypnosis during the period of labor. Through suggestions of rest and relaxation, fatigue can be lowered. Furthermore, unlike some chemoanesthetics, it does not lower uterine activity. Several writers (August, 1961; Kroger, 1963) reported that in the primipera the period of labor is shortened on the average by some 2 hours. Erickson et al. (1961) hold that when chemical anesthesia can be reduced or eliminated there is a reduction of the risks of respiratory and circulatory infection in the mother and baby, such as often results in anoxia. This reduction can be achieved when there is a less prolonged labor. If tension in the patient has been reduced through relaxation, there is less likelihood of the necessity for a breech delivery because of malpresentation of the fetus.

A potential use for hypnosis has been suggested by Rice (1961), who claimed that it is effective in inducing labor and that the process can be speeded or slowed by such suggestion. Once labor has started, the patient's attention can be distracted from pain by asking her to count the average time of each labor contraction by seconds, such as "101, 102, 103," and so on. Another device that may be useful, and that can be related to deepening trance or inducing anesthesia, is to have the patient clasp a wrist tightly and squeeze, especially during the contractions. This mechanism, if it is to be used, should have been established previously as a posthypnotic suggestion (e.g., "Every time you squeeze your wrist you will sink into a deeper hypnosis where you will not suffer discomfort").

Suggestions of relaxation in hypnosis can be effective in preventing a premature onset of labor. If the patient has been responsive to the doctor's voice, both the induction and the relaxation suggestions can be administered over the phone.

In general, a patient who has been trained in hypnosis, who has learned to enter trance rapidly by a prearranged signal, and who can induce an anesthesia in herself can respond much better to the doctor for the reduction of her discomfort and the handling of unforeseen contingencies.

Hypnosis During Delivery

If the previously suggested hypnotic procedures have been carried out, then the control, which they afford, can be extended to facilitate the delivery and reduce or eliminate pain. Cheek and LeCron (1968) suggested the use of ideomotor signal questioning, during labor and delivery, to ensure maximal understanding by the doctor of the patient's doubts, fears, and hopes.

The delivery represents the time where the total of all previous hypnosis training is used. If a patient is a somnambule, one who goes into hypnosis so deeply that she emerges totally amnesic as to what took place, she should be asked whether she wishes to be conscious at the time of the delivery. Some women feel cheated if they are not aware when their baby is born; they wish to participate in the event.

Some obstetricians who use hypnosis do so primarily during the period of labor and during the initial stages of delivery, in which anesthesia has been transferred by the patient to the perineal area from a previously conditioned glove anesthesia on her hand. A local chemoanesthetic is then used for the episiotomy. Others recommend the combination of a pudendal block with hypnoanesthesia. Most practitioners prefer a combination of hypnosis and chemoanesthesia and report few deliveries with hypnoanesthesia alone. Several, however, apparently are able to secure sufficient pain control and use it with a large number of their patients. August (1961), for example, listed some 1,000 deliveries performed with hypnosis as the sole anesthesia. No data have been reported differentiating the number of deliveries accomplished with glove anesthesia versus those in which the dissociation technique was employed. The alteration of what is subject and what is object, and how these can be hypnotically manipulated, has been described elsewhere (see our Volume II). Such changes occasionally occur spontaneously.

In this respect, some precautions should be made concerning the complete safety of hypnoanesthesia. On the surface, the pain has been suppressed or repressed. However, John Watkins and Helen Watkins (1979–1980), working with unconscious ego states, discovered that although the conscious person overtly felt no pain, the "hidden observers" (which they see as equated with ego states) reported underlying anger and fear. As in the case for chemoanesthesia, hypnoanesthesia seems to be quite effective at the conscious level. However, we do not know whether some internal psychhological trauma is suffered. Further research with the hidden observer phenomena might shed more light on this question.

Childbirth by Hypnosis: The McCarthy Method

Patrick McCarthy, a physician living in Wellington New Zealand, developed and individualized a structured approach to teaching hypnosis for childbirth. The training program is completed in just five, 30-minute sessions conducted in the very final few weeks of pregnancy. To date, he has used the procedure successfully with well in excess of 600 New Zealand women seen individually (McCarthy, personal communication to A.F.B., January 2003; McCarthy, 2001). He emphasized that hypnosis is not necessarily therapeutic. Consistent with our (A.F.B. and J.G.W.) conceptualization, hypnosis is a means of communicating therapeutic and helpful comments to the patient, a way of being with a patient. The program is highly individualized, but the specific content of the obstetric hypnosis-training program is of course crucial to the overall effectiveness of the program. It is not a specific set of words that are used in hypnotic trance to some marvelous effect for all pregnant women. It is more important to recognize the fundamental principles required to use hypnosis to good effect in childbirth. This of course requires the therapist to have knowledge and experience in hypnosis, obstetrics, and psychology. The approach is designed around the precise language that women have used to describe their experiences of delivery, such as the following: (a) "The contractions seemed to last forever and I thought the labor would never come to an end"; (b) "The contractions seemed to be tearing me apart"; (c) "I felt so exhausted, I just couldn't push any longer"; (d) "The contractions were just awful, I was helpless, I was out of control"; and (e) "I seemed to be floating away from my body, I couldn't do anything, I was looking at the doctors and the nurses from far away."

McCarthy recognized that a woman may forget many things such as the name of a best friend or a long-time lover, but a woman never forgets that she has given birth. Unfortunately, although recollections of giving birth seemed to be recalled with amazing sharpness, they are often frequently inaccurate when compared with records of the event taken at the time by the mother herself. McCarthy made a special point of listening to the language of women, particularly those who have had bad experiences of labor, as keys to possible pathology such as the diagnosis of PTSD. As we (A.F.B. and J.G.W.) discussed earlier in this chapter in the section on posttraumatic stress and high hypnotizability to hypnosis for childbirth, high hypnotizability can be a double-edged sword, where a patient's dissociative capacity, fantasy proneness, and PTSD can make a highly hypnotizable woman inherently vulnerable during labor. McCarthy recognized that although childbirth can be a momentous milestone in life, it can also produce an indelible memory that could weigh a woman down for the rest of her life. Some women vow never to be pregnant again, only to find themselves pregnant again and again. McCarthy reported that contrary to notions of the glory of childbirth, such symptoms are not uncommon during childbirth, on the basis of his experience with more than 2,000 deliveries.

The training program assumes that for each negative sequelae, it should be possible to teach an equal and opposite positive and constructive hypnotic response. McCarthy's training is prophylactic to childbirth PTSD. Although hypnotizability is not accessed using a standardized scale, the procedure teaches women to recognize and generate a large number of phenomena, which are common to the gold standard of hypnotizability measurement, the *Stanford Hypnotic Susceptibility Scale*, Form C, and the shorter *Stanford Hypnotic Clinical Scale*. Phenomena that go beyond the scale that are specific to childbirth such as anesthesia are also included, as are ideosensory responses and time distortion. The responses emphasized in training include the following: (a) muscle relaxation, (b) catalepsy, (c) age progression, (d) amnesia, (e) anesthesia, (f) dissociation, (g) hallucination, and (h) posthypnotic suggestion. McCarthy stressed the importance of planning hypnotic responses for uses in birthing that are tailored from the special abilities talents of each individual woman. Practice and mastery of this usually comprehensive list of hypnotic phenomena make it possible for the patient to readily alter her perception of reality and, thereby, make it possible to have the best possible experience of childbirth. Rather than starting training early, as in most other programs, the training program is planned to be completed as close to the actual delivery as possible. The idea is to enable each woman to use self-hypnosis proficiently during her labor. Much in the same way an athlete is prepared for a championship, the patient intends to peak her hypnotic performance during her labor.

Typically, the prehypnotic induction discussions take place 6 to 8 weeks prior to the expected delivery date. The proposed training protocol is discussed, which will normally take four additional sessions, typically once a week, each lasting about 30 minutes. Sessions are audiotape recorded, so that the woman can use the tape to aid her in her daily practice with hypnosis and hear aspects that they may have forgotten. It also allows her partner and her friends to hear the content, if she so wishes. It is emphasized repeatedly that she will always be in control of her mind when she uses hypnosis.

McCarthy emphasized that one should never make promises that one cannot keep, such as that the patient will have pain-free labor. He believed the best clinical tactic is to always underpromise, and then overdeliver in the teaching of hypnosis to her. The benefits of completing the program as close to actual delivery as possible are discussed with her and she is invited to choose the date for her final training session. This is consistent with always keeping her in control of what is going on. The preinduction discussion is aimed at developing rapport by listening to her, assessing her hypnotic capacity in a clinically sensitive way so as to help her to achieve hypnosis. The practitioner should recognize and be concerned about the patient's wishes, desires, and needs, and be careful to inform her about the process, to seed realistic expectancies and excitement about the delivery process. The patient will then be eager to return to learn more about hypnosis.

Session 1. The first hypnosis session introduces hypnotic trance, in a manner as adopted to the individual person as possible. In general, the session is intended to make the hypnosis experience as simple, effective, soothing, and reassuring as possible. Most frequently, the session includes some form of directed eye closure, with very permissive and empowering language. The concept is to use a simple induction method that will be easy for the patient to remember and repeat in self-hypnosis, such as the progressive muscular relaxation method. Use of the induction protocol from the *Stanford Hypnotic Clinical Scale* would be close to what McCarthy uses, working slowly from the feet and various muscle groups on up throughout the body. As almost directly stated in the *Stanford Hypnotic Clinical Scale,* the person's current state of mind at the end of the muscular relaxation procedure is known as hypnotic trance. The patient then is asked to indicate what she notices about her body now. The notion of "the body" is introduced, rather than "your body," to begin to promote dissociation.

Next, the index finger attraction method of self-hypnosis is employed. She is asked to hold her hands in front of her chest with palms touching, as if praying. She then is told to intertwine her fingertips, and let them rest against the back of the knuckles on "the" other hand. Then she is asked to extend "the" index fingers until they are parallel, separating them by about 2 to 3 centimeters (1 inch). Then she is told to use her conscious mind to look at the gap between the fingers and that if she is ready to go into hypnosis the subconscious mind will close the fingers spontaneously. It is indicated that the point at which the fingers touch is the point at which she can simply close her eyes and take a deep breath, and as she breathes out go back into the same relaxing trance that she experienced with the longer version of the muscle relaxation induction. Each exhalation is intended to allow her to take her deeper and deeper into trance. She is then reminded that she can take herself out of the existing trance simply by counting back from 10 to 1, at which point she will be wide awake, alert, and feeling just fine. She is then congratulated on her hypnotic talent, told to practice what she has learned using the tape of the session that has been provided to her. It is then explained that there is a difference between talent and ability. The point is that she has the talent and that she will learn how to develop it to make it work in practice to help her achieve her goal of a pleasant and rewarding childbirth experience.

Session 2. This session begins by emphasizing the expectation that she should have practiced her self-hypnosis during the previous week, by asking her to put herself into trance using the index-finger attraction method. Then the therapist uses the initiation of trance by the patient as a beginning point to deepen hypnosis with any of the standard deepening techniques employed. Once this has been accomplished, an image of a beach scene is constructed, with waves crashing onto the shore and tumbling on to the beach as they recede. The notion behind this imagery is that the sensations from her contractions can be used as an aid in the visualization of the wave. The incoming wave is a representation of the rising contraction while the wave crashing on the beach is the peak of the contraction, and the wave receding represents the fading of the contraction. The patient is invited to feel the range of sensations that coincide with the images.

Other sensory modalities are also raised, such as the patient's ability to feel sunshine on her face or notice the breeze of sea wind, the sound of the waves crashing and splashing. The olfactory sense is also evoked as she is invited to smell the sea, the sense of touch as the spray touches her lips, and the gustatory sensation of the taste of saltiness. The imagery is intended to fit as closely as possible to the expected physiological inputs, rather then trying to create some idyllic relaxation scene, such as lying on a beach on a calm day. It contrasts sharply with traditional hypnotic procedures, or simple natural childbirth techniques, which emphasize relaxation in face of the need to be involved in contractions. The patient is also told that she can forget that the wave has passed, calling on her ability to produce an amnestic response, assuming that she has demonstrated the ability for amnesia. In so doing, she has amnesia for the associated contraction. As the visualization is well developed, she might even be asked to view the beach and see the high-tide mark, and note that the tide is coming in and that the process is inevitable and cannot be slowed down or sped up in reality. She can simply use her imagery to alter perception of the duration of the contractions and of the resting phases using time distortion. The transition phase of labor involves major contractions at the end; these can be reframed as surfing waves. The patient, of course, is then reminded that there are but a few of these and they mean that it will soon be time to start pushing. She is reminded that she has control, that she can "take the chance if you want, to get on your surf board and ride those waves all the way up the beach."

Because the second stage of labor is characterized by pushing, the desired phenomena can be mimicked in hypnosis using catalepsy, such as the arm catalepsy we discussed earlier in chapter 4. McCarthy suggested that the best imagery he found to approximate the physiological aspect of the second stage of labor is that of "squeezing a tube of toothpaste to empty it completely." Time permitting in this session, she can be asked to use age progression to imagine holding her baby in her arms in the very near future, surrounded by excitement, happiness, and how wonderful she will feel emotionally. Prenatal bonding may also be encouraged by asking the woman to mentally communicate with the fetus and to notice her baby's response. It seems important to ask the woman to practice these skills daily, including communication with the baby. Frequently, women report that if they communicate in such a way, they can feel the baby kick.

Session 3. This session is devoted to mastery of the skills of anesthesia and dissociation. After inducing trance, the woman is invited to simply imagine looking at herself in a full-length mirror. Her attention is drawn to how identical her reflection looks in the mirror, by specifying her eye color, clothes, hair, and so on. Her attention is then drawn to the fact that her rings, for example, are on the opposite hands just as they would be in a real mirror. At this point, the therapist asks her to step into the mirror and change places so that she is the reflection and looks out at herself. Once she is able to image her dissociated, out of body reflection, she is then encouraged to float off to a wonderful idyllic forest with a gurgling stream. Then just beyond the forest is the same beach that was practiced in the previous session. Thus, she can experience the beach and the waves, but as if looking at them from a dissociated point of view. She can observe her physical body from a distance so that if there are complications or special difficulties with labor she will be able to spontaneously or deliberately use this additional skill to dissociate the pain and take herself away from it.

McCarthy taught the woman how to come back into her body and to hyperassociate. The patient is told to place her hand on her thigh and to simply notice the texture of her clothing beneath her finger tips, then the feeling of her skin, and then the feeling of her underlying muscles. She is even asked to go further by imagining the feeling of the femur and to even go on to imagine the bone marrow within the femur and what it feels like. McCarthy stressed that this concept of hyperassociation seems to make complete sense to almost every woman. It is explained that if she hyperassociates like that when having a contraction, she will be able to more fully experience the intensity of the contraction and get more from it.

Anesthesia is then taught using the glove-anesthesia technique. McCarthy simply asked, "Imagine yourself wearing a weird-colored glove, a glove that has been soaked in a powerful local anesthetic solution." Then ask whether the patient is already beginning to notice the changes in the hand. Use hypnotic suggestions to intensify the hypnoanalgesia. She is then told that she is given the option of two alternative hypnotic suggestions, either that she is wearing a pair of tights made of the same material or that she simply step into a hot tub or a pool spa, which is filled with an anesthetic liquid that is the same color as the anesthetic glove. Referring to the history of the patients' prior birth experiences, the therapist may know that the patient had an epidural for some previous birth. If that is the case, the therapist simply asks her to access that memory of the epidural to augment the anesthetic reaction. The procedure often produces excellent lower-body anesthesia. Another technique of inducing glove analgesia that we (J.G.W. and A.F.B.) find to be effective includes the following wording:

"Concentrate on your left hand. As I [or you] stroke the back of that hand, all of the hand including each finger will become increasingly numb. The hand begins to feel like it was made of wood. Sensation is being withdrawn from it, so that when it is pinched you can feel no pain. It feels like it is made of wood and covered with a leather glove. Your arm above the wrist is normally sensitive to all touch, but not the hand. It is almost as if it was no longer a part of you."

Such hypnotic suggestions should be repeated many times. Anesthesia used to be tested by pinpricks applied both to the hand and to the other hand or to the arm above the hand to demonstrate to the patient the reality of the loss of sensation. A far safer method is to use a disposable Wartenberg pinwheel. You can hold the handle in your hand and roll the little wheel of sharp little pins on the patient's alternative hands. The Wartenberg pinwheel points are pointy enough to test sensation to pain but unlike actual pins not sharp enough to puncture the skin. A new version of the Wartenberg wheel tests pain by electrical stimulation using a Violet Wand as used in the cosmetology industry. Electrical stimulation is produced through a Tesla coil, thereby precluding the need for practiced technique to preclude skin punctures as can occasionally occur with the traditional wheel. Another alternative is to use a pair of surgical forceps with rubber tips. Such demonstrations are important and should be performed several times before the patient enters labor so that she will have developed a solid conviction of her ability to shut out pain. Inability to establish an anesthesia after several sessions suggests that hypnosis cannot be relied on to be of much help during the time of labor and delivery. Adequately, hypnotized patients typically should, after training, demonstrate the ability to remain in hypnosis after slowly opening their eyes. This can be another useful test of ensuring at least some hypnotic depth.

We (A.F.B. and J.G.W.) find that a number of obstetricians who use hypnosis favor the more gentle methods, involving relaxation, rather an authoritative approach. This is especially true with the woman who has fewer feminine dependency needs and may have a stronger masculinity component, which is more common today than even 20 years ago. The woman shows considerable resentment, among several of her ego states, against being dominated by men. Inititially, she may appear submissive, but during the period of their relationship the gravida will usually let her doctor know how she feels about her significant other, the kind of relationship they have, and whether she feels controlled by him, and if so, whether she still accepts it or resents it. If she seems to have strong strivings for independence from masculine control, an authoritative manner in the doctor may stimulate resistance to hypnosis and lead to failure in the critical moments of giving birth. At least in one case I (A.F.B.) know of, the mother gave up hypnotic control of pain during delivery when the dominating father was present. An effective although painful punishment for both parents was the result. Once he left the room, hypnotic pain relief was reestablished. The more active hypnosis techniques that reflect the birthing process are much more effective than relaxation-oriented methods, even with patients who have a strong basis for independence. As always, the key is the relationship with the therapist.

Session 4. This session is the final session before the onset of labor, preferably scheduled within 24 hours of giving birth. Unlike the other sessions, this session is first intended to review and clarify any specific details about techniques, rather than to teach new techniques or new hypnotic phenomena. McCarthy's intention is to lessen the pressure of training just before the birthing event. The patient is realistically and honestly praised for her accomplishments and for her disciplined practice of the techniques that are anticipated to show her hypnotic ability in labor. Typically, it is the last time the patient is seen before giving birth. Simple posthypnotic suggestions are given during this session relating to lessening the physical effort of labor and rapid recovery thereafter. The ease of breast-feeding and making adjustments to the role of mother can also be given, as well as suggestions about being able to achieve sound sleep patterns and resume sleep when disturbed. She is encouraged to continue use her hypnotic procedures after delivery for relaxation and anxiety reduction and when breast-feeding to strengthen the emotional bond with her baby.

Normally, at least 10% to 15% of women giving birth experience postnatal depression (MCarthy, 2001). McCarthy taught the patient optimistic thinking to protect against the development of depression. McCarthy also emphasized to the patient that if she continues to practice regular self-hypnosis, the self-discipline of regular practice would be an excellent achievement. At the same time, McCarthy did not overemphasize the importance of practice or give the patient a heavy workload. The idea is that lack of success, therefore, will be entirely due to the doctors failing and not hers. To assess postnatal depression, McCarthy administered the *Edinburgh Postnatal Major Depressive Disorder Scale* (Cox, Murray, & Chapman, 1993; Schaper, Rooney, Kay, & Silva, 1994). He noted that in the 7 years (600 follow-ups) that he had been teaching the program, there was only one brief case of fairly mild, postnatal depression. This is a dramatic result compared to the 10% to 15% normal occurrence. It is also a particularly impressive finding because this special type of depression may be initiated by the enormous changes in hormones that occur soon after birth. Yet numerous researchers have studied the variety of hormones and found no direct link between the incidence or severity of postnatal depression in hormone levels. The problem seemed to occur with attitudes relating to loss of autonomy, loss of personal boundaries, issues of control, pessimism, demands on time, and lasting negative changes in their relationships with their significant other as well as the dramatic lifestyle changes that arise from motherhood. McCarthy recommended a review of Michael Yapko's (1997) work on hypnosis for depression.

Childbirth by Hypnosis: The Oster Method

Unlike the McCarthy procedure, psychologist Mark Oster has developed a method intended to assist patients in their preparation for medical procedures rather than to eliminate any medical aspect of the procedure, such as chemoanalgesia or other medications. However, the reduction in such a need can be expected as a benefit of the approach. The procedure is intended to give the patient a greater sense of self-control and to increase her participation in the entire process so she can better assist her physician when needed. It is also aimed at making it an easier and less complicated recovery without the use of medication. Typically, patients are able to transfer what they learn in the 1-hour sessions to other situations. The total time involved in using Oster's procedure is 6 hours rather than the typical 2 hours involved in the previous procedure. However, Oster pointed out that after about four sessions, the patient is usually quite adequately prepared for the procedure and has mastery in the use of self-hypnosis when required. The entire procedure is intended to empower the patient so she can ask questions of the doctor as needed and to discuss any issues with any other health care personal relating to test procedures and any examinations being conducted. Of course, a major goal is to reframe the patient's perspective from "what is being done or happening to me" to "what are we doing together."

Session 1. In this session, Oster is primarily concerned with establishing rapport as well as interviewing the patient about her personal interests, hobbies, beliefs, and values. This information is used to individualize hypnosis and to help develop the metaphors and images that are created for the patient. The initial assessments are intended to determine the suitability of hypnosis for the patient. The interview is intended to rule out contraindications for hypnosis and to provide the opportunity for formal hypnotic assessment if appropriate and other psychological assessments as necessary. The patient can be introduced to hypnosis in this session or early in Session 2. The patient's questions about hypnosis are answered, common myths about hypnosis are dispelled, and information on the patient's previous personal experiences with hypnosis, if any, is sought.

Next, the focus is on neutralizing any problem perceptions acquired through negative views about hypnosis or past experiences with hypnosis, which more frequently then not have been with a lay therapist. However, if past experiences were positive, inquiry is made of those experiences; this information is then used to help further establish a positive relationship with the patient. It is emphasized that hypnosis is a cooperative, interpersonal process that exists between the doctor and the patient, rather than something that is done to the patient. Self-control and active versus passive participation, for both the hypnosis experience and the procedure, should be emphasized, as well as cooperation that extends to asking the patient to provide feedback regarding any phrases or methods that might be particularly useful or particularly unpleasant. The content of the phasing is then, of course, adjusted accordingly.

Session 2. This session is used to finish preparation of the patient for hypnosis. This session is devoted to the initial hypnotic induction, including deepening and termination. The session is intended only to address the experience of hypnosis, without any therapeutic demand or introduced expectations. Ratification of the experience of hypnosis includes hypnotic suggestions for alteration of hand temperature and limb or body anesthesia using the typical methods discussed elsewhere in this book. Catalepsy can also be induced and opening of the eyes, while talking in trance and posthypnotic suggestion can be tested. The patient is also introduced to dissociation by means of the notion of "parts" of the unconscious mind, where each part has a specific hypnotic function.

Session 3. This session emphasizes use of parts of the mind introduced at the end of Session 2. The first part of the mind is the one that the patient uses to induce trance and terminate trance. Commentary reinforces the patient's awareness of changes in her ability to control various sensations in her body. Part two of the mind is devoted to creating a special place where she can retreat from her concerns. The special place induction certainly could be similar to the procedure reviewed in the McCarthy protocol. Oster emphasized that the patient can choose whether to share what she might have previously used for such a place. The special place imagery is enhanced by using many different sensory modes, including visual, auditory, olfactory, gustatory, and kinestheic, as well as emotional, as in the McCarthy approach we reviewed in detail earlier. Finally, each modality is noted as serving as a special signal for deepening the experience and as a cue for extending to the next mode. This unique and clever technique serves as a way of enhancing the experience and deepening the hypnosis at the same time.

In part three of the mind, the patient is told that the unconscious mind engages further in the deepening process. This includes age regression to locate positive memories. The focus is intended not to be psychotherapeutic but merely to identify positive past memories that might be used to promote a form of adaptive dissociation during the childbirth process, if required. Ideomotor signals are used so the patient can cue the therapist as to her movement through the process. Touch is used to deepen the trance. Once part four of the unconscious mind is solicited, further deepening is suggested so that in the next session the fourth part will have the capacity to begin the preparation. However, in the current session, part four of the mind is used to begin various trance ratification exercises. Suggestions for self-hypnosis are also provided. Termination is begun by moving back through the process and back through each of the parts of the mind. It is the first part that induces hypnosis, and now it is used to terminate hypnosis for her. Following termination of hypnosis, the experience is reviewed with the patient in the alert wakeful state.

In this third session, the patient's experiences from the previous session are first discussed. Problem areas, if any, are addressed and modifications for the next induction are considered. In this session, the induction begins as in the previous session, allowing for implementation of the modifications as needed. Hypnosis involves a patient proceeding through the second and third parts of the mind as in the previous session, but in a briefer manner. Deepening is a primary goal of third part. The fourth part of the mind then engages in hypnotic rehearsal, beginning the day when the patient wakes up in the morning, rather than at arrival at the hospital where the procedure will take place. Each event is intended to serve as an activation signal for the hypnotic process and to enhance the deepening process. If at any time during the process the patient becomes uncomfortable or anxious, she is then encouraged to quickly and effortlessly return to her special place. The patient signals that she has done so, using an ideomotor signal such as moving a specific finger agreed upon in advance. Each event that occurs is intended to serve as a signal to enter the trance, deepen the trance, or create relaxation. The idea is to foster a sense of mastery and to help maintain a sense of calm throughout the procedure. A sense of emotional control comes with a knowledge and understanding of what is happening as it happens and what will be happening next.

Session 4. This session begins like the third session. There is a discussion of the previous session and any modifications necessary to increase the quality of the hypnotic experience for the patient are recorded by the therapist. These modifications are then used to further improve upon the hypnotic training.

Sessions 5 and 6. These sessions are shorter in length, usually 30 to 60 minutes. The intention is to proceed as in the previous two sessions, but to proceed more quickly and with greater flexibility so that the patient can create her own experiences. These experiences are recorded so that they can be brought to bear, if needed, during the birthing process. The session is also intended to provide a kind of "fine tuning" of the hypnotic procedures in preparation for the birthing event.

The period of questioning and desensitizing is followed by relaxation exercises accompanied by simple inductions such as eye fixation or arm drop (see chapter 5). The aim is to help the patient to raise her pain threshold and to teach her to be able to establish a glove anesthesia.

Suggestions to induce a glove anesthesia following an induction might be administered as we described earlier.

Such hypnotic suggestions should be repeated many times, especially during the early training sessions. Oster tested anesthesia by pinpricks applied both to the hand or arm to demonstrate to the patient the reality of the loss of sensation. Such demonstrations are important and should be performed several times before the patient enters labor so that she will have developed confidence in her ability to control pain. Inability to establish anesthesia after several sessions suggests that hypnosis cannot be relied on to be of much help during the time of labor and delivery. Typical patients with moderate or better hypnotizability will, after training, demonstrate the ability to remain in hypnosis while opening their eyes. This can be another useful way of assuring the patient that they are at least experiencing a moderate level of hypnotic "depth."

Obstetricians who use hypnosis frequently favor the more gentle method, involving relaxation, over an authoritative approach. This is especially true where the woman has many aggressive needs, may have a strong masculinity component, or shows considerable resentment against being dominated by men. During the period of their relationship, the gravida will usually let her doctor know how she feels about her husband, the kind of relationship they have, and whether she feels controlled by him and, if so, whether she accepts it or resents it. If she seems to have strong strivings for independence from masculine control, an authoritative manner in the doctor may stimulate resistance to hypnosis.

Hypnosis During the Postpartum Period

Assuming childbirth by hypnosis has gone well as expected and little if any chemoanesthesia has been used during delivery, it is usually quite possible for the patient to get off the delivery table and return to her room. This experience will provide her with a deep sense of accomplishment and mastery of the situation. Thus, morale is improved and the speed of recovery enhanced. More important, she retains the ability to induce anesthesia in the perineum, which she can use to lessen discomfort during this period.

Hypnosis can also be used to promote or suppress lactation even within the first 48 hours in those women who wish to nurse. Kroger (1963) reported the only study published to date was conducted in Russia, which claimed 95% success in stimulating milk production in some 77 women. Hypnosis can be used to stimulate lactation by the patient's using visual imagery of holding the baby in her arms and feeling its head against her breast. Imagery can be further enhanced by inducing the sensation that the milk is flowing. Research is needed to determine whether hypnosis secures better results than the hormones that are commonly used.

Summary

Whether Rank's (1952) hypothesis that the birth trauma is the original source of an individual's anxiety (because of separation from the mother) is true, the addition of chemoanesthesia, which drugs the child and the mother, can certainly add to the hazard the infant faces upon entry into this world. Childbirth, when traumatic to the mother, is very likely to be traumatic to the child. Such trauma can affect the child's emotional and intellectual development. The beginning of the mother-child relationship is certainly critical. If childbirth can be accomplished without undue pain, the mother's attitudes toward the child may be substantially more positive than if birth was accompanied by much suffering. The positive effects of hypnosis for childbirth have been well documented in clinical situations. As Patrick McCarthy (personal communication to A.F.B., January 2004) pointed out, "It is a lot more easy and enjoyable to use hypnosis to treat a dozen very pregnant women who are a bit anxious than it is to use hypnosis to treat one very anxious woman who is a bit pregnant."

Chapter 12
Mind–Body Interaction I:
Hypnosis in Internal Medicine

Mind and body interaction has become a matter of increased interest to health practitioners and the public. The National Institutes of Health (NIH) established the National Center for Complementary and Alternative Medicine (NCCAM) in 1996. The NCCAM gives national recognition to the role that psychological factors play in producing tangible and physical manifestations of illness. Of course, Freud's discoveries led us first to consider mind-body interactions and the terms "psychosomatic" and "psychophysiologic," which were employed to indicate such conditions in the practice of medicine.

F. Alexander (1939) embraced the psychophysiological perspective from a psychoanalytic point of view. Others, such as Flanders Dunbar (1938), took a more eclectic approach. However, in all of the approaches in the era, psychogenic factors were usually perceived as contributory only to the primary physiological etiology of such disorders as bronchial asthma, peptic ulcers, hypertension, and so on. Before the NIH (1996), recognition of hypnosis and other specific psychological approaches as efficacious psychological treatments were considered by most internists and general practice physicians as secondary or at best adjunctive to the various drugs. The recent attention to the application of psychological techniques in the problems of general practice, highlighted by the creation of the NCCAM, is in no small part due to the U.S. government's revelation that Americans spend about 23 billion dollars a year on alternative medicine.

The Effects of Psychogenic Factors on Organic Illness

More than four decades ago, Raginsky (1963) tried to bring attention to the fact that half of all medical illnesses are probably functional (psychologically caused) and that an enormous range of emotions are expressed through physiological processes. Furthermore, psychogenic factors are being increasingly recognized as playing a significant role in the etiology of various organic diseases. Fatigue may often be psychological, as intrapsychic conflicts exhaust the patient's energies. Worry and depression can result from a patient's concern about his or her poor health, and the depression by itself may cause physical symptoms. Sometimes anxiety is channeled into psychosomatic symptoms, and the patient remains unaware of the underlying conflicts that are creating the anxiety. Patients of this type are often uncooperative and refuse to listen to their doctors. They do not wish to face the underlying emotional meaning of their symptoms. Such meanings can be primary to their symptoms, contributory, maintaining, or a consequence of them. In fact, patients can have a number of unconscious fantasies connected to their illness, which can be discovered through hypnotic uncovering such as can be rapidly acquired by ego-state therapy (Emmerson, 2003; J. Watkins & H. Watkins, 1997). (Hypnotic interventions are explained in our Volume II, *Hypnoanalytic Techniques*. When underlying psychogenic conflicts have played a significant role in creating an illness, patients who recover because of the impact of medication may not welcome their return to health but instead compulsively seek some other crippling disability. This is why it is important, even in the treatment of ostensibly organic disorders, to understand just what the illness means to the patient. Otherwise, the doctor's efforts at cure may be like swimming upstream. The motivational current within patients will be opposing the treatment. Entire individuals, not merely their symptoms, must be treated. It is possible that many reported side effects of drugs may actually be symptom substitutions by patients who are psychologically resistant to treatment.

Even though a disorder is psychogenically caused, it may result in physical stresses, which in time initiate permanent organic damage. An individual with a hysterically paralyzed hand was relieved of his paralysis by hypnotherapy (J. Watkins, 1949). However, he had held it for some 14 months in a tightly clenched manner, resulting in considerable atrophy in his fingers. Much of the atrophy became permanent, and despite extensive physiotherapy only partial motility could be restored.

Precautions in the Use of Hypnosis

Some general policies regarding the use of hypnosis in general medical conditions are in order here. It is usually appropriate to deal with minor symptoms first and to evaluate the response. However, major symptoms might be more likely rooted in significant psychological conflicts and, therefore, will be more resistant to change. If the minor symptoms respond readily, one can then move to hypnosis to ameliorate or eliminate the more important ones.

Far too much has been made about the potential hazards of symptom suppression through hypnosis, but the prudent therapist will always consider this factor. Hypnotic suggestion is an intervention into psychological (and hence physiological) processes that alters disease–health equilibriums. Such interventions may be permanent. The underlying meaning to the patient of his or her illness and the meaning of the intervention will interact to determine its efficacy. When the disease process is circular and self-reinforcing, for example, depression as a reaction to a physical symptom may aggravate the symptom, and the hypnotic suggestion may successfully alter the malevolent cycle by providing the patient with coping methods. Hypnosis, framed correctly for the patient, can be used to give the patient choice. The patient, by virtue of training in hypnosis, is given a new option. He or she can experience the negative symptom or choose not to experience it. Alternatively, the patient may simply choose to modulate the symptom as needed. The point is, if handled correctly by the therapist, patients have a new level of control over their lives.

The concept that physical treatments such as drugs and physical exercise are appropriate for psychological symptoms like anxiety and depression is widely understood. Because of the cost constraints of managed care in the 21st century and the long periods required for many psychotherapeutic treatments, psychiatrists are returning to the more somatic approaches in therapy. With the dawn of brief and effective interventions such as ego-state therapy, psychoanalytic approaches are finding a resurgence in acceptance. However, for decades classical long-term psychoanalysis has suffered because of the immense amount of time and effort required of a highly specialized therapist. The search for briefer approaches is being recognized more and more widely as having been answered by hypnoanalytic rather than standard psychoanalytic interventions.

The ability of hypnosis to influence physiological functioning has been clearly supported by numerous studies. Since this work is centered primarily on hypnotherapeutic technique, we (A.F.B. and J.G.W.) do not try in any comprehensive way to review the enormous amount of literature, which has shown that many cardiovascular, cutaneous, gastric, and many other physiological functions are subject to influence by hypnosis.

Hypnotherapeutic techniques have long been recognized as being effective in the management of psychogenic illnesses. But only recently (see

Hebert, 1998, for a review) has it been recognized as effective in helping to manage organic disorders. A few studies from our lab at Washington State University are illustrative. For example, in the national award-winning research of Ruzyla-Smith, A. Barabasz, M. Barabasz and Warner (1995) the effects of hypnosis, relaxation, and control conditions were tested on the immune systems of 65 healthy university students who were stringently divided on the basis of hypnotizability. Only the hypnotizable participants in the hypnosis condition showed significant alteration of the immune response as measured by B cells and helper T cells. Using A. Barabasz's alert induction procedure (A. Barabasz, 1985; A. Barabasz & Barabasz, 1996), hypnosis also has been shown to facilitate neurotherapy for attention-deficit/hyperactivity disorder (Anderson, Barabasz, Barabasz, & Warner, 2000; A. Barabasz & Barabasz, 1994b, 1995, 1996, 2000; A. Barabasz, Crawford, & Barabasz, 1993).

Curiously, all of this began nearly half a century ago. In 1958, the second author (J.G.W.) attended a meeting of the Academy of Psychosomatic Medicine in which a paper was presented by a physician who was using hypnosis to treat carcinomas — not the pain but the cancer itself. There was much skepticism among the physicians attending. Decades later, research funding from the NIH made it possible for David Spiegel and his colleagues at Stanford University to demonstrate convincingly the effects of hypnosis on cancer. Their 10-year follow-up of nearly 100 cancer patients revealed that self-hypnosis training in group therapy not only reduced cancer pain but also extended life by an average of 1.5 years for terminal patients. Further detail and hypnotic interventions appear later in this chapter, in the section "Hypnosis in the Treatment of Cancer." It is in such ways that hypnosis has proven valuable by increasing resistance to disease, potentiating drug effects, and perhaps stimulating the immunological system. It has been employed throughout a wide range of physical disorders.

Hypnosis as an Aid to Diagnostic Procedures

Many diagnostic procedures that involve penetration of body orifices can be painful. These include such instruments as the gastroscope, bronchoscope, laryngoscope, nasoscope, vaginoscope, and proctoscope, as well as a range of procedures in interventional radiology. The relaxed cooperation of the patient is greatly desired during such procedures. If the patient tightens up, he or she may prevent insertion of the instruments and cause tissue damage. In extreme cases, local or even general anesthesia maybe required, if hypnotic intervention is unavailable.

One of the greatest values of hypnosis is relaxation, reduction of anxiety, positive attitudes, and willingness to cooperate. Furthermore, because hypnosis permits a focusing of attention (or inattention), the hypnotic suggestions can be directed toward or away from a specific body area. One can suggest to hypnotized patients pleasant reveries that can effectively dissociate their attention from the site of the diagnostic exploration. It is wise for the doctor to inquire about fantasies or memories that are associated with pleasurable and relaxed feelings. On the basis of this information, hypnotic suggestions, which correspond to these specifics, can be formulated. The patient is encouraged to continue experiencing the described scenes or fantasies during the time the diagnostic procedures are being undertaken. Using deep hypnosis, amnesia for the entire experience can be suggested, thus setting aside painful or potentially traumatic memories, which can be dealt with more easily, if needed, after the patient recovers.

Even the more comfortable and painless diagnostic procedures, such as an echocardiogram, may precipitate anxiety because of conflicts over the regions of the body under exploration or fears as to what might be found. A patient suffering from a respiratory disorder may be tense because of fears of suffocation. Then even the sight of the bronchoscope will initiate a paralyzing fear or a complete lack of cooperation. Violent gagging may follow attempts to do a gastroscopy. In some cases, the individual will not relax the glottis sufficiently to permit introduction of the gastroscope.

Proctological examination may precipitate anxiety in patients who have conflicts over bowel and anal function. Various hypnotic techniques may be of use here. For those patients capable of a deep level of hypnotic trance, the procedures can be conducted as if they were under a general anesthesia. One can suggest that the patient relax, show no physical response, and be amnesic to the entire procedure upon emerging from hypnosis. It is not necessary to achieve an extremely deep state for hypnosis to be of assistance. General suggestions, using light trance, of calmness, lowering of anxiety, and relaxation of sphincters can aid greatly in completing a satisfactory examination. However, in some procedures, patients may complain of pain. In such instances, hypnotic analgesia for the relevant areas may be sufficient to ameliorate it.

In one case, an internist wished to use a string test to assist in locating the site of the gastrointestinal hemorrhage. The patient could not tolerate the string and went into continuous gagging. However, using only light hypnosis, she became calm, relaxed her throat muscles, and permitted the string to remain for enough time to locate a duodenal ulcer. For the extremely tense and anxiety-ridden patient, hypnotic relaxation may accomplish as much or more than medicinal sedation without any of the side effects often associated with such drugs. The usual principles applying to hypnotic suggestion, as we described in the earlier chapter, should be employed.

Poor cooperation of patients in some diagnostic procedures may be due to a deep, unconscious meaning or conflict. For example, insertion of a speculum may precipitate rape fears, whereas in males the proctoscope can initiate images of homosexual rape. In male individuals who have latent homosexual tendencies, this sometimes results in a panic reaction. If the patient shows evidence of such a disturbance, no attempt should be made to continue the examination until reassurance and hypnotic relaxation have reestablished the patient's self-control. The clinician who is intent on the physical examination and who ignores the signs of psychological distress may create a psychologically traumatized patient. Even internists trained in dealing with rape fears are very unlikely to be trained to treat the condition of "latent homosexuality." This task requires the skill of experienced psychotherapists. However, their awareness of the possibilities for trauma to such patients can have much to do with averting the creation of a new psychiatric problem.

Hypnosis in the Treatment of Cardiovascular Disorders

Cardiologists have learned not to reveal undue concern to a patient upon listening to a heart murmur. Such concerns can become readily apparent to the patient. Audio amplified echocardiograms can be disconcerting to the uninitiated patient, even without the appearance of a disorder. If the patient becomes alarmed, a fixation may be established on the cardiac region, and a mild or nonexistent heart condition can be elaborated into a cardiac neurosis.

More than half a century ago, Kline (1950) described the case of an individual who reported "heavy pressure around the heart" accompanied by much anxiety. In hypnosis, Kline regressed his patient back to a previous medical checkup, during which the examining physician, after listening with the stethoscope, called in another doctor to do the same thing. This triggered an anxiety reaction. After the patient had recalled and relived the incident using hypnotic regression, the symptom ceased. This technique can be useful in any case of suspected iatrogenic symptom fixation.

Heart rate can be influenced by a number of psychological factors. Hypnotic suggestion can be combined with biofeedback procedures to slow down heart rates. The attentional process of concentration, particularly in the early stages of a hypnotic induction itself, usually increases heart rate. Heart rate can also be increased by direct hypnotic suggestions, such as having the patient imagine being in a car accident, or by indirect hypnotic suggestions tailored to the patient's personal history.

Efforts to reduce blood pressure through hypnotic suggestion have, in general, been unsuccessful. However, three decades ago Deabler, Fidel, and Dillenkoffer (1973) reported that they were able to decrease both systolic and diastolic pressures using hypnotic suggestion. A year later, Brady, Luborsky, and Cron (1974) described a metronome induction procedure to reduce blood pressure in patients with confirmed essential hypertension. Audiotaped instructions emphasized hypnotic suggestions for relaxation with the verbalizations synchronized to the metronome ticking at 60 beats to the minute. Given such little supporting data, we can only conclude that this area needs further investigation. Obviously, hypnosis may be considered as a possible approach, perhaps as an adjunct to medication, when other methods have not been effective. In these cases, the patient should be taught relaxation and self-hypnosis because he or she may need to use self-hypnosis several times a day to accomplish and maintain a set medical goal.

One patient I (A.F.B.) saw was a Royal New Zealand Air Force pilot who had a phobic reaction to the inflation of the blood pressure cuff. This produced false high readings. He managed to "barely pass" his medical reexaminations after a course of 10 sessions of systematic desensitization, followed by daily practice (in vivo exposure) using the sphygmomanometer to check his blood pressure. The more he practiced the better he became at producing normal range blood pressure readings. However, as time went on the anxiety reduction became specific to the patient's or therapist's measures of blood pressure. His response no longer generalized to readings taken by the examining physicians or nurses. The pilot's *Stanford Hypnotic Clinical Scale* score was at the average level, but this was more than sufficient to facilitate his response to the direct suggestion that "it will be easy and natural to remain as relaxed as you are now when you take your own blood pressure or when others take it for you. In fact, it will be easier without having to bother with the reading, bulb squeezing, and cuff inflation." In this case, a single session of hypnosis was more effective than the whole course of systematic desensitization had been previously. His medical exams for the entire follow-up period of 18 months remained in the normal range. Let us remember that in this case, we were dealing with a simple phobic reaction rather than treating a blood pressure–related disease process.

Relaxation in cardiac patients can be facilitated best by using hypnosis to initiate fantasies, such as lying on a beach, relaxing on a grassy hillside, and so on, rather than direct verbal suggestions such as "You will relax." Picturing scenes in which relaxation comes indirectly as a consequence of vivid imaginal involvement is much more effective. Kroger and Fezler

(1976) indicated that hypnotic suggestion of warmth paired with relaxation may improve compromised coronary circulation in cases of angina pectoris. They also report success in using hypnotic age regression to ameliorate and relieve arrhythmias due to rheumatic fever in childhood. Again, controlled experimental research is still lacking.

The effect that hypnosis can have on a cardiac patient was dramatically illustrated in a classic case by Raginsky (1963). A patient who had previously suffered cardiac arrest during an operation was induced under hypnosis to relieve his anxiety about that procedure. During this experimental episode, his heart ceased for some four beats as measured on the electrocardiogram. This case illustrates that hypnosis can be a very potent technique and can produce serious consequences. It must be employed with professional skill if harmful side effects are to be prevented.

Buerger's and Raynaud's diseases result in restricted flow of blood to the extremities. There are a number of reports of hypnotic treatment of these conditions (A. Barabasz, 1977, pp. 24-28; Crasilneck & Hall, 1985; Jacobson, Hackett, Surman & Silverberg, 1973; Norris & Huston, 1956). Suggestions were given in hypnosis aimed at increasing flow of blood to the arms, hands, or legs. We have found that having hypnotized patients visualize putting their hands into a basin of warm water significantly increased skin temperature in the fingers an average of 4° F in a group of eight patients. Vivid descriptions by the therapist and clear imaginings by the patient are essential for success with this technique. E. Hilgard (personal communication to A.F.B., 1992,) observed that if "the Hypnotizability Scales do not predict responsiveness to this form of imagery, a light trance will work."

Because being overweight is associated with heart conditions, treatment of obesity in the cardiac patient is frequently indicated. Fortunately, hypnotherapy has been found to be of considerable value. A meta-analysis of 18 studies of hypnosis as an adjunct to cognitive-behavioral psychotherapy (Kirsch, Montgomery, & Sapirstein, 1995) showed that patients who underwent hypnotherapy showed greater improvement than at least 70% of clients receiving nonhypnotic treatment. The effects, recognized as efficacious by the NIH, were particularly pronounced for treatments of obesity (see also M. Barabasz & Spiegel, 1989; Kirsch, 1996). We describe hypnotic techniques for dealing with this problem in chapter 14.

Hypnosis in the Treatment of Respiratory Disorders
Breathing is a function normally under conscious control. But in certain conditions, such as an asthma attack, it is closely related to fear and anger.

A highly emotional experience can be sufficient to set it off. Afterwards, fear of dying may continue and reinforce the attack. A vicious cycle is thus set up. The disease is considered to be psychosomatic, because either or both the presence of chemical allergens plus emotional conflicts can serve as the triggering mechanism. Allergic reactions may also result from learning or conditioning. For example, some sufferers who have an allergy to roses may produce an asthmatic attack upon being brought into the presence of paper roses.

Because hypnosis is able to produce relaxation and lowered anxiety, its efficacy in the treatment of such conditions has been reported in many clinical reports for more than half a century (A. Barabasz, 1977; Collison, 1975, 1978; Marchesi, 1949; Van Pelt, 1949). Raginsky (1963) explained that asthmatics are characterized by conflicts related to the suppression of any sort of "intense emotion" and by threats to dependent relationships and to the security based upon them. Asthmatics have often learned to use their symptoms to control and force significant others to reinforce their dependency needs. French and Alexander (1941) described the asthmatic attack as a "cry for mother." Accordingly, a direct suggestive assault on the main symptoms often results in worsening instead of amelioration. Rather than use direct hypnotic suggestion to suppress the symptoms, doctors should make it possible for the patient to ventilate fears and develop the relaxation response to help him or her gain ego strength.

A variety of special hypnotic suggestions for relieving asthmatic attacks and reconditioning the breathing habits of asthmatic patients have been tested in clinical settings. Vivid imagining in hypnosis can be a valuable technique. Thus, the Spiegels (H. Spiegel & D. Spiegel, 2004) used hypnosis to help their patients to create a vivid image of tubes in the lungs slowly opening up. This is followed with hypnotic suggestions that the patient will experience "cool, fresh air entering their lungs." However, most are aimed at providing an option for the patient to control the attack with some form of relaxation.

One of the most effective approaches, which has stood the test of time, emphasizes that it is quite important for the clinician to time hypnotic suggestions so that some are given while the patient is inhaling and others during the patient's exhalation (Jencks, 1978). The goal is to reverse the asthmatic patient's tendency to increase the period of inhalation and shorten that of exhalation. She presented a series of respiration exercises and accompanying fantasies as follows:

1. *Long breath* for relaxation and a slower breathing rhythm imagine that the inhaled air enters at the fingertips, goes up the arms into the

298 • Hypnotherapeutic Techniques

shoulders and chest, and then, during exhalation, down through the trunk into the legs and leisurely out at the toes. Repeat a few times.

2. *Warm shower* to counteract tension in the shoulder and neck region, imagine water from a warm shower streaming pleasantly over the back of the head, shoulders, and neck. Feel the warmth and relaxation during exhalations.

3. *Imagined pathways* for easing the breathing or relieving pressures, imagine that the breathed air streams in and out easily at any of the places where relief is needed. Asthma patients found relief by "breathing through the small of the back;" tension headaches may be relieved by "inhaling or exhaling through the top of the head or the temples;" and "breathing through the holes under the chin" opened up the sinuses.

4. *Opening flower* to counteract anxiety and feelings of tightness in throat, chest, or abdomen, imagine during exhalations a flower bud opening at the right place, as in time-lapse (computer controlled) photography. Repeat and feel the opening for several exhalations.

5. *Bellows* to ease the breathing or to increase the vital capacity, breathe as if your lungs were bellows, which draw air in and push it out. Imagine that the air streams in and out freely and easily.

6. *Golden thread and clothes hanger* for a well-aligned posture with an alive yet relaxed feeling, imagine a golden, energizing thread all the way up the spine and through the crown of the head. Imagine being held from above by this thread, so that straightness is achieved effortlessly. Imagine during inhalations that the thread is pulled from above and invigoration streams into the spine from below. Imagine during exhalations that the tissues of the shoulder region are soothingly and loosely draped over the shoulder blades or over a suspended clothes hanger.

7. *Toad* for ego strengthening, inhale and imagine blowing yourself up to an enormous size, like a toad does. Let yourself stay this size in your mind while you relax during exhalations.

Readers with a background in meditation or yoga will no doubt recognize some of the similarities between Jencks' procedure and Taoist "Microcosmic Orbit Meditation." If your patient has an interest in meditation, as a number of patients who seek out hypnosis often do, you may wish to adapt the relevant aspects of the process to your hypnotic induction for relief of asthma. We discuss meditation-based hypnosis and Taoist-based induction, developed by the first author, in chapter 14 in the section titled "Meditation and Hypnosis for Health."

Hypnotic abreactions can also be quite effective. In this technique, the effort is made to release bound-up tension and provide other outlets for rage and fear. Abreaction borders between a symptom-manipulation technique and a hypnoanalytic one, in which the goal is resolution of psychogenic conflicts. It can be effective in bringing great relief to the over-controlled patient. Our Volume II, *Hypnoanalytic Techniques,* reviews several alternative techniques for achieving abreactions that can produce profound and lasting results in very brief periods of therapy.

It is critically important to remember that studies reporting on the efficacy of hypnotherapy are not valid unless careful attention has been given to the manner in which the induction was conducted, the exact wording of the suggestions, and the manner in which they are presented. Two hypnotherapists could read off the same script of words, but by their manner of rendition and by the way in which they relate to their patients, they can produce very different treatment outcomes. Experimentally controlled EEG event related potential brain studies have clearly shown that even slight wording differences in hypnotic suggestions can produce bi-directional results (A. Barabasz et al., 1999) and that the induction can make an enormous difference in outcome and effects on the organism (A. Barabasz, 2000).

Relaxation. Most people who are knowledgeable about asthma treatment stress the need for relaxation and the slowing of breathing. Fortunately, hypnosis is an extremely effective method to induce such a reaction when the patient is at least of average hypnotizability. It thus becomes the method of choice, even though all too frequently the patient arrives at the office of a hypnotherapist only as a last resort, after inhalators and drugs have not proven to be effective or have been of limited value.

Asthma frequently involves a secondary reaction to even a slight breathing difficulty. The patient needs to feel that he or she can induce and stop an attack. One approach I (A.F.B.) have found to be effective with a significant number of patients is to couple the onset of an attack with the posthypnotic suggestion to enter trance, as soon as circumstances allow, just by rolling the eyes up and then silently repeating the hypnotic suggestions found to be effective in heterohypnosis. Frequently, this can simply involve repetition of the word *calm* at each exhalation while imagining working freely and normally.

Crasilneck and Hall (1985) described to their young asthmatic patients a television fantasy of horses that are running fast and, hence, breathing heavily. When the horses slow down and walk normally, their breathing becomes calm and they wheeze less. As the breathing of the horses slows, the young patients are taught to slow their own breathing likewise. They then suggest that the patients will have this same experience (e.g., the slowing of rapid breathing) each time they enter a hypnotic trance. I (A.F.B.) emphasize, "Breathing will be normal when awakening from hypnosis and when fully alert, wide awake, calm, and confident — normal good breathing."

Crasilneck and Hall (1985) also reported a case of coughing that accompanied an ulcerative mucosal lesion on the tracheal bifurcation. The coughing continued even after the ulcer had healed. The patient was given the suggestions that "Your throat muscles will be relaxed and at ease. The itchy irritability will decrease. Your breathing will be normal and easy." After 5 days of hypnotherapy, his cough ceased.

Desensitization. Kroger and Fezler (1976) reported a number of studies in which the behavioral technique of systematic desensitization combined with hypnosis (see also A. Barabasz, 1977) was effective in reducing wheezing. Unlike the behaviorists who were uninformed about hypnosis, they noted that highly hypnotizable patients tended to make the best response. They view asthma as a conditioned reflex and perceive the therapeutic task as one of reconditioning. The patient is taught in hypnosis to reexperience a relaxing episode from the past when he or she senses an attack coming on. For some unexplained reason, few clinicians use this approach today, but Kroger and Fezler indicated very good results a quarter of a century ago. The approach remains worthy of use and further research.

Hypnosis in the Treatment of Gastrointestinal Disorders

As an organ system, the digestive tract is especially sensitive to emotional influences. One does not have to accept the classical Freudian view that "oral" activities represent the first and most elemental stage of personality organization to recognize that the giving of food and drink is a common sign of affection. We take people we like out to dinner. We buy them a drink. We eat when we are disturbed or unhappy. We imbibe alcoholic beverages to quiet our nerves or to relax with our friends. We refer to an individual as having a "sweet" disposition, and to a loved one as a "sweetheart." A person who impresses us unfavorably may be called "sour," and an angry individual is described as "bitter." A manner of personality may be termed "salty," and an individual close to us may be called "honey." Sometimes we can hardly "stomach" dealing with another person who "gripes" at us, and it is "shitty" when we are treated badly. A courageous individual may be described as having "guts," whereas the colloquial term for the anus is used as a sign of derision. No wonder the gastrointestinal system is imbued with such a rich set of meanings and emotions. It makes sense to expect that tangled interpersonal relationships, struggles between love and hate, problems of fear and rage, could be translated into disturbances of the digestive tract in whole or part from entrance to exit.

Swallowing problems. Resistance to oral intake may begin even before the act of swallowing. Probably first to address the difficulties some people have in swallowing pills was Secter (1973), who described an interesting imaging subject-object technique to alleviate the problem. The patient is told to visualize another person who is trying to swallow a pill, but who chokes on it. The patient is induced to identify with this individual and then told in hypnosis to observe that after "our friend" has been given a signal to relax his or her throat muscles, he or she can calmly take the pill. The patient is then induced to see himself in the place of the previously imagined individual and prepare himself to relax on signal so as to be able to swallow the pill.

Anorexia nervosa is one disorder that appears to be directly related to psychological problems. Raginsky (1963) described the successful treatment of such a case by "nonspecific suggestions for relaxation comfort and hope." However, a family conflict was also revealed that involved dissension between the patient's parents. Agreement of the mother for hypnotherapy, followed by a request from the patient that his mother "feed him," when fulfilled, reversed the process of food avoidance. Although the patient was close to death when first seen, he recovered and eventually became a physician. It is important to note that hypnosis worked only when the family's emotional problem was treated simultaneously. This indicates that suggestive hypnosis alone may need to be supplemented by at least some relationship or insight therapy. Hypnosis may be critical to treatment success, but it is best to be thought of as an adjunct to comprehensive treatment rather than a treatment in and of itself.

The *dumping syndrome* was participant to a substantial amount of study decades ago. It is characterized by sweating, diarrhea, anorexia, nausea, and weakness. Although the origin may be organic, it has a strong psychological component. Progressive relaxation enhanced by hypnosis has been found to be effective in relieving its most acute symptoms.

Dorcus and Goodwin (1955) reported previous studies that had shown that duodenal ulcer patients who developed dumping syndromes following subtotal gastrectomies tended to score high on the *Taylor Scale of Manifest Anxiety* and on the "Neurotic Triad" scales of the *Minnesota Multiphasic Personality Test* (MMPI). In an application of these findings, they employed hypnotherapy with four such patients. The hypnotic suggestions were directed towards reducing tension, removal of fear of this condition, and enhancing the olfactory qualities of food and the feeling of comfort with food or liquid intake. All four patients responded favorably.

Doberneck, Griffen, Papermaster, Bonello, and Wangensteen (1959) combined hypnosis with group therapy in the successful treatment of chronic dumping syndromes. Bonello, Doberneck, and Papermaster (1960) reported symptomatic success in some 56% of 36 gastrectomy patients.

Although all of these studies employed hypnosis as the primary technique, it is important to consider the possible meaning of the dumping syndrome as involving anger, hate, and resentment, which have been symbolized in the rejection of food. Accordingly, other approaches, which aim at externalizing and releasing such feelings, might be found to be effective without the need for comprehensive psychotherapy.

Compulsive vomiting. Lait (1972) reported an interesting case in which he temporarily relieved compulsive vomiting symptoms in a 31-year-old woman, first by using simple suggestions for relaxation and relief. When the symptoms returned later, he traced their source through hypnotic regression to an experience when the patient was a child. Her drunken father would beat her and her mother. He often became nauseated after drinking bouts and would vomit into the bathtub. The patient hoped he would die, and in fact prayed for his death at those times. Her episodes of nausea as an adult would occur following times in which her husband came home intoxicated. After seeing herself as a 6-year-old girl involved in that experience and "forgiving" herself under hypnosis, she apparently lost the nausea permanently.

This indicates the likelihood that more complex hypnoanalytic techniques may be required when simple suggestion achieves only temporary results. The case also highlights the seriousness of the underlying psychopathology that one faces when confronted by an alcohol prohibitionist mentioned in chapter 13 on dermatological disorders. Such rigid-thinking individuals go beyond the legitimate decision of choosing not to imbibe alcohol for themselves. They attempt to control significant others in their life by evoking guilt over even the most responsible use of alcohol and by demanding promises to abstain. Such pseudomoralistic behavior is most frequently a defensive maneuver because of their own underlying childlike dependency, inadequate ego strength, and fears of losing self-control. Rigid and closed-minded in their maladaptive desperate defensive posture, such individuals are unlikely to change. They are resistant to psychological interventions, including hypnosis.

The fact that gastrointestinal symptoms are likely to have meanings and, hence, require more than hypnosis for their permanent resolution is exemplified in a classic case reported by Crasilneck and Hall (1985). Complaining about her husband, a woman suffering from globus hystericas stated that she "could not stomach the crap he puts out!" This statement turned out to be related to his pressuring her to provide oral sex.

Many clinicians focus their therapeutic strategies around the use of hypnosis to inculcate calmness and relaxation and to reduce excessive gastric motility. Used in this way, it would seem unlikely that any severe sequelae would be induced. However, the therapist must be prepared to employ more comprehensive psychotherapeutic approaches should symptomatic relief turn out to be only temporary. Careful follow-up of patients is essential.

Constipation. In such cases, proper dietary and exercise habits must be a major and primary focus of treatment. Hypnosis provides an excellent adjunct to the development of such healthy habits. Specific hypnotic suggestions for treating constipation involve "teaching" in hypnosis the physiology of peristaltic movements, followed by suggestions aimed at the relaxation of anal sphincters (Cooke & Van Vogt, 1956). The hypnotic suggestions can be linked to the act of sitting on the toilet to precipitate defecation. Erickson, Herschman, and Secter (1961) reported "discussing" with the constipated patient in hypnosis "the possibility of setting aside a certain time each day" for "emptying the bowel." They also recommend allowing the patient to use the same period to "to merely sit and speculate whether the bowel movement will be a full one or a partial one." (See also the section on irritable bowel syndrome in chapter 16.)

Hypnosis in the Treatment of Neurological Disorders

Ambrose (1963) found hypnosis valuable in the treatment of petit mal in children. He has his young patients ventilate their grievances, express aggression, and deal with underlying fears and guilts while in hypnosis. He believed they can also be taught auto-hypnosis for self-suggestion, but he presented no specific data to support this later contention. J. Smith et al. (1996) demonstrated experimentally that children as young as 4 years of age could be taught self-hypnotic procedures for pain control, but this has yet to be attempted for epileptiform seizure disorders.

Frankel and Orne (1976) described a case of "phobias and temporal lobe epilepsy" they treated at the Beth Israel Deaconess Medical Center and the Harvard Medical School. Onset of the disorder dated from a traumatic episode when the patient was 12 years old. He was alone in a boat rowing away from the shore of a lake when he became very frightened and disoriented. At that time, he was diagnosed as having petit mal. His fears generalized to all sailing, flying in planes, and being caught in traffic jams and crowded tunnels. Seizure activity increased over the years and was characterized by a blank stare and feelings of depersonalization. The electroencephalogram showed "paroxysmal left temporal discharges." The treatment strategy "was based on having him imagine (in hypnosis) that he was experiencing the situations he had been avoiding. Each situation was dealt with and mastered in a separate session." The hypnotherapy here employed tactics involving abreactions and behavioral systematic desensitization techniques. Frankel and Orne noted, "After a few months he reported no further seizures and an absence of strange feelings related to visual stimuli."

Raginsky (1963) hypothesized, "A patient suffering from organic epilepsy may have a convulsion precipitated in hypnosis, but that once started it cannot be terminated by hypnosis." John Watkins confirmed that hypothesis in one case. A patient who had a seizure at the dinner table three nights earlier reexperienced the seizure when he was hypnotically regressed to that same meal. The EEG seizure signature was recorded on the electroencephalograph.

Raginsky also reported a case in which a patient who had been experiencing one to four epileptiform seizures daily was completely relieved in three, 45-minute sessions of hypnotherapy during which the only goal "was to relax the patient and to set the stage for him to express himself without fear of reprisal." The patient remained free of seizures during a 19-year follow-up.

Kroger (1963) was able to eliminate all further needs for medication in a 32-year-old woman suffering from grand mal seizures. She had suffered this condition, involving two or three seizures a week, for some 25 years. Without detailing his procedures, Kroger stated that he taught her to become "proficient in autohypnosis and sensory-imagery techniques." He reported that striking personality changes occurred at the same time.

Perhaps the best current psychological alternative to medication in the treatment of a variety of neurological disorders involves the adjunctive use of hypnosis to facilitate patient self-modulation of EEG (A. Barabasz & M. Barabasz, 2000; Sterman, 2000). An alert hypnotic induction to facilitate attentional focus developed by Arreed Barabasz (A. Barabasz, 1985; A. Barabasz & Barabasz, 1994a, 1994b, 1995, 1996; A. Barabasz, Crawford, et al., 1993) has begun to be tested in controlled settings, with promising results thus far (Anderson et al., 2000; Warner, Barabasz, & Barabasz, 2000). The field of neurotherapy is advancing rapidly. Cutting-edge findings, beyond the scope of this book, appear regularly in the *Journal of Neurotherapy*.

Hypnosis in the Treatment of Cancer

Perhaps one of the most intriguing hypnotic interventions involves its use in the treatment of carcinomas. As highlighted in the introduction to this chapter, John Watkins attended the 1958 meeting of the Academy of Psychosomatic Medicine in which a paper was presented by a physician who was using hypnosis to treat carcinomas — not the pain, but the cancer. The doctor presenting made no claims of "cures" but reported that his patients lived much longer than would be expected for the types of cancer they had. When asked why, he replied, "I increase the resistance of the host."

Despite this report, years went by while clinicians and researchers focused primarily on the secondary effects of cancer: pain, anxiety, depression, feelings of hopelessness, and so on. In this area, the most moving story is of "David" by Gail Gardner (1976), now a classic in the literature. Gardner, by her sensitive interaction, enabled this 12-year-old boy to master his fears, to live his remaining months to the fullest, and to die with dignity. The paper is a "must" for every therapist who works with dying children (see chapter 17). Nonetheless, hypnosis has not until very recently been recognized as an important part of the comprehensive treatment of those suffering from cancer.

The defining research in the field was completed by David Spiegel and his colleagues at Stanford University Medical School. The NIH funded this 10-year follow-up of 86 cancer patients. Those who received self-hypnosis training and group therapy had 50% less pain and survived a year and half longer than did the patients who had had standard medical care (Kogan, Biswas, & Spiegel, 1997; D. Spiegel, 1991, 1997; D. Spiegel & Bloom, 1983).

Hypnotic visualization and imagery techniques have been reported by Margolis (1982–1983), Rosenberg (1982–1983), and others in directly treating the cancer and controlling the side effects of cancer therapy. The patient's motivation is stimulated by direct hypnotic suggestion. The aim of hypnosis is to mobilize the patient's own physical resources to fight the cancer. Imagery can involve visualizing the cancer in a form of the patient's own choosing. It might be perceived as a black mass, or perhaps symbolically as a castle that is being attacked. In a direct or symbolic manner, this cancer will be attacked by the patient's own powerful antibodies, and these patients will "bite away" pieces of the cancer and imagine these pieces being carried away by their own normal eliminative processes. For younger patients or those that particularly enjoy their personal computers, doctors may wish to use imagery involving typing the word *black* on the screen. Then image issuing the command or using their favorite search function "to search, find, and destroy (delete, send to the trash, empty the trash) the cancer cells one by one." Emphasize calmness and confidence (e.g., "As simple as pressing a few keys, the cancer program running in your body is deleted forever"). Doctors can reinforce the emptying of the trash with an auditory hallucination by asking patients to hear the sound their computer makes when emptying trash is commanded.

A team of therapists at the Newton Center for Clinical Hypnosis in Los Angeles also focused on the use of hypnosis in treating patients with cancer for more than 8 years (Newton, 1982–1983), but once again control conditions and follow-up was less than ideal. The doctors used hypnosis to relieve incapacitating symptoms such as pain, nausea, insomnia, and loss of appetite, and reported substantial success in the treatment of some 105 cases seen for at least ten, 1-hour treatments over 3 months as contrasted with 57 cases, which were "inadequately treated" by those criteria.

As in Gardner's classic case of David, treatment emphasis was placed on improving the "quality of life" rather than aiming to reverse the disease process, although the latter did occur in a substantial number of their cases. Simple and direct induction techniques were used, aimed at building ego strength and enhancing coping. In some cases, intensive hypnoanalytic therapy was employed. Visualization techniques were used but not forced or imposed, and confronting patients with responsibility for their illness was found to be counterproductive.

Once hypnosis has been induced, and at least a moderate level of depth achieved, visualization and imagery that goes beyond adapting to the disease process, instead focusing on the body's ability to produce inner healing, might go something like the following:

> Of course you already know that the body has the ability to heal itself, you've had wounds and cuts, and burns throughout your life, and other injuries, and your body was able to heal itself, was it not? Your body completely replaces all of its cells from time to time, matter of fact virtually all the cells in your body are renewed and changed over the period of several months or sometimes years.

> The body knows how to regulate itself, how to regulate heart functioning and so on, your body regulates the way your heart operates, it regulates your breathing for you, it controls your blood pressure, and your temperature, when you are cold your body restricts blood flow to the extremities so that your inner core stays safe and warm, and when you're very, very warm, your body knows how to bring blood to the very, very tips of your fingers and the tips of toes, and to the very, very surface of your skin to help you regulate your temperature, through other mechanisms such as perspiration, all of these happen automatically to maintain your health, your body knows how to regulate itself. It regulates its blood chemistry, it regulates its hormones, and it's all aimed at healthy functioning, mind and body.

Amazingly, or not so amazingly, your body does this without any kind of extra special effort or overstimulation. For years, your body maintained its immune system automatically, hoarding off invading organisms before they ever had a chance to take a foothold. The body knows how to make those good T cells and B cells, and helper and suppressor cells to build those antibodies, to build those white blood cells. Those white blood cells are like strong white horses, galloping to surround any invading viruses or bacteria. Your body and mind have the ability to work for health, to work for healing, and to then maintain healthy functioning once again.

This inner life force is strong, and cancer cells are weak and confused. Normally, when invaded by carcinogens, cancer cells are quickly destroyed by the immune system; now if they reduce rapidly, they can form a tumor, but, as you know, your body has the ability to conquer those cells, to surround them, to regulate them, to cast them out; the body is strong, cancer cells are weak and confused. You can let your life energy circulate throughout your body to tell your immune system to release strong and more effective white blood cells, more strong powerful white horses that can gallop to protect you. You can even think of them, streaming through your blood stream full of energy, sure of their purpose to surround, dissolve and destroy any unhealthy growth they may find. And as you think about those things, and you imagine them on their own, no doubt you will come up with other images that will even be more personal to you. You of course can also thank your immune system for doing such a wonderful job for you in the face of a challenger or ask your immune system if there is anything you can do to help speed your healing.

The immune system is strong and getting stronger, the powerful white horses can gallop, surround and overcome any unhealthy growth, the area can heal, heal completely, and then those white horses can patrol through your body at a leisurely prance, in a loving protective and graceful way, so you can begin to see yourself being restored, to your ideal health and appreciate and love yourself for taking the time to work with your body in this way, your mind and body working to protect you.

Although still viewed with skepticism by a few oncologists, the substantive work by David Spiegel's group at Stanford has gone a long way to reverse previous rejections of hypnosis for cancer. Some hypnotherapists have reported remissions of the cancer, whereas others have noted an arrest in its development. Although it is to be doubted that psychological interventions will take the place of the usual surgical, pharmacological, and radiological treatments, the attempt to mobilize and improve natural physiological resistances to neoplasmic development suggests yet another approach that may be of value. Because controlled experimental research has clearly demonstrated that the modality of hypnosis can influence and alter many physiological processes such as color processing in the brain (Kosslyn, Thompson, Constantine-Ferrando, Alpert, & Spiegel, 2000) and the immune system (Ruzyla-Smith, Barabasz, Barabasz, & Warner, 1995), it appears that further experimentation in this area is warranted.

Summary

We have come a long way since the French Royal Commission, headed by Benjamin Franklin, declared Mesmer's cures to be a fraud because they were produced by imagination. Given that both physiological and psychological processes mutually interact with each other, we can conceptualize most illnesses as "psychosomatic." Under the umbrella of complementary medicine, this concept has at last been recognized by the NIH and by the ever-increasing numbers of health care facilities in the United States.

Through its effect on perception, motivation, and covert processes, hypnosis can assist in the treatment of many "physical" disorders, if one considers therapy as a way of helping patients to mobilize their own capacity for recovery. A wide variety of conditions have been found responsive to favorable influence by hypnosis, and greater numbers of general practitioners and specialists are showing interest in the possibilities for hypnotic techniques in their therapeutic armamentarium. Research is being conducted that will test and develop improved treatment approaches and that will determine which of the various disorders respond best to hypnotic interventions. The acceptance of complementary medicine is essential to providing the best care for patients and opens new opportunities for psychologists trained in hypnosis to work in hospital settings.

Chapter 13
Mind–Body Interaction II: Hypnosis in the Treatment of Dermatological Disorders

Mrs. R. L., aged 44, was referred to us with acute neurodermatitis of the neck, involving the upper portion of the chest and the back. The patient was refractory to all medicaments. Glove hypno-anesthesia was employed for relief of intractable itching. Post hypnotic directions were given for the patient to feel sensations of warmth and coldness over the involved areas. Direct hypnotic suggestion for the improvement in her skin was not given at any time. The neurodermatitis had developed immediately after her daughter had announced her engagement to a young man of another faith; this upset Mrs. R.L. terribly. The daughter was referred to a psychiatrist in attempt to delay the marriage; she was able to work through her feelings toward the young man and finally decided it would not be feasible marry him. The mother's neurodermatitis promptly improved. However, during the period that her daughter was receiving psychotherapy, hypnosis afforded Mrs. R.L. relief from her itching, nervous tension, and anxiety. Hypnotherapy was employed as an adjunctive procedure. (Horan, 1950, p. 43).

Our skin is an organ most expressive of emotions. In the face of fear, it can turn white. Rage may redden it. Blushing demonstrates embarrassment or sexual arousal. Weeping of the skin may act as a substitute for lay-chrymal crying. Irritations in relationships with others can cause attacks of neurodermatitis. The scratching to relieve itching has been shown to stimulate pain receptors. And psoriasis has been known to break out in resentful wives to keep the unwanted attentions of husbands at bay. We even use terms such as "irritated," "burned up," "hot under the collar," and "itching for action" to describe emotional feelings. Our skin is, indeed, reactive to emotional stimuli.

Dermatological diseases are caused by many things, but most frequently they are related to bacteria, fungus, allergens, external stimuli, internal biochemical balance in the skin, and emotional stress. This interactive effect of physical and psychological factors in stimulating dermatitis was first clearly demonstrated by Ikemi and Nakagawa (1962). The suggestion to patients that they were passing near noxious laquer trees caused a breaking out of the skin very similar to that observed by actual contact or proximity to such trees. Most practitioners recommend that, to treat such disorders, doctors should combine the appropriate medical treatment with some form of psychotherapy. Accordingly, hypnosis should be considered as adjunctive to the overall management of the disorder.

The skin is the boundary between the organism and its environment and serves as a protective and defensive organ. Scott (1960) reported that hypnosis has been found effective in treating a wide variety of skin disorders including pruritis, numular exzema, neurotic excoriation, warts, and especially so in cases of neurodermatitis. He notes that hypnosis can often achieve permanent results in disorders that are organically determined. Perhaps in no other general medical condition has hypnotherapy been so rewarding as in the treatment of dermatological disorders.

Because the skin is such an expressive organ, the "meaning" of a symptom here becomes especially important if it is to be removed or alleviated. Ambivalent as he was, a middle-aged war veteran alternated in reporting to the dermatology and psychiatric clinics. Psychotic symptoms were finally relieved by the rather extreme approach of electroconvulsive shock therapy, whereupon severe dermatitis would break out. His skin problem would then receive aggressive pharmacological treatment in the dermatology clinic, and as the skin cleared, hallucinations would reappear. Such cases require deeper psychotherapy and are not cured by symptomatic treatment, hypnotic or otherwise. If funding for only brief therapy is available, hypnosis could then be used in an ego-state therapy approach with abreaction as a way of getting to the root of the underlying conflict (see our Volume II *Hypnoanalytic Techniques* and J. Watkins & Watkins, 1997). Although some cases of skin disorders have shown rapid improvement using hypnosis, it appears that a general reduction of their severity, step-wise by spaced suggestions, is desirable. In some cases, it may even be prudent to leave the patient with a residual symptom—a small patch that does not entirely heal up. Strenuous attempts to remove the last vestige of a psychogenic skin disorder by hypnosis alone may result in a reprecipitation of the entire condition. Gradual improvement through regular hypnotherapy also has the advantage of permitting the practitioner to detect early adverse reactions. We believe it is important to always bear in mind that the symptom served a protective function for the patient at the onset of the disorder. If it is still needed at some level or by one or more of the patient's ego states, its complete removal will reverse the gains of therapy.

Itching. One of the most difficult problems in dermatological disorders is the sensation of itching and the compulsion of the patient to scratch the afflicted area. This is a behavioral consideration and is one of the first aspects in which hypnosis can make a significant contribution. A number of alternative hypnotic approaches have been reported by various therapists.

When the scratching is employed by the patient primarily to relieve emotional tension, suggestions of relaxation, maintained posthypnotically, can be sufficient. Occasionally it is possible to suggest that the scratching will be displaced to other areas of the body, those that are not afflicted, leaving the lesions free to heal without continuous excoriation. As in the treatment of pain (see chapter 9), at the most simplistic level the patient, while in hypnosis, is presented with the concept that he or she may well be aware of the itching but that it is not a bother, and thus "there will be no desire to scratch it."

Itching can also be relieved by changing the nature of the sensation. Thus, a hypnotized patient might be told to imagine that cold compresses were being placed on the afflicted areas and that the feeling of coldness will bring a cessation of the itching feeling. Katalin Bloch-Szentagothai (personal communication to A.F.B., 2004) suggested an image of taking a shower to comfortably lower the skin temperature, leaving a "nice cool skin." Jencks (1978) suggested controlling itching with hypnosis by using the hypnotic suggestion that the patient is "imagining breathing through the afflicted skin area, thinking cool and still, while inhaling and calm or relaxed while exhaling." Another helpful image involves floating in the ocean or diving into cool water in a diving bell. Another technique we have found to be effective in the relief of itching for some patients is essentially the same as the glove-analgesia technique used for pain control (see chapter 11).

Itching sometimes has a masturbatory quality (J. Watkins, 1987, p. 260). In cases of urticaria (hives), pruritis ani or vulvae, it becomes a way of satisfying erotic needs, particularly when fixed patterns of maladaptive guilt are underlying. Exploration of the patient's sexual history and current sexual activities are usually indicated in such cases. It may be particularly valuable to assess the patient's repertoire of sexual fantasies. Rather than investing the time and energy needed to accomplish this by means of Freudian free association or dream analysis, which can lead to over interpretation, I (A.F.B.) have found the "Self-Scoring Questionnaire" (Wilson, 1978) to be useful. It was developed on the basis of research by Glen Wilson and Rudie Lang at the Institute of Psychiatry, University of London. The questionnaire makes it possible for patients to evaluate their own fantasy life in relation to that of a sample of other reasonably normal people. The data obtained can be incorporated in hypnotherapy, but the function of the questionnaire for patients can be remarkably freeing of fantasy guilt as they learn that their fantasies are typical of most people rather than bizarre and worthy of the control that guilt can have over one's life. In at least three cases, itching was relieved completely within hours of the session without recurrence or the need for extended therapy.

Approaches to simple organic itching reported by Kroger and Fezler (1976, p. 347) involved displacing the scratching to a doll. They described a case in which skin picking at night was turned toward a toy doll with which the patient was induced to sleep. This represented a displacement of anger from the self to an external object. The patient was also asked to indicate which area she wished to have relieved and to remove any doubt that such would be the case. This gave her the option we favor in hypnosis—that is, giving the patient a choice. Kroger and Fezler have also employed finger twitching as a substitute activity for scratching. After this substitute was well established, the twitching was progressively reduced and then eliminated by hypnosis.

Direct substitutions, a form of sublimation, can be made for scratching as well as for other needs. Painting, sculpture, working with tools, and strenuous exercise may provide distraction from itching sensations and constructive activity of the hands, so as to inhibit destructive self-excoriation. Inquiry should be made about possible interests that the patient has in such activities. These can then be reinforced with hypnotic suggestion once an adequate level of trance depth has been established. We see such distraction methods as merely a stopgap type of intervention that can be employed when time is needed to explore and resolve underlying conflicts that may be involved.

In a classic case involving hypnosis for psoriasis, Kline (1954) suggested that the afflicted areas would change sensation, first by becoming warm, then cold, feeling light, then heavy, feeling larger, then smaller, and so on. Surprisingly, the skin soon cleared, although no direct suggestions were given for its improvement. He used a similar technique with considerable success in the treatment of neurodermatitis (Kline, 1953). One might hypothesize that the therapy lay in "teaching" the patient control of skin reactions. If then motivated to secure relief from the itch, he or she would be able to achieve it. Helping the patient learn how to "control" such autonomic reactions is apparently an important factor in eliminating symptoms. Erickson, Herschman, and Secter (1961) employed this technique in the treatment of a child's hives (urticaria). The youngster was taught to turn them on and off, the same way in which biofeedback is intended to work.

However, patients with strong masochistic needs unmet due to inhibited guilt-ridden sexual interactions (and many dermatological patients have exactly this) might not respond favorably. Patients who have strong self-destructive impulses should have these resolved through insight therapy. Sadly, many of these individuals, who are most frequently women, may meet these needs by entering into relationships with jealous, immature significant others who further reinforce their underlying guilt. A patient's often legitimate but unmet underlying needs are further frustrated as she becomes further subrogated to the maladaptive needs of her significant other. A patient may exhibit occasional angry outbursts lending to more feelings of guilt. As the cycle repeats itself, she becomes more and more dependent on her partner to the point of making it difficult to break off the relationship that inhibits her personal growth. Her true needs may be met by impulsive behaviors, which can become secretive and sometimes desperate attempts in cases when the controlling rigid partner is severely pathological.

The maladaptive (it no longer serves the person's needs) underlying guilt frequently has childlike qualities or a history of strict religious, absolutistic qualities of right and wrong, which can function as a mechanism whereby a woman rejects potential partners who have the maturity to accept and appreciate her as a worthy unique person without the need to try to control her. In other words, the very persons who are most likely to provide her with healthy unconditional nurturing and help to build her self-esteem to adapt to the world maturely are the ones most likely to be rejected by such guilt-ridden individuals.

Despite some self-insight that manifests itself ambivalently, such a patient cannot accept such a mature partner because at conscious and subconscious levels she believes she is not worthy, she "doesn't belong with such a person." Her immediate dependency needs seem met by pathologically controlling individuals, and preconsciously she believes she deserves no better or she fantasizes that "he will change overtime." Of course, all of this childlike thinking can simply become a roadblock to her own growth. She repeats the same self-defeating, childish, romanticized behaviors over and over again.

J. Watkins and H. Watkins (1997, p. 97) described a case in which the woman married a series of eight alcoholics before eventually seeking help from an ego-state hypnotherapist. By then, much of her life had gone by, her youth and energy given away to pathological controlling partners. Of course, the pathology expression would be no different, if not even more serious, if she had married eight alcohol prohibitionists who, in the process of exerting control over her, for example, played on her guilt for her responsible use of alcohol in social interactions. Obviously, such cases can enter a wide variety of symptomatic expressions of itching beyond the domain of dermatology.

An expressionistic organ. The skin is the organ most displayed to the world. It is not surprising that it can easily become a means of expressing exhibitionistic impulses. Being noticed (even if not admired) is better than being ignored. Patients with such adolescent-like needs will often express them through gaudy or unusual dress, loud speech, or other attention-getting behaviors. The physician or therapist who suspects these motives will do well to inquire into the feelings of inferiority and lack of acceptable recognitions in the patient's life before attempting to remove unsightly skin blemishes through hypnosis alone. Constructive substitute activities, which permit the patient to achieve notice, acceptance, and praise from others, can go a long way in making disfiguring skin blemishes unnecessary. If through some form of athletic, economic, artistic, creative, or scholarly achievement the needs for attention can be met, then psychotherapy, with or without hypnosis, has a much better chance of succeeding.

Warts. One of the first methods developed to evaluate the possible effect of hypnosis per se was to direct it first only toward certain specific areas of lesion, ignoring others. Sinclair-Geben and Chalmers (1959) induced hypnosis and gave 14 patients the suggestion that their warts on one side of the body would disappear. Nine of 10 patients judged to be hypnotized showed a complete disappearance of warts from that side in less than 3 months. The untreated side of the body showed no change. This approach permits the practitioner to evaluate the effect that hypnosis may have in the case of a given patient, without trying to remove all the symptoms at once in case there is an underlying need for them.

In what must be the most dramatic first example of the effectiveness of hypnosis to be recorded photographically, Mason (1952) found that aiming suggestions only at one area at a time was very effective in treating a case of congenital ichthyosis erythrodermia. Nearly every square inch of the patient's skin was warty and elephant-like. Because the condition is grotesque and physically uncomfortable, the patient was scheduled for surgery. The young and inexperienced Dr. Mason was to assist. Upon seeing the patient's dreadful condition, the surgeon indicated that the patient was inoperable. Mason, who had recently completed a workshop on hypnosis, said something on the order of "I could just hypnotize him [to make his skin normal]." The deprecatory surgeon reportedly said in a laughing voice, "Well you just go ahead and hypnotize him then." And that is precisely what Dr. Mason did, using a series of targeted hypnotic suggestions aimed at one area of the patient's body at a time. It remains of interest today that the patient became completely unresponsive to hypnosis just when all that was left of his symptom was a patch of warty skin on one ankle. Apparently, the symptom served some unconscious need and, therefore, could not be relinquished.

Barabasz's technique for warts. In a rather less dramatic case I (A.F.B.) saw while at Massachusetts General Hospital/Harvard Medical School, a 13-year-old girl presented with hundreds upon hundreds of warts all over her neck. She scored at the upper limit of the *Stanford Hypnotic Clinical Scale* for children (Morgan & Hilgard, 1975) and especially seemed to enjoy the hypnotic image of floating on a cloud. So after determining her depth of hypnosis by asking her to "give me a number any number" and she indicated the number 10, I asked her then to indicate when she had gone to a depth of 20 by simply raising a finger on one of her hands. After she raised a finger, I returned to the cloud image. Once confirmed that she was feeling and floating on a billowy cloud, I explained to her, "You are dressed warmly, in a coat and gloves and a wonderful warm fuzzy hat. All so nice and warm but your neck, of course, is completely exposed to the cool air and as clouds do, sometimes, the cloud continues the rise up and as it goes up, the air, of course, becomes cooler and cooler. Now your body is just warm all over, but the neck itself becomes very cool, very cool." I asked her whether she could feel this feeling, and without being told to do so she indicated by simply raising a finger on her left hand, rather than nodding. I took this as a "yes" answer without further inquiry, and continued the image of coolness. I asked her to relax her thoughts and to just listen to me, and I said, "The warts are ready to leave, if you are willing to let them go on their way, just let them leave, one by one, you can let them leave. We have already shown you how your mind can control your body, and the warts are ready to go away and leave, you can leave them way up in the air, as you descend back down to the earth. Your skin will feel slightly cool around the area of the warts, for a day or so, and as the coolness begins to fade, the warts will begin to fade too." She was scheduled for another appointment in just over 2 weeks. I waited to see the results of our work together and wondered whether hypnosis would be effective. The patient and her mother failed to show for her scheduled appointment. I called her home and her mother answered. I inquired as to what the reason was for missing the appointment. Her mother indicated they did not show up because her daughter was "absolutely frightened to death" about hypnosis. "Yes, she liked the cloud and all that, but the warts are gone you see, all that's left is one little one on the back of her neck." After further discussion, I then talked with her daughter on the telephone and reassured her about reactions. Recognizing her daughter's comfort level, the mother agreed to bring her in for another session.

In that next session, we confirmed that the warts all over her neck had faded almost completely, and all that remained was a single wart at the back of her neck. She was asked if she could go into hypnosis again, saying that she was no longer frightened of it, after realizing that she had control. She went back into hypnosis once again, and this time I left her with the image that the only wart she needed was that small one on the back of her neck, and she could keep that wart as long as she wished, until her mind and her body were ready to let it go. "That's the only wart you need to keep, the others have gone and they will never return, you can keep that wart as long as you wish, your body and mind will know when to let it go." I continued with several suggestions for relaxation, relief of tension, and calm confidence about her ability to enter hypnosis and to always control it. At the time, I was unaware of the function that the warts had in the patient's life. It became evident that the patient's younger sister had been receiving what the patient reported to be essentially all of her mother's attention and love, and it seemed that once that younger sibling was born the patient felt that she no longer really mattered to her mother. I saw her mother in therapy for two or three sessions and was able to deal with a number of the home situations in short order. This case was another lesson in subconscious needs not being met when symptom removal is the only focus of therapy.

In reflection on this particular patient, I might have improved the comprehensiveness of my treatment by using the child's apparent ability to use ideomotor finger signals to inquire of her subconscious mind regarding the meaning of her symptoms and why they were important to her. I also might have employed ideomotor signals to inquire about her resistance to their removal by the wide range of techniques that had been tried earlier, including medical freezing and number of "suggestive techniques" that her parents had attempted before seeking hypnosis.

Watkins' technique for warts. A 9-year-old girl that I (J.G.W.) treated used the "magic-finger technique." The child was brought in by her mother during a hypnosis workshop for treatments of warts on the left hand. Her index finger was anesthetized by stroking it. I told her, "If you will lightly touch the warts on the back of your left hand each day with the magic numb finger, they will go away." In this manner, she was taught how to self induce the numbness by rubbing the finger in the other hand and release it by squeezing the finger with the opposite hand. Although the case involved but one treatment, her mother reported that the warts, which had been in existence for a long period of time, completely disappeared shortly after the session.

Tasini and Hackett's technique for warts. Tasini and Hackett (1977) used a simple relaxation hypnotic induction to achieve the hypnotic state and simply asked the child to imagine doing something that he or she likes to do to have fun. They stressed long deep breathing and imagination about developing relaxation with each breath out. In one example, they asked the child to simply "feel his hand and that it will begin to tingle, and it will start to feel light like a feather, and so it will begin the rise up, let it go." In so doing, they coupled the simple relaxation induction with an arm-levitation procedure to determine some level of hypnotic depth without actually inquiring about depth. They stressed the point that as the hand rises, the child will begin to feel ever so relaxed and good, and the child is asked to let it stay up for awhile and then let it come down. As it comes down, the child is asked to "continue feeling so relaxed and good" and then is told that the warts "will feel so dry and they will turn brown and fall off, the warts will not trouble you anymore." Tasini and Hackett reported seeing such patients for a total of three sessions.

Ewin's technique for genital warts (condyloma acuminatum). Dabney Ewin (1974), professor of surgery and psychiatry at Tulane University, has been treating this condition for decades. Recognizing that the sites of the warts are rich in blood circulation, he emphasized the opposite of the suggestions we discussed previously. In cases of penile and vaginal warts (human papillomavirus or HPV), he suggested that the affected areas feel warm and produce a dilation of blood vessels to, thereby, enhance the supply of blood. He specified that he generally uses only a light trance and tells the patient, "Now in your mind we will lock in on this and maintain this warmth until the warts are healing and your skin becomes normal in everyway. You can forget about the warts and turn your conscious thoughts to other things, because your natural healing processes will cure the warts without you having further concern about them." Ewin then explains, "Your blood vessels will dilate to bring in more antibodies and white blood cells to fight infection and prevent cancer while bringing more protein and oxygen to help build normal tissue when the wart has gone away." The ideomotor signal of raising a left index finger is used to determine whether the patient perceives feeling the increased warmth. He noted that after implanting such hypnotic suggestions, conscious attention can be taken away from the area and that "unconscious motivation" is generally more potent than one that the patient is fully aware of. In so doing, he is taking responsibility for the treatment rather than transferring responsibility for maintenance of this imagery to the patient by some sort self-hypnotic procedure.

The procedure of hypnotically influencing a blood supply to specific areas has been used for many years (see A. Barabasz, 1977, pp. 3-28; A. Barabasz & McGeorge, 1978). Let us recognize that ideomotor signaling is convenient method of communicating with a person in hypnosis, although Kihlstrom (personal communication to A. Barabasz, 2004) believes that there is absolutely nothing in the literature that suggests that ideomotor measures are better than verbal measures at tapping implicit (unconscious) memories or emotions. Contrarily, Ewin (2004, personal communication; see also Ewin, 1990) explained that he had found ideomotor for signaling to be a key with several patients who refused a necessary surgery until he reframed something "they" believed they had heard under anesthesia. Another had been confined to a chair for 2 years by constant pain following a spinal operation, and after reconstructing a "memory" and reframing it with hypnosis, he entered a work-hardening program and returned to work.

None of Ewin's patients had a waking memory of hearing during surgery, and in trance none of them responded to verbal requests for what they might have heard. It was only after nonverbal ideomotor reviews that they came up with the key material. Ewin acknowledged that skeptics will say there is no confirmation that what was retrieved was actually said in the operating room, but what they said was what was in their minds (it was not implanted), and the clinical course changed when the expressed idea was changed. He considered this a clinical experiment when the same patient is the control, reports no waking memory and no memory in trance, and then comes up with a life- changing memory after ideomotor reviews. Anbar (2001) employed a computer word processor with his patients and found responses with typing are consistent with those that patients provide by answering "yes," "no," "I don't know," or "I don't want to answer" with ideomotor finger movements.

HPV of the genital tract is a highly contagious disease with a number of ramifications that go beyond simple penile warts, the most serious of which can be, depending on the type of HPV infecting the patient, progression to cervical cancer. Current medical treatments for HPV consist of invasive procedures including burning, cutting, freezing, or applying acidic substances to the skin. Because of the resistance many patients have to these painful treatments, including poor follow-up treatment compliance, hypnosis can make a very special contribution.

The only study extant to provide experimental controls testing hypnosis against standard medical procedures was conducted in two phases (A. Barabasz, M. Barabasz, Higley, & Christensen, in press). The first phase of the study was conducted at Massachusetts General Hospital and Harvard Medical School, while the second phase was conducted at Washington State University. In the Massachusetts General Hospital phase, seven female HPV patients were treated with hypnosis and were compared with seven patients' hospital records using standard medical procedures. One of the seven patients in the hypnosis treatment showed no change, whereas the remaining six showed an average decrease in the number of warts by more than two thirds and nearly a 90% reduction in the area of infected tissue. In the second phase of the study conducted at Washington State University, six female HPV treatments were treated medically with freezing or medication, whereas six patients were treated with hypnosis. In general, the routine medical treatments average about 50% to 70% response rate. In the second phase of the study, the medical treatments produced a 51% reduction in the number of warts and a 72% reduction in the area of tissue involved. The hypnosis patients showed a 67% average decrease in the number of warts and a 67% average reduction in the area of infected tissue. Although both treatments were effective, statistical analysis showed no difference in treatment outcome between the medical treatment group and the hypnosis treatment group. It seems on the basis of these findings that hypnosis should become the treatment of choice for HPV considering the high patient drop-out rate and poor patient compliance with treatment using the typical medical procedures. Hypnosis offers an excellent noninvasive alternative, which, unlike the majority of standard medical interventions, is also safe for pregnant women.

Barabasz's hypnotic suggestions for HPV. A. Barabasz (A. Barabasz, 1984b; A. Barabasz et al., in press; Russell, 2002) first establishes a moderate level of hypnotic depth and then provides suggestions such as the following:

> Your body has the capacity to overcome the wart virus and heal this infection. Focus your attention on the involved area and soon you will notice a sensation of warmth in the surrounding area. Your

blood vessels will dilate to bring in more antibodies and white blood cells; more lymphocytes and natural killer cells. The virus will be totally and completely destroyed and carried away. Your body and your mind are more powerful than the virus, your body will annihilate the virus and it will be gone forever. Protein and oxygen will then increase to help build the new, normal, and healing tissue when the warts have disappeared. When you feel the increased warmth, your right index finger will rise ... good. ... Now your inner mind will lock in on this and maintain this warmth until the warts are healed and your skin becomes normal in every way.

Watkins's technique for rash. For decades, practitioners (Bowers, 1976; Frankel, 1976) have employed guided fantasy and induced hallucinations to influence skin reactions. One of my (J.G.W.) own cases may be illustrative of this approach.

A nurse in her early 30s requested hypnotherapy for neurodermatitis, which she had suffered for some 8 or more years. Although her dermatologist was highly skeptical of the effectiveness of hypnosis, he agreed to respect her wish for this type of treatment. This condition would especially flare up whenever she had a controversy with the chief nurse, whom she despised.

Although the evidence of a transference conflict related to mother figures was strong, I (J.G.W.) hypnotized her and used the following hallucinatory fantasies: "Imagine yourself taking a warm bath in which has been placed a soothing, healing lotion. You can feel the gentle, soothing relief to your irritated skin." I asked her to "visualize and experience this situation for a few minutes" and then told her, "Imagine now that you have emerged from the warm bath and that you are taking a brisk, cold shower, which has a toning effect on your skin and your entire body. It makes you feel very much alive." I asked her to alternate several times between the "warm, soothing bath" and the "brisk, cold shower." This constitutes a variation of Kline's procedure, but it is implemented by specific images rather than simply the words "warm" and "cold," and so on.

After she had bathed and showered several times, I asked her to visualize a self-image using a subject-object technique:

Look at yourself in the full-length mirror that is on the door of the bathroom. Notice that the woman there looks exactly like you; she has your hair and your features. However, her skin is pink and clear. There are no lesions. As you look at her, the mirror seems to fade from view and she appears like a replica of yourself standing in front of you. You wish to have clear, pink skin like her, and so you decide to join her. You move over in front of her, turn around, and back into the space she occupies until your body and hers coincide. Your head and hers are the same; your arms and legs are in the same space as hers. You and she are one and the same, now you look down at your body and you see that the skin is pink, healthy, and free of lesions. A sense of great happiness comes over you.

Twice a week, for 6 weeks, the same visualizations were used. The dermatitis rapidly cleared.

Two years later, I (J.G.W.) was accosted in the hall by a hospital staff physician: "What did you do with Miss X?" he inquired. "I have followed her case for many years. Her skin is now clear and has been so for some time." Rather taken aback, I (J.G.W.) asked, "What did she tell you that I did?" "Why, she said that you told her to quit scratching." What does one say at this point to a practitioner who had little understanding of the psychological factors of disease, and no scientific grounding in hypnosis? Do we describe hallucinated baths, subject-object self-transpositions, and so on? "Yes," I replied, "I told her to quit scratching." He smiled, seemingly satisfied with my answer, and proceeded on down the hall.

Summary

Given that upon the onset of a disorder patients develop symptoms to protect themselves, we must always bear in mind that their complete and rapid removal could produce adverse reactions or reverse the gains of therapy. The skin, in particular, is an especially expressive organ, so extra caution is warranted when hypnosis is focused only at the symptomatic level. Dermatological diseases are typically precipitated by biological stimuli, yet we must always remain aware that there is an interaction between the skin and the autonomic nervous system. Unresolved emotional issues and overt emotional stress can initiate or exacerbate the disease process. Hypnotherapeutic interventions are meditated by personality type and the specific psychopathological skin disorder present. Emotional issues should be treated with an appropriate psychotherapeutic intervention either with or without hypnosis. Hypnotherapy can be central to psychotherapeutic intervention or it can be used as a strictly adjunctive technique. The great effectiveness of hypnosis in treatment of dermatological disorders makes it especially rewarding for both the patient and the practitioner.

Chapter 14
Meditation and Hypnosis for Health

Classical hypnosis and concentrative meditation are similar in the attentional and concentration practices employed that result in altered states, in the phenomenology of those altered states, and in the neurophysiology associated with those states. Both hypnosis and meditation begin with attempts to relax and concentrate the mind by focusing attention. Instructions from 2,000-year-old texts read, "[The monk] trains thus: 'I shall breathe out tranquillising the body' (lit. bodily formation)" (Nanamoli & Bodhi, 1995, Sutta 118). Buddhist texts list many targets (*kasinas*) for focusing the attention: colored disks, elements in nature, and so forth. (Nanamoli & Bodhi, 1995, Sutta 77). Meditators today most commonly focus on the breath. In hypnosis, focusing and sustaining attention might mean staring at a spot, watching a swinging pendulum, or focusing on the suggestions themselves. (If the suggestion is that one's arm is becoming lighter and lighter, attention is focused inward to an almost subliminal experience of physical movement.)

The process used to reach the state has been described in the hypnosis literature as not attending to competing stimuli (Crawford, 1994, 2001), or suppressing competing thoughts (David & Brown, 2002). In the meditation literature, Ayya Khema (1997) described it as letting go of thoughts and perceptions (Holroyd, 2003, p. 109).

Jean Holroyd's (2003) article "The Science of Meditation and the State of Hypnosis" discussed how the attentional focusing procedures used in hypnosis are similar if not identical to Buddhist, Christian, Hindu, and Jewish forms of meditation. Attentional focus, characteristic of both hypnosis and meditation, produces similar mental state alterations (Cardena, in press; Venkatesh, Raju, Shivani, Tompkins, & Meti, 1997). The emphasis is on letting go of thoughts or as termed by the Buddhists, "mindfulness practice." The concept is that practicing concentration focuses attention and shifts it to a more qualitative experience to let go of thoughts. In meditation, one learns to observe rapidly shifting sensations, thoughts, and emotions that can be described in great detail (Shear & Jevning, 1999; Wallace, 1999). One form of meditation that very closely resembles deep hypnosis is termed *samadhi* concentration, which produces altered states of consciousness. Such altered states, termed *absorptions* (or *jhanas*), closely resemble those that correlate significantly with hypnotic states (Tellegen & Atkinson, 1974). As absorptions are practiced, they increase in depth (Bucknell, 1993). Holroyd pointed out that mindfulness, or *sati*, is intended to produce insight, or *vipassana,* by the process of observing one's own mental processes and altered states of consciousness. Such meditation has been used in pain management programs to produce less reactivity to painful stimuli.

Ainslie Meares (1982-1983) described a form of intensive meditation that is characterized by intense simplicity and stillness of mind rather than directing the patient to focus on increasing awareness of such processes as breathing. Although Meditation is now recognized by the National Institutes of Health (NIH), such was not the case back in the 1960s. Meares was ahead of his time by recognizing the benefits of the intervention. He became so taken with the effects of meditation as an avenue to the hypnotic state that he was rejected by his Australian medical colleagues and gave up his medical license rather than reject meditation.

Meares (as in Zen Buddhist meditation) helped his patients "not to try" but rather to let themselves effortlessly slip into an altered state of consciousness. He reported considerable success with certain patients.

The Zen method, embraced by Meares, involves a good deal of silent sitting or facing something vacant until the mind "becomes blank." The idea is to practice sitting until the moment of "pure awareness" takes hold, even if it takes practicing for decades to arrive at that point. Curiously, this approach as well as many other meditation methods includes key elements of restricted environmental stimulation (REST). Flotation REST, where the individual floats effortlessly supine on a 20% Epsom-salt solution heated to skin temperature in a light-free, sound-attenuated enclosure for about 1 hour has been demonstrated to serve as a hypnotic induction approach without a formal induction (A. Barabasz, 1993). Chamber REST, consisting of 6 hours on a bed in a well-lighted, sound-attenuated chamber where individuals wear Ganzfeld goggles, has been shown to increase hypnotizability (A. Barabasz, 1982).

An alternative common meditative approach involves the Mantra. This involves literally thousands upon thousands of repetitions of sounds and images. The mediator becomes involved with "energies" thought to be beyond that of normal sensory processes or functions of the mind.

Taoist Meditation

In contrast to Zen approaches, the Taoist approach is the one most concerned with physical health and is, therefore, the one we concern ourselves with here. I (A.F.B.) have found a Taoist-based procedure to provide an alternative induction method that facilitates a new sense of self-control for the patient without the need for anything more than a light to moderate the level of hypnotic depth. The Microcosmic Orbit–based induction illustrated here is a structured method of self-hypnosis for patients who fail to respond well to the methods we have discussed earlier in this book.

Instead of attempting to create the impression of an absence of all thought, the practitioner of the Tao focuses on circulation of energy referred to as *chi* along certain pathways inside the body. The belief is that such routes can be opened to direct the chi (also known and *prana* or ovarian power; in India, *Kundalini* power) to higher upon higher centers known as *chakras*. The U.S. NIH lists meditation in its short list of complementary medicine interventions that have health benefits. The practice of circulating the chi has been practiced for thousands of years in Tibet, parts of India, and China where it has reportedly brought extraordinary improvements in health and longevity because of its focus on prevention of illness and immune-system enhancement rather than on the treatment of illness after it occurs (Chia, 1983, pp. 103–110). Taoist rejuvenation using internal power chi first appeared in the Yellow Emperor's text on internal medicine.

Chi is conceptualized as the primordial life force. Ancient writings point out that chi begins with the fertilization of an egg by a sperm cell, and from this original fusion, of course, a highly complex human being evolves. Chi energy is believed to enter the human fetus at the navel. It circulates in what is known as the "Microcosmic Orbit," which is sometimes also referred to as the "Heavenly Cycle." It is a continuous flow of energy that is reputed to involve all the various tissues, brain functions, and organs unified into a person. It is also thought that it is a key to linking people to their environment.

Ancient researchers recognized that the human fetus inside the mother's womb grows about its mother's navel point and through the umbilical cord, exchanges nutrients for waste products all the time, in a sense "breathing through the umbilical cord, into its own navel, down to the perineum, and up through the head, and then down from the mouth (later discovered to involve the tongue) to begin once again at the navel. Therefore, the Taoists believe that the starting point for all of this chi begins and ends at the navel, in not only the child but also the adult.

In a sense, we may conceptualize Taoist meditation as a rejuvenation of the human life force through a form of age regression, where one focuses on the approximation of some sort of return to the primordial self. Meares's many publications on hypnosis explained meditation as a regression to preverbal levels. Obviously, once removed from the safe, warm, soothing, flow enhancing womb of the mother, our marvelous equilibrium that was once so nurturing has been cut from us. According to the Tao, as we age, from the very moment when the neonate enters the world, our life energy begins to settle into the back, hot, *yang* parts of the body and the front, cold, *yin* parts of the body. So then what was once a balanced, warm mixture becomes imbalanced, as hot yang energy rises to the upper part of the body, including the liver, lungs, heart, and brain, while the cold yin energy settles in the legs, the genitals, the kidneys, and the lower stomach. It is thought that if we fail to practice the Tao, to keep the energy routes open, we slowly but surely develop premature sickness, imbalances, and the classic signs of old age.

The energy routes when kept open, are believed to bring vital power to our internal organs and enable them to function. But without efforts to live a healthy lifestyle and keep the routes open through Taoist meditation, they are thought to become blocked by both physical and mental tension, all of which is linked as the primary cause of weaknesses, poor health, and fatigue. The remarkable energy circulation enjoyed by the fetus carries us through our younger years. To about the age of 20 years, the body usually has sufficient energy to maintain the major health functions because it has sufficient energy to keep the routes less obstructed.

Remarkably, a small fraction of 1% of adults decades and decades old have, most likely because of genetic makeup, managed to keep routes (nadi) less obstructed. Western medicine reveals that although apparently aging in certain features of appearance, a sign of wisdom in non-Western cultures, their endocrine systems can rival that of 20-year-olds. There still is little data available from personality inventories, but clinical lore indicates such individuals seem to be universally characterized by above-average intelligence, creativity, openness to new ideas, and flexibility in thinking. They are frequently as adventure seeking as adolescents, albeit with the mature judgment of an experienced adult. As alluded to in ancient Chinese writings, pairing such individuals with young adult practitioners of the Tao greatly enhances the life energy for both persons when produced by this form of meditation as it flows through the bodies. Chang (1977) noted that these ancient masters recognized a long list of factors, both psychological and sexual, as to why a mature man in good health (25 to 35 years older) and a younger woman are a "superb combination." Except for the peasantry, this arrangement remains a norm in parts of the world where this tradition is practiced.

Practice of the Microcosmic Orbit is intended to reawaken the undivided balanced healing power that was once an accepted fact of our being before birth and in early life. This is accomplished by harmonizing yin and yang energy. Taoist practice focuses on the two primary energy channels that are thought to provide the strongest current. The "Functional" channel begins at our perineum. It is then thought to flow upward past the sexual organs through the stomach, the heart, and the throat. The other channel is referred to as the "Governor" and starts in the same place, but it flows from the perineum upward into the tailbone (coccyx) and then up through the spine into the brain and back down to the roof of the mouth, where the tongue is thought to be like a switch that connects these two currents when it is touched to the roof of the mouth. The energy cycle is said to flow in a circle, up the spine and back down the front of the body. When the energy flows in a loop around the body through these two channels, the Microcosmic Orbit has been achieved. Acupuncture and acupressure, now both recognized by complementary Western medicine, focus on opening blockages to this energy loop to promote healing and correction of dysfunction. But again, this form takes more of a Western medicine approach, where it is only explored and tapped once illness occurs rather than maintained and opened at the routes to prevent illness from occurring in the first place.

Clearing the obstructions that stop the flow of chi energy in their natural paths is referred to as "opening the routes" The obstructions are thought to be due to emotional tension, mental stress, or some form of physical impediment. The notion is that when the natural forces are tapped to help the body clear itself of such obstructions, natural energy flow is restored and the healing power is then available as it was when the body was younger. The Taoists also believe that all of these energy routes in the body are somehow grounded in the larger balancing forces of nature, which probably explains why Taoists have been known for centuries to be environmentalists with respect for all living beings and living things, both plant and animal.

Once the routes are joined and cleared of obstructions, the power and energy flow in a circuit, linking the vital organs of the body in this Microcosmic Orbit circulate around the trunk and head of the body. By opening these main routes, the greatest possible reserve of warm chi can flow into every bodily organ to bring health and vitality. Taoists believe that the whole process of harmonizing yin and yang, balancing physical, mental, and emotional aspects can take place automatically once the blockages have been removed.

The obvious hypnotic intervention that flows from this practice goes along the lines of hypnotically suggesting to the person that the body has known all along how to heal itself. The hypnotic suggestion could be as follows: "You know your body has healed itself from cuts, scrapes, burns, and fractures, it knows how to do it." Keeping the channels (nadis) open using the Taoist approach provides an induction procedure that can be particularly acceptable to those new to hypnosis but interested in the benefits of meditation. It offers an avenue to those who are otherwise closed-minded about hypnosis. The therapist can help the person "let the warm current of chi wash away any blockages that may be there, massage and nurture internal organs and restore health to damaged and abused tissues. Dreadful diseases can be prevented and the effects and toll of anxiety, stress, and tension are flushed out of the system." Because of the emphasis in typical Western medical practice, to focus only on diseases after they occur, many of us have yet to recognize our own built-in ability to heal ourselves and prevent illness simply by using the energy that we can help unite between the fronts and backs of our bodies.

The following is an example of a hypnotic induction using the Microcosmic Orbit meditation as its basis, which I (A.F.B.) conducted with a volunteer. This sample induction is not intended to be used verbatim. It is merely a basic guide. For greatest effectiveness, the therapist must tailor the induction to the individual responses and idiosyncrasies of the individual patient. Specific hypnotic suggestions directed at your patients needs may be inserted, as appropriate, at points of your choice.

> Let yourself be calm to the very best of your ability Let your body sink into the [couch], relaxing ... relaxing ... [pause]. I see your eyes are already closing. If you're ready [patient gives slight nod], we can begin to concentrate on what we call the "first energy center." That's usually the navel. As you let your body become calm, to

the best of your ability, see if you can focus your concentration on your navel, let your mind go right down to your navel [pause]. Focusing and concentrating at the navel ... focusing and concentrating ... as you keep focusing you will find it easier and easier to focus your concentration on your navel.

Continue to remain as relaxed and focused as you are now, but see if you can let your focus sink about an inch and a half beneath the skin, inside you, let your mind focus right there [pause]. When you begin to feel something a little different, just raise a finger on this hand [therapist touches right hand, which is by Buddhist practice already placed over the left hand]. Focus and concentrate your energy beneath your navel all the time going deeper into hypnosis, and your body becomes calmer and calmer. All of your concentration and focus right there, one and a half inches inside your body at your navel. As you begin to focus even more on that, let it go deeper [upon observation of an appropriate reaction], and there it goes [pause].

OK, now just take this hand [therapist touches right hand], and place your thumb on your navel. While remaining deeply hypnotized and comfortable, spread your fingers out downward. Notice where your little finger is. As you notice where your little finger rests, press down a little with your finger there. See if you can move your focus to that place. That is the next energy point. Just as you did at your navel, put your mind there. Let your mind go there, and just like before, let it go right inside your body, about an inch and a half, inside your body. Focus and concentrate ... and again, like at your navel, you may begin to feel something. When you do, lift a finger to indicate that to me. Remember, this is only an experience you can have; such feelings feel different for everyone [pause]. Focusing ... concentrating ...focusing. Your mind, down from the head, and inside your body. Focusing, and concentrating. Good [upon observation of the finger lift ideomotor signal].

See if you can let the energy travel right to your perineum, as if touching it without actually doing so. Try to focus there, as if you were pressing on your perineum. ... Good. ... Continue with your mind at your perineum, and as if pressing, ever so gently concentrating the energy there [pause]. Squeeze your muscles, squeeze, hold it there, and now relax. At this particular stage, you may begin to feel your energy coming right through the front channel of your

330 • Hypnotherapeutic Techniques

body, right to your perineum. Keep your mind there, focusing and concentrating. Squeeze again. Notice whatever you are feeling … the energy, right there at the perineum [pause].

And now, if you are ready, like before, using your focus, you can direct the energy to the next energy center. Focusing and concentrating, pleasantly hypnotized [pause], calm. You can begin to move your focus point up to the fourth energy center, your tailbone, which is at the base of the spine [ideomotor finger signal confirms]. Slowly let the energy go up from the perineum to your tailbone, it's called the coccyx. This point is very important because it is here that the power is returned to your body but it can also get lost. When the generative power is returned, it passes through this canal and into the spine and then right up to the brain. It is here that the warm current is said to enter the central nervous system. Now, as you have been concentrating for some time, you may feel a sensation of pressure or perhaps warmth rise up into the coccyx. As it moves up, it moves up into your spine [pause]. Let yourself go deeper and deeper into hypnosis. Let me know if you can feel it. … Good [patients typically raise a finger on their right hand to indicate recognition of the sensation].

Now that you have felt the warmth of your energy caressing your spine, if you are ready, see if you can move your focus to that lower curve of your back — your lumbar — while remaining deeply hypnotized and relaxed. You may notice it is exactly opposite the navel but on the back of your body, your spine, the middle of your lumbar. This is a very special safety valve of sorts. It allows cool excess energy to be dissipated. Allow your focus to be there, as you go deeper and deeper into hypnosis. Your mind is there, aware of this energy. You can go deeper into a pleasant hypnotic state if you wish, deeper. Yet, you are always able to hear me clearly and distinctly, no matter how deeply you take yourself. Good.

While remaining pleasantly and deeply hypnotized, let your focus and concentration move your chi further up. This is opposite the center of the abdomen, adrenal glands, opposite the solar plexus, on the spine, opposite the abdomen, on your back. Let all your focus, all of your concentration be there, put your mind there [pause]. Feel the warmth of your body's energy. [The following should be said upon observation of what is usually some small bodily movement.] As you feel it, some parts of your body may move a little ... as it has just done. Going deeper now, you may notice your lips will part a little as you go deeper and deeper into hypnosis [pause]. You might have an increase in salivation; just swallow normally, its just another good sign of going deeper and deeper into hypnosis as you concentrate the energy on the point between your adrenal glands [observe for such signs] [pause].

While continuing to listen to my voice and remaining deeply hypnotized and relaxed, see if you can move your focus, your concentration, to the next energy center up ... slowly take it up ... control it ... focused and concentrated, moving the energy, slowly up to the seventh energy center ... the back of the neck, your cerebellum. I will touch the spot so you can feel exactly where it is. This is where your brain controls breathing, heartbeat, and other functions that are associated with the autonomic nervous system. As your chi energy passes up your back to this point, many changes may occur ... perhaps you may notice different breathing patterns. At this particular energy center, if you have had any discomfort or pain in your upper back, this is a very good opportunity to let your energy spread throughout that portion ... let the energy soothe the discomfort to make those feelings comfortable. ... You may already begin to notice how different those areas feel now ... very different from before [pause].

When you are ready, let us try to move your focus and concentration to the eighth energy center, right up to the crown of your head [Cz, central vertex] [pause]. I will now touch the center of the top of your head so that you know exactly where that is ... concentrate it there for just a moment ... concentrate it there. The chi energy, right at the crown of your head, concentrating your power ... the energy ... all of it totally under your control, focused and concentrated at the crown of your head. The energy to focus your attention! The energy to heal yourself!

Now, you can go deeper and deeper in hypnosis as you let your energy and focus flow right down to the point between your eyebrows. This point is the master endocrine control gland regulating growth and so on. According to the Tao, it is believed to be the seat of love, compassion, knowledge, personality, love of humanity, and devotion. All of this, plus intelligence, memory, reading, thinking, studying, and abstract conceptual thinking.

This pituitary- and pineal-gland point is very important to our opening and completing the routes. As you focus and the energy flows through, some people enjoy a pleasant odor as the hormonal glands carry impurities out of the body. If you feel a little pressure there, it is due to the pent-up resistance to the normal purifying flow of energy. The pressing feeling will gradually go away and you can pass the energy on.

When you are ready, try to begin to return the energy back down to the front channel, focusing your mind on returning the energy. Focusing and concentrating on returning the energy to the front channel. ... Using your present level of deep hypnosis, you can easily control the energy to now connect the back yang and front yin energy channels. The way to connect those two channels is to gently press your tongue to the roof of your mouth. ... [Sometimes people have difficulty doing this. If the patient is inexperienced say, "If you find this difficult or uncomfortable, you can start by putting your tongue at the back of your teeth, but if you are comfortable and ready, the most effective way is to press your tongue to the top of the roof of your mouth."] This is a very important step because we don't want to let all the energy stay up in your head. Just press your tongue there and your chi energy will begin to flow right back down ... down the front to the cool yin channel [pause]. Stay there with your tongue gently pressed to the roof of your mouth [or the back of your teeth]. ... Focusing and concentrating ... focusing your mind on returning the energy back to the front channel ... continue to do so until you feel the energy release downward, and then release your tongue ... your tongue back to normal with the energy released down to your throat. In this level, we are bringing together the warm yang energy from your back to the cool yin energy in your front channel. Many people notice a release of stress as this occurs. You may notice yourself becoming even more calm and able to concentrate more easily. All of the energy centers are linking together.

The heart center is the key center. This vital point revitalizes love and joy. It's usually easy to focus on and bring your mind there. Because concentrating there feels good as stores of energy are released, it's tempting to stay there too long. Staying there too long will cause the energy to be reabsorbed into the tissues around the heart. So, as soon as you feel the warmth you can tell me by moving a finger [upon observation of the ideomotor signal]. Good.

Now above your navel is your abdomen. It is time to let your energy travel there ... your mind there. ... This energy point is the site of many energy centers [use the word *chakras* for those familiar with the Microcosmic Orbit]. By circulating the energy in this way, you are opening the channels to well-being, self-healing, and health. You can achieve this by doing this special form of self-hypnosis. You can open your channels. Ones that have become blocked can be opened. You open the channels in self-hypnosis by letting the energy flow around your body in this Microcosmic Orbit.

Eventually, as you begin to bring the energy up the back, you will notice that you can experience each and every vertebra in your spine, one after the other, as the energy moves up your back. Just be sure to pause ... as long as you need to. Let your mind be there! Feel the chi as you go to each point ... starting down from the navel.

When you move the energy up to the back of your neck and the crown of your head, always remember to touch your tongue to the roof of your mouth [or the back of the teeth]. Then let the energy channel down the front to your navel, an inch and a half deep inside your body, and then to the point a hand-width below your navel ... pressing there ... feel the energy deep inside. Then to your perineum when you're ready. Always remembering you are in total control ... you can control the energy cycle to open all the channels and all the routes to health, well-being, calmness, and confidence. From the perineum move the energy up to the coccyx, up to the point opposite the center of the abdomen ... up to the back of the neck, and then to the top of your head, your heart, and back down to your navel, all the time going deeper and deeper into hypnosis. ... The organs of your precious body collect only the energy they need.

To complete your hypnotic Microcosmic Orbit, ground yourself. Complete the route by collecting and storing the energy in your navel. Now, if you are ready, let's do that. Make a fist with your right hand and place it at your navel [pause until the patient has complied]. Good. Now, make a small circle with your fist. Go around and around your navel [For males, go 36 times clockwise; count to 36 softly as the patient rotates his fist. Collect the energy by going counterclockwise 24 times. Slowly make the circle smaller and smaller. For females, collect the energy by first rotating counterclockwise 36 times and then clockwise 24 times, slowly making the circle smaller and smaller].

[For both males and females] And now that you have completed the cycle and grounded your energy, the routes of the channels are more and more and free of blockages. Now, as I count from 10 to 1, just let yourself come out of hypnosis, your eyes opening at 5 but not fully alert until I reach 1. At 1, you will be wide awake, alert, calm, and feeling fine. 10, 9, 8, 7, 6, 5, 4, 3, 2, 1 ... wide awake, alert, and calm.

Summary

The commonalities in focused attention and regression processes found in meditation and hypnosis have become more evident now that meditation has found a recognized place as part of psychological science and complementary medicine. We emphasize the health benefits of the Taoist meditative approach and its potential use as a hypnotic induction. Such an approach can often be the induction of choice for patients skeptical about hypnosis yet interested in meditation and for those who are of low hypnotizability who have failed to respond well to the procedures we described in the earlier chapters. The sample Microcosmic Orbit induction presented is not intended to serve as a substitute for traditional meditative practice. It is an approach we have found to be highly effective, on the basis of clinical trials, as a hypnotic induction in certain resistant individuals. Practitioners should endeavor to tailor the induction to their individual patients and to employ specific hypnotic suggestions aimed at each patient's therapeutic needs.

Chapter 15
Dental Hypnosis (Hypnodontia)

In psychoanalytic theory, the oral cavity is assigned the most significant role in the development of a child's personality. It is the primary "love organ" of the body during infancy. Through the mouth, the neonate receives life-sustaining food provided by the mother, and in this process establishes the first relationship with another individual. The meaning of love and the fear of its loss are reflected in the frequency and way by which the mother feeds the child. Many psychoanalytic studies trace the later development of dependent and aggressive behaviors to the imprinting that the individual received during this early oral stage of his or her growth. Fixations at this level or later regressions to it often occur when the child is unable to cope with more mature demands (J. Watkins, 1987, p. 315).

A Brief History of Hypnodontia

In view of the great psychological significance of the oral cavity, the dentist must know more than the anatomy and physiology of this area of the body. He or she should be very aware of the stress that procedures in this region can induce in a patient and be prepared to cope with the consequences when those procedures are painful, anxiety provoking, and disruptive to reparative efforts.

Dentistry is associated with pain, and, therefore, many patients come to treatment burdened with anxieties, tensions, and fears. Despite the great strides in maintenance of our teeth brought by 21st-century dentistry, some individuals needing dental treatment still continue to avoid regular visits. The result is, more often than not, tooth decay, which can potentially lead to tooth loss. Rodolfa, Draft, and Reilley (1990) noted that at least 10 to 12 million and up to 30 to 40 million people in the United States alone receive inadequate dental care or avoid dental treatment altogether, entirely because of feelings of anxiety about dental procedures.

Since the first use of ether by a dentist, Morton, in 1846, practitioners have developed and used a number of different chemoanesthesias. However, hypnosis has proved to be a valuable adjunct to dental therapeutics and surgery, which has not yet realized its full potential. The emphasis in research on hypnosis for dental applications has fluctuated greatly (Nash, 2000; Nash, Minton & Baldridge, 1988) but on average, about 150 articles on hypnosis in dentistry appear each year in medical, psychological, dental, and interdisciplinary journals, but recently there has been a decline in the overall numbers of papers published (Finkelstein, 2003). Interestingly, professional organizations of dentists using hypnosis predate the formation of the larger societies involving physicians and psychologists. Because we as psychologists wrote this book, our treatment of dental hypnosis reflects only a small fraction of our independent-practice cliental. However, we report the major uses and techniques as described by major workers in this field.

Psychological Importance of the Oral Cavity

A few reflections on our language direct us to the emotional significance of many terms related to the mouth and to eating. The word *sweet* applies equally to a taste and to personality attributes. "Putting teeth" into a project, a "biting" remark, "swallowing" one's pride, translate oral terms into descriptions of behavior. Furthermore, one loves one's "honey." A relationship can go "sour," and one may have to learn a "bitter" lesson. An old-timer can have a "salty" personality. We take a person we like to dinner. We kiss each other with the lips, and we can "spit out" angry words during an argument. It is obvious that the mouth cavity is established very early in life as an organ of the greatest emotional significance. It is, therefore, not surprising that manipulations of this organ, such as the repair or extraction of teeth, can provoke primitive fear reactions in many people.

Although the technique of inducing hypnosis can be learned with a minimal level of sophistication, the practitioner who crudely intervenes with his or her patient psychologically can cause considerable emotional harm. Accordingly, it is recommended that the use of hypnotic techniques be learned in a general setting of personality dynamics and psychopathology. Such instruction, which is highly recommended for the hypnodontist, is almost equally recommended for the dentist who does not yet use hypnosis, because he or she, too, whether recognizing it, is evoking psychological reactions. Some dental schools have understood this importance and are providing psychology courses. However, because many of the brief workshop courses in hypnosis offered by professional societies have little time in which to teach the broad psychological background desired, the dentist who studies hypnosis is advised to supplement such workshops with classic readings, such as Coleman, Butcher, and Carson (1980) and Derlega and Janda (1978). Books of this type can help the dental practitioner who intends to use hypnotic techniques to practice them with a broader psychological understanding. The study of psychopathology and personality dynamics is to psychological treatment as the learning of anatomy and physiology is to surgery (Wald & Kline, 1955). Much of this can, at first, seem overwhelming to the dentist in practice who is paid on the basis of coded procedures that do not include hypnosis. However, highly effective direct, indirect, verbal, nonverbal, or simple strengthening of an already extant dissociated state can be accomplished in fewer than 5 minutes (Finkelstein, 2003).

Dental Problems Relevant to Hypnosis

In what areas could hypnosis be of help to the dentist? All of the following have been included in publications on dental hypnosis as reported by various hypnodontists:

1. Patient relaxation
2. Alleviation of fears and anxiety related to dentistry (dental phobia)
3. Dealing with objections patients have to necessary dental work
4. TMJ dysfunction
5. Getting patients accustomed to orthodontic or other prosthetic devices
6. Treating bruxism
7. Correcting faulty habits such as nail biting and thumb sucking
8. Anesthesia and analgesia during painful procedures
9. Amnesia for painful procedures
10. Premedications
11. Treatment of gagging and nausea
12. Taking impressions
13. Reducing excessive salivation
14. Reducing bleeding
15. Assisting postoperative recovery

Precautions and Contraindications

Before discussing hypnotic techniques that can be employed in dealing with these problems, we should consider the conditions for which a dentist should not employ hypnosis. These conditions fall into two categories: (a) restrictions of hypnosis to the necessities of dental practice, and (b) precautions that should be observed in dealing with certain problem patients.

Hypnosis involves an in-depth intervention into internal personality processes. As such, it is not a field for amateurs. Accordingly, it is assumed that the dentist who would employ hypnotic techniques has acquired not only the skills of inducing hypnosis but also the instruction in normal psychology, psychodynamics of personality, and emotional disturbances that result in psychopathology and other disorders. The dentist is not expected to be a psychologist or psychiatrist, but he or she should be acquainted with major psychopathological syndromes, such as schizophrenia, borderline states, and severe neuroses. The dentist should be able to recognize when anxieties are within the normal range, and when symptoms are sufficiently severe as to warrant referral to a mental health specialist.

Although the possibilities of actually harming an individual simply by the induction of hypnosis are slight, in general, it is not wise to use such procedures on patients who are borderline to a psychotic break or who demonstrate paranoid ideation. In the first case, a severe anxiety attack can be stimulated in the person who is close to a schizophrenic break with reality, and improperly applied hypnosis might trigger such a break. Although such a break is not very likely, it is probably undesirable for the dentist to employ hypnosis with patients who show emotional instability. In the case of individuals who present with paranoia (i.e., those who exhibit suspicion, secrecy, ideas of reference, and feelings of persecution), an attempt to induce hypnosis might cause them to feel they are losing control to another person. Freud believed that if the patient's state of mind is the result of repressed homosexual impulses, then he or she might regard the induction of hypnosis as an attempt at sexual seduction. In this case, the patient can become angry and litigious. These cases are rare, but the dentist should be aware of the existence of such situations. If patients have verbalized suspicions and veiled hints that they think other people are "out to get" them, the dentist would be wise to discontinue attempts at hypnosis and have the assistant close by when working with that patient. Borderline personality disorders pose an even greater threat to one's practice with or without the use of hypnosis. Unfortunately, borderlines are sometimes difficult to diagnose, even for the experienced clinician. When in doubt, refer to or consult with a psychiatrist or psychologist skilled in hypnotherapy.

Occasionally, a patient will react to hypnosis, or to some fantasy activated by hypnosis, with severe anxiety. Again, these situations are very infrequent but must be dealt with if they occur. It is of the greatest importance that the practitioner not panic under these circumstances. Such reactions are commonly transitory, even if they are severe. Reassurance should be given in a calm and firm voice: "There is nothing to fear. You are in complete control of your mental processes. As I count down from 5, you will become alert, wide awake, feeling calm and relaxed. 5, 4, 3, 2, 1, wide awake!" Letting the patient discuss his or her experiences for a few minutes before returning to dental work can be most helpful in the reduction of any possible residual anxiety.

When experiencing hypnosis, patients are especially sensitive to cues presented by the practitioner. If the dentist is overawed by the powerful effects of the hypnotic modality or filled with doubts and anxieties about its use, he or she should resolve them before beginning any procedures. Attendance at advanced workshops, supervised experience with skilled workers in the field, or further reading and study usually provides sufficient desensitization so that novices can overcome any uncertainties they may have. The cues then transmitted to patients will be those of calmness, certainty, and competence. Hypnosis is, in essence, no more daunting than many of the procedures the dentist learned while training for the dental profession, and it is far safer than most physical interventions.

The greatest criticism about the majority of brief training workshops in the field is that there is usually inadequate time to provide the experience of performing hypnosis so as to desensitize the beginner in the field. A high percentage of those who attend introductory workshops do not leave with sufficient confidence in their newly acquired skills. They do not follow through and begin to employ the hypnotic modality in their practices. Hypnosis, more than most other therapeutic procedures, tends to activate emotional processes within the practitioner and in the patient. If the dentist (as well as the physician or psychologist) who has completed a course in clinical hypnosis does not immediately start to apply those skills,he or she can become like many former students we know. Follow-up questionnaires showed that participants stated that they enjoyed the course and learned a great deal about psychological functioning, but they never actually used hypnosis in their practice.

Perhaps one of the greatest obstacles to the use of hypnosis in dentistry is the time-cost factor. A few patients are not responsive to hypnosis, or at best achieve only light trance states. In such cases, the use of hypnosis is likely to be discouraging to the practitioner and the patient. This is some-times offset in that once a patient has been hypnotized, the state can be easily and quickly reestablished for future procedures. However, it is not economically sound to employ hypnosis with resistant patients when the procedures are minor, and they can be handled effectively with chemoan-esthesias. Nonetheless, much can be accomplished with the majority of patients in no more than 5 minutes (Finkelstein, 2003).

Techniques of Hypnotic Induction and Deepening

Many of the procedures we described in the earlier chapters can be used by the dentist and the psychologist or physician. However, certain proce-dures are better adapted to the physical conditions surrounding the practice of dentistry. Variations peculiar to the dental chair and dental office equipment become possible. Finkelstein (2003) recommended the following:

1. Establish the clinical relationship (a context of care, attention of the patient, and a focusing of the patient's attention)
2. Determine the need for hypnosis that might rule out other forms of anesthesia (consider trauma, pain, fear, anxiety, or tension)
3. Assess the capacity of the patient for imagery in any or all of the five senses
4. Determine patient motivation for the use of hypnosis
5. Assess the patient's belief that something can be accomplished using hypnosis
6. Assess the patient's belief in the skill of the therapist (recognize that patients are very sensitive to the confidence and familiarity the den-tist has with the procedure)
7. Recognize the patient's need for ego strengthening, reassurance, positive reinforcement, and a feeling of remaining in control

Finkelstein (2003) recommended relaxation-based brief induction proce-dures such as the following:

1. *Eye closure/touch.* The therapist asks the patient to stare at the back of his or her own hand and gives suggestions for relaxation as the thera-pist strokes the forearm from the elbow to the wrist. This is repeated and suggestions added, noting that the patient can close his or her eyes upon the therapist's noting signs of hypnotic involvement.
2. *Eye closure/breathing.* This exercise focuses on the patient's exhala-tion as part of a natural relaxation process. The therapist instructs the patient to take a deep breath, hold it, and relax as he or she

exhales. Repeat the process, suggesting eye closure if it does not happen spontaneously. Advise caution to prevent hyperventilation.

3. *Guided imagery.* This exercise focuses on using fantasies. The sound of the drill or of the saliva ejector can be tied into an image of flying in a jet plane, perhaps in travel to a tropical island. Music can be integrated into the hypnotic procedure as follows: "As you relax deeper and deeper, you will find yourself immersed into beautiful music, concentrating on it, swimming in it, as you sink into a more and more pleasurable state in which you can now only feel sensations of comfort." The induction and office music are combined with suggestions aimed toward anesthesia by dissociation. (Use caution with adolescent patients who wish to use their portable CD player and earphones. Hard, pounding rock may aid dissociation but at the same time prevent communication between doctor and patient.)

4. *Instant alert hypnosis.* As we describe in chapter 17 (see also A. Barabasz, 1994), instant alert hypnosis is quite effective for rapid induction with both adults and children. The therapist asks the patient to roll his or her eyes up, as if looking at the forehead. Lead the patient's eyes to this position with instructions to focus on the therapist's thumb. The therapist moves the thumb slowly from 10 to 15 centimeters in front of the patient's nose to the approximate center of the patient's forehead. At this point, the shift is made to the requirements of dental analgesia. Once the patient's eyes are rolled up, the therapist can perform an eyes-open catalepsy test. He or she tells the patient, "The eyes are rolled up and they cannot close; try to close the eyes [pause only long enough to see evidence of an attempt to open them]; stop trying." If the patient's eyes have not closed, the therapist instructs the patient by saying, "OK, you can roll your eyes down now, and as your eyes roll down you can let your eyelids close; they are so much more comfortable closed than they are opened as the relaxation comes over your entire body." This method when used in dentistry transfers the instant alert induction to a relaxation effects procedure. Alternatively, the eye-roll technique described by the Spiegels (H. Spiegel & D. Spiegel, 2004) can also be used for a fairly rapid assessment of hypnotizability and a rapid induction.

Although a deep state of hypnosis is desirable for long and painful surgical procedures, not all patients can achieve a deep trance. However, many patients can attain light and medium states sufficient to reduce discomfort significantly for most dental work. Failure of a patient to reach a deep trance is not contraindicated for using hypnosis. In many cases, the amount of Novocain necessary to have a numbing effect can be greatly reduced when the patient is in a light hypnotic state, even though the need for chemoanesthesia is not entirely eliminated. The dentist who employs a firm and confident tone to his or her suggestions can expect much better compliance than one who gives them in a hesitant, vacillating, or tentative manner. When about to inject a local anesthetic after hypnosis has been induced the dentist can say, "You may feel a slight pinch, now." Confidence is essential and will come with experience.

A patient (one who waits) is usually regressed to more childlike attitudes and may be "waiting' to be taken care of, to be treated, to be told by his or her "doctor parent" what must be done to alleviate suffering. These patients must feel that the doctor knows what he or she is doing. Hypnodontia, like hypnotherapy, requires that the dentist be more verbal than usual. Practitioners who prefer to work in silence will not find the hypnotic modality congenial to their practice.

Use of Hypnosis by Dental Assistants

There has been considerable controversy among hypnosis specialists as to how much latitude should be granted in training dental assistants to use hypnosis. The more conservative position in the hypnosis societies requires that its use be restricted to psychologists, physicians, dentists, and, more recently, nurses with advanced credentials. However, in the field of dentistry, it is already restricted to hypnosuggestive procedures directly related to dental practice. The Society of Psychological Hypnosis (Division 30 of the American Psychological Association) 2003 Annual Convention business meeting began to "rethink overly restrictive notions of limitations on practice (personal notes, A.F.B.)." In the future, a wider group of registered health-care providers will no doubt be allowed to obtain workshop training in hypnosis from the recognized societies of hypnosis currently restricted to MDs, PhDs, EDDs, and DDSs as well as those with advanced degrees in clinical social work and nursing. Nonetheless, hypnoanalytic probing is contraindicated in the dental setting. Although the majority of patients can benefit from rapid inductions, to others it can be time-consuming. In those cases, the time of the dentist may be more economically employed in direct treatment, it seems that hypnotic conditioning might be entrusted to a good dental assistant, well-trained in hypnosis, who is under the immediate supervision of a dentist also trained in hypnosis. His or her services in hypnotically relaxing the patient and then transferring rapport to the dentist might improve the efficiency of the office practice and encourage the use of hypnosis more frequently. The assistant should have had instruction in the handling of untoward reactions, and the supervising dentist should be immediately available if any of these occur.

Reassuring Patients and Reducing Their Fear

If hypnotic procedures are to be employed, no attempt should be made to disguise that this is hypnosis. Patients are usually aware that they are being hypnotized. Authenticity is the best policy. The patient should be told either that hypnosis could be of help or the possibilities should be elucidated. We have found it effective to describe the procedure to be used as "a natural, hypnotic relaxation, in which the use of drugs can be eliminated or reduced, a state in which it is possible to reduce discomfort." Orientation of the dental patient in this way usually avoids the anxiety and resistance that some patients can develop if told, "We will now hypnotize you." Words are very important, and those used to describe a procedure may well determine the patient's reaction. For example, "I will now put some Novocain in your teeth" is not as frightening as "I'm going to inject some Novocain."

Integration of Hypnoanesthesia With Chemoanesthesias

Induction techniques can easily be combined with the administration of nitrous oxide. Suggestions of deep relaxation by a light hypnotic induction technique given at the same time as a diluted mixture of nitrous oxide and oxygen can have just as much effect in pain reduction as a greater concentration of nitrous oxide without hypnosis. When this can be done, the patient recovers more quickly and avoids the side effects that can occur in some cases. It should be recognized that the administration of the gas is a form of suggestion. A placebo effect is, therefore, secured over and above its pharmaceutical properties. This effect should be constructively used and maximized: "As you inhale, you will feel yourself sinking into a deeper and deeper state of comfortable relaxation, where nothing unpleasant can bother you." Some dentists have found that by combining hypnotic relaxation with nitrous oxide, they not only get a potentiated effect with both but also increase their own skill and confidence in employing hypnosis. They can gradually reduce the concentration of the nitrous oxide while increasing the potency of the hypnotic verbalizing.

Fantasy techniques of induction and deepening, which are effective in the dental office, can involve the vivid description of baseball games, picnics in a meadow, hiking in the mountains, relaxing on the sand at the seashore, walking through an art museum and looking at the pictures, attending a musical concert, going fishing, or reliving a pleasant episode in one's life. The skill lies in picturing these situations so vividly that the patient becomes involved in them and completely dissociates from the procedures that the dentist is using on his or her teeth. In a real sense, his or her "self" has left the dental office and is experiencing the fantasy, not the uncomfortable dental procedure. A brief inquiry concerning the recreational activities of the patient may enable one to depict an image into which this patient can throw oneself most completely. The person who never goes fishing and has no interest in this activity will scarcely respond to attempts at initiating such a fantasy. The dentist should find out what the patient enjoys and build the induction and deepening techniques around that.

Dealing With Resistance

When patients are resistant and enter only light hypnotic states after much effort on induction, do not attempt to accomplish a great deal of dental work during early sessions with hypnosis as the sole pain reliever. The dentist can employ the principle of fractionation, put patients into the light states and take them out, perhaps several times during the first session, and follow with several sessions. Time may be required to reach a state deep enough as to permit dental work to be done without anxiety or discomfort, but in the case of a severe dental phobia, it can determine whether patients get the needed work done or lose their teeth.

If a dentist employs hypnosis with several patients, it is wise to record their reactions to hypnotizability tests, induction techniques, and deepening. These records should include the kinds of inductions employed and the time involved in reaching a desired state. A note on a patient's idiosyncrasies, such as anxieties at descending a staircase, slowness of hand levitation, or the description of any untoward reactions may greatly shorten the time for successful induction during the next session. Immediately following an unsuccessful dental procedure the patient is likely to be more resistant. This is not a good time to suggest using hypnosis. It is better to schedule another appointment and initiate this procedure later. Dentists' sensitivity to the feelings and moods of their patients will determine the difference between practitioners who are successful in the use of dental hypnosis and those who find it unsatisfactory and give it up.

Specific Problems and Techniques

Patient Relaxation. One of the most common impediments to the dentist's work is the inability of many patients to relax and remain quiet. Fidgeting, moving about, scratching the nose, and general restlessness can slow up dental procedures considerably. Therefore, relaxation techniques of initiating a hypnotic state not only will induce hypnosis but also will result in the quiet, passive type of involvement, which is most desirable to the working dentist. These can involve eye fixation and closure plus deepening procedures, which combine lowering of muscle tone with stimulation of inner fantasies. Although ordinarily we do not use the word *sleep* when inducing hypnosis for psychotherapy, the word can facilitate relaxation in the dental chair. Even though we know that hypnosis is not the same as ordinary sleep, the similarity of sleep to a passive trance state as experienced by the patient renders use of the word legitimate in this case.

The first use of hypnosis in dentistry is simply to promote such relaxation. This is closely related to the method of progressive relaxation (see chapter 5). In fact, such relaxation techniques, which involve teaching an individual to relax progressively different muscle groups, are sometimes used as a preinduction conditioning. The procedure involves first tightening a group of muscles, such as those in the leg, concentrating for a few moments on the feelings in that limb, and then letting go. Other muscle groups are then treated progressively in the same way until the whole body is relaxed. In this way, patients compare the sensations of tension with those of relaxation. The procedure operates similar to biofeedback technique. By identifying physiological reactions, patients bring them under control. Progressive relaxation suggestions given to hypnotized patients can be carried out more affirmatively than when administered in the conscious state. A reduction in the patients' muscle tension allows their minds to become calmer, and the patients can ignore external stimuli. This is not unlike what happens when we go to sleep.

Even if the hypnotic modality did no more than help patients to maintain a quiet and relaxed attitude in the dental chair, it would be making a considerable contribution. To induce such a state, the hypnodontist or trained assistant might voice repetitiously such phrases as "You may feel a beautiful, warm feeling coming over you. Your eyes are relaxing, your face is relaxing, the muscles in your neck are relaxing, you can feel a sense of relaxation moving down through your arm, the trunk of your body, and into your legs. The tension is melting away. Relax, relax deeply." After an apparent state of quiet and relaxation has been achieved, the patient can be told, "You will enjoy remaining in this relaxed, calm state. You need not pay attention to the procedures I will use. Perhaps you would like to think of pleasant matters or remember some pleasant experiences. You can focus on your relaxation and the enjoyment of your thoughts while I work." Many people who are not deeply hypnotizable will respond sufficiently to such hypnotic suggestions as to reduce their discomfort and make the dentist's work easier.

Anxieties and Dental Phobias. Some individuals are so frightened of the dentist that they become dental cripples. They avoid all contact and often end up losing their teeth. Even if their friends and relatives can induce them to visit the dentist, they are so easily traumatized that at the slightest pain their fears are reinforced. They often fail to return for a second visit. Almost every dentist has contacted such individuals who have a mouth full of rotting teeth that have been neglected over many years. They need a great deal of dental work, yet they can hardly tolerate even one minor filling. In such cases, hypnosis has a great deal to offer. Something must be done to counteract previous unpleasant experiences and raise the pain threshold. Their first visit must also be handled so that they will return for further necessary work. One 36-year-old woman I (A.F.B.) recently saw from northern Idaho had teeth so rotten that she had been on liquid foods for years. Sadly, when her spouse sought out hypnotic intervention for dental phobias and pain control, it was only to have almost all of her teeth removed. If only she had sought hypnosis decades earlier. She responded well to hypnotizability testing and was entirely able to dissociate herself from Wartenberg wheel and ischemic pains in preprocedure hypnoanalgesic testing.

A procedure that some dentists have found useful is to have the patient squeeze the arms of the chair whenever the drill is being applied. For normal individuals this can be helpful. For the patient suffering from a severe dental phobia, it will probably prove inadequate, as it is nothing more than crude distraction. With such people, the possibility of being helped through hypnosis can be broached by asking them, "Would you like to have your fear removed?" If this opens a way for the dentist to discuss hypnosis with them, and if they agree to try it, then the first session or two should be devoted only to orientation, hypnotizability tests, and induction. It is inadvisable to do more, or at most, undertake only a very minor dental procedure. If the patient can begin with a period of confidence and relaxation, dental work can be performed later.

A behavioral technique used by psychologists to eliminate a phobia can be applied here (A. Barabasz, 1977). It is called *systematic desensitization.* The patient is first deeply relaxed and given suggestions of comfort. Although in that state the feared stimulus is applied, it is in such a minor intensity that the fear reaction is not evoked. In hierarchical fashion, the stimuli are suggested to the patient in temporal contiguity with the state antagonistic to anxiety until he or she has learned to tolerate that which he or she could not stand. In applying this principle to the deconditioning of dental phobias, the hypnotic state is induced and intensified, and then a very small bit of dental work is done. At the slightest sign of anxiety and fear the dentist stops the procedure and goes back to the hypnotic induction, reinstating and deepening the hypnotic state, giving suggestions aimed at inculcating a sense of pleasure and confidence. Obviously, little will be accomplished in restoring the teeth during the first session, but if patients can leave without being traumatized, feeling they have mastered this first session, they will return, with their pain threshold higher. The patient is given ego-strengthening suggestions such as "When you return next time, you will feel stronger and more confident. You have not suffered this session, and you know that you can handle the next one. You will have no fear. You can relax calmly in the chair and focus your mind on pleasant things."

More can be accomplished the next session, when as little as two minutes might be needed for the hypnotic induction. Dentists using this procedure have reported that they were able to complete needed work on many patients who previously would never come to see them, or if they did come, would not return after the first session.

Patient Comfort. Closely associated with the reduction of fear and anxiety is the maintenance of comfort in normal patients, those who do not exhibit overt fears but who could be happier and more cooperative if they felt more comfortable during the dental work. Holding one's mouth open for long periods of time, or keeping the tongue out of the way, particularly when work is being done on the molars, can be fatiguing. Because the hypnotized patient is more responsive to suggestion, hypnotic suggestions aimed at relieving fatigue in the lips and facial muscles or in holding the jaws open can be quite helpful: "Your facial muscles are becoming soft and relaxed. They feel good. All the tension is going out of them. It is easy to open your mouth and to hold it open. It just naturally stays open. You do not need to pay any attention to the muscles which hold your jaws apart." This is partly suggestion and partly hypnotic dissociation because through suggestion the feeling of "selfness" is being directed away from the jaws and the facial muscles. It can be desirable to suggest to the patient that time spent lying on the dental chair is a period of rest and relaxation, and that he or she will look forward each time to the opportunity to set aside worries, cares, and tensions. Some individuals under such hypnotic suggestions not only are able to exclude painful stimuli from the dental procedures but seem to resent completion of the session and cessation of the pleasurable hypnotic state in which they find themselves. This maintenance of patient comfort is especially desirable during a long and arduous procedure.

Anesthesia and Analgesia. The greatest contribution hypnosis can make in dental practice is the reduction of pain. The same principles regarding pain control in dental problems apply to those used in the medical field of anesthesiology (see chapter 10). However, certain considerations unique to the practice of dentistry need to be added. In most cases where some degree of hypnotic trance can be secured it is usually possible to reduce the amount of chemoanesthesia, such as Novocain or nitrous oxide, required to secure a desired condition in the patient. When the individual is highly hypnotizable and is able to enter a profound hypnotic state, chemoanesthesia can be entirely dispensed with. Direct suggestions can be given the hypnotized patient to the effect that "You will completely ignore any unpleasant sensations in your mouth. The entire region of your mouth will be completely numb. It will have no feelings of discomfort." Strong, positive suggestions like this, administered while the patient is in a deep trance, are usually effective. Hypnosis can also be used to replace chemoanesthesias when they are medically contraindicated. However, the dentist should be prepared to administer the chemoanesthesias, when not contraindicated, if the patient shows signs of emerging from the hypnotic state. This cannot always be ascertained by the patient's apparent behaviors. E. Hilgard and J. Hilgard's (1983) research showed that pain can be registered at unconscious levels even though it is not overtly experienced. Accordingly, the patient might show signs of movement or response and still emerge from the hypnotic state reporting that he or she "felt no pain." When such movements do appear, it is probably best to interrupt the dental work and deepen the hypnotic state before continuing. Some clinicians recommend suggesting amnesia to the patient before bringing the patient out of hypnosis: "When you are alert you will have no recollection of discomfort during this past hour."

It is important to ensure that all hypnoanesthesia has been removed before the patient leaves the office (except such analgesic suggestions as might be given to alleviate discomfort during the postsurgical period) and to permit the patient to sleep that night. When it can be used, hypnoanesthesia has certain specific advantages over chemoanesthesia in the practice of dentistry. For example, it can be highly localized. A large area need not be made numb when the work is to be done within a specific region. Areas anesthetized hypnotically do not need to correspond to those innervated by specific nerves. Any area touched by a finger can be rendered insensitive. Hypnoanesthesia can be applied without the necessity of any abstention from premedication or food. It can be initiated and terminated at the suggestion of the dentist and need not be continued for some time once administered. There is no nausea or sickness stemming from the anesthesia during or after a procedure. Once hypnoanesthesia has been induced, it can be reinduced very rapidly. Furthermore, because suggestions can be given to render it effective postoperatively, the need for postoperative medication may be eliminated, or at least greatly reduced.

The disadvantages of hypnoanesthesia in dentistry stem primarily from fact that it cannot be applied to all patients. Wookey (1938) held that 35% of his patients could be hypnotized deeply enough for painless dental surgery. Given the new hypnotic procedures available now, the number is certainly much higher. However, the issue of time can limit its use, especially if the clinician is at the stage of gaining experience with the modality.

Hypnotic suggestions to produce anesthesia might proceed as follows: "I shall press down on this tooth, and you will feel a sense of pressure in the gums. The more I press, the more numb the gums will feel. I shall count backward from 10 to 0. By the time I reach 0, all feeling will be gone from the tooth. Ten, you are beginning to sense the numbness. Nine, the numbness is increasing. Eight, 7, 6, the feeling is going away from this tooth. Five, 4, all you can feel is a slight sense of pressure. Three, 2, the tooth is becoming almost totally insensitive. One, 0. It is completely numb; it can feel almost nothing. It is completely anesthetic. You will feel completely comfortable during the dental work. Relax deeply. You need not be disturbed in any way."

Half a century ago, Moss (1952) suggested that the dentist should then press the points of an instrument lightly into the gums while stating firmly, "See, it's completely numb." He then followed this by contrasting the sensation with a probing of another, nonanesthetized area, stating firmly, "I shall now press this pointed instrument into the opposite side of your mouth. This time you will feel the usual sharp pain and draw away." It is our feeling that, although this test is very definitive and quite convincing to the patient when deep anesthesia has been obtained in the anesthetized area, the probing into the nonanesthetized region should not be so severe as to bring the patient out of hypnosis. Perhaps this second part of the test might be verbalized as follows: "I shall now press this pointed instrument into the opposite side of your mouth. This time, you will feel a definite pain and draw away. However, it will not disturb your deep hypnotic calm. You will continue to remain in the same state." One precaution should be noted. Because the deeply anesthetized patient may make no response to drilling, the dentist should ensure that the tool does not overheat and that consideration for brief rest periods be given, as usual. Remember, the hypnotizable patient will not react like the nonhypnotizable patient if the usual cooling water stream is interrupted.

With training, patients can be taught to use hypnosis to produce anesthesia in any part of their bodies. This is most easily done by having them focus on the hand or a particular finger and suggesting a numbness there. Once numb, the anesthetic feeling can be transferred to any part of the body simply by massaging that part with the anesthetized hand or finger. Thus, the index finger can be anesthetized and the patients can then be instructed to make the gums adjacent to a given tooth insensitive by rubbing their anesthetized finger over that area. In many cases, this will be sufficient to permit operative work without further anesthesia. In others, where the numbing is incomplete, the effect will at least be such that the patients will feel no discomfort from the needle during injection of a chemoanesthesia, and less chemoanesthesia will be needed. Hypnoanesthesia makes the problem of suturing gum tissue much less painful or even painless.

Once the patient is hypnotized and suggestions of anesthesia are administered, it is advisable for the dentist not to question a patient about possible feelings of pain. Assume that the patient is not present and proceed with the dental work unless the patient questions or complains. When in doubt, use chemoanesthesia. However, hypnoanesthesia should be tried first. Some dentists have found hypnosis useful for premedication, especially during short operations.

Postoperative Care. Postoperative sequelae, such as pain and bleeding, can often be mitigated by hypnotic suggestion. There are many reports on the effectiveness of hypnosis for the relief of bleeding. Most clinical studies are positive (Newman, 1971, 1974; Stolzenberg, 1955). However, Crasilneck and Fogelman (1957) were unable to secure significant effects on clotting time. Even though there may be exceptions for certain patients (particularly those using aspirin or vitamins E and A supplementation) the frequency of successful reports suggests that hypnosis should definitely be considered for bleeders, both during surgery and postoperatively. The different effects may be due to lack of adequate hypnotic depth and the idiosyncratic characteristics of deep trance participants (Barrett, 1990). The patient should be informed while in the hypnotic state that "there will be no bleeding" during the operation. Some practitioners have had patients visualize their vascular bed and "see" the blood vessels constricting and the flow of blood being restricted. Moss (1952) held that bloodless tooth extractions can be generally performed on somnambulistic patients (those who can enter a very deep trance state,) and that they are successful in some 20% of patients.

To aid in postoperative recovery, the practitioner should say that, while the patient is in hypnosis, healing will be rapid and there will be no pain. There is considerable new interest in the extent to which psychological intervention in general and hypnosis specifically can stimulate the healing processes. Such influences are thought to have a mobilizing effect on natural physiological restorative processes.

Gagging and Nausea. Gagging is a natural reflex that is developed to protect the soft palate from harmful contact. In some individuals, it becomes so strong as to prevent any dental procedure, even to the point that it will begin when the dentist's hand is simply approaching the oral region. Severe gagging can make taking impressions impossible. A number of techniques have been proposed for controlling this response. Strasberg (1960) taught his patients how to control the tongue as a way of inhibiting gagging. He had them notice that whenever they gagged, they would thrust their tongue up and forward, almost out of the mouth. By bringing an instrument into proximity of the oral cavity, he would initiate the gagging and call their attention to this tongue response. He then explained that if they held their tongue back, low in the mouth, and almost swallowed it, they would be unable to gag.

Secter (1960) tied the gag reflex to control of the abdominal muscles. Patients were instructed to hold their breath and tighten these muscles. Attention was called to the fact that if there was any lessening of this tension, then they were "leaking" air, and that they must not leak air. Secter used the direct stare induction method combined with an authoritative manner and maintained that the hypnotic suggestions must be given very firmly with no hesitation or doubt by the dentist.

A commonly used procedure is to induce anesthesia (as we discussed earlier as a treatment for acute pain) in some other part of the body, such as the hand or a finger, and then transfer it to the entire oral cavity. The patient is then told, "Your mouth is numb all over, therefore, you cannot gag. It is impossible to gag." Secter added the phrase "Try to gag and take pleasure in failing." The gagging may not be inhibited directly by the numbness. However, a clear demonstration of hypnotic influence to the patient by the induction and transfer of the anesthesia establishes confidence in the potency of hypnosis, before attempting to deal with the vagaries of the gag reflex. Accordingly, the following suggestion of "It is not possible for you to gag" is believed and followed.

Henry Clarke (Clarke, 1996, 1997; Clarke & Reynolds, 1991) has worked for many years in hypnodontia. As part of his research and practice, he developed a unique imagery technique to treat gagging (Clarke & Persichetti, 1988). Once hypnotized, the patient is asked to imagine "breathing through an opening in the neck" (cricothyroid region). The concept at play is that it is not difficult for patients to focus on the pharyngeal area during a procedure when they are focusing on breathing, thereby bypassing the "gagging" area. The image is designed to fulfill the patient's primary concern with maintaining the ability to breath. The hypnosis continues with the suggestion of "cool fresh air flowing in and out of the hole with no effort whatsoever." Obviously, some patients are rather turned off by the image of breathing through a hole in the neck, but that can be overcome by the use of hypnosis to "numb the throat" or by breathing in some other creative way that is more acceptable to the patient.

Clarke & Persichett (1988) also recommended combining desensitization with hypnosis to familiarize patients with procedures that are to be completed and to reduce or eliminate potential anxieties Patients are asked, usually by use of a home audiotape approximately 5 minutes in length, to practice rehearsals of the various procedures that will be used in their cases.

Accustoming Patients to Prosthetics (Dentures). The problem of accustoming a patient to new a prosthetic device can be approached in another way. In hypnosis, a memory of the patient's original teeth is suggested. This is done by regression, going back to the period when he or she still had teeth. The patient is instructed to run his or her tongue over the teeth in fantasy and to recall just exactly how they felt. Next, the patient is told that every time he or she moves the tongue over the new dentures, he or she will reactivate a memory feeling of the original teeth. In this technique, the tactual memory of the original teeth is hypnotically activated. Then the touching of the new dentures by the tongue is made to constitute the stimulus cue, which reactivates that familiar memory. The dentures begin to feel like the original teeth as the contact stimulation is fused with past memory experience. This same procedure can be used to secure adjustment to any new formation in the mouth, such as a crown, bridge, or orthodontic appliances that might feel initially strange. Ament (1955) used the principle of time distortion to suggest to the patient that he or she had been wearing these dentures for a long time already and that within a short period it would be experienced as if a long period of time had passed.

Gagging can result from deep-seated unconscious conflicts related to the oral region. In such cases hypnoanalytic therapy is effective. Sometimes it is essential when none of the more suggestive or directive hypnotic approaches succeed in the face of powerful underlying motivations to the contrary. However, hypnoanalysis is not a procedure that will ordinarily be used by the dentist. It should probably be employed only when these simpler procedures have failed.

Salivation. The dentist's suggesting to the hypnotized patient that the mouth will feel as if it is full of dry crackers can inhibit excessive salivation. The principle involved here is to suggest a condition associated with a physiological response and allow that response to emerge indirectly as a consequence.

Dental-Phobic Patients. Goodman (personal communication to A.F.B., 2004) explains that although "scrubbing and gloving," a time when the patient is most likely to be in spontaneous hypnosis, metaphoric and subliminal suggestions are given for relaxation, comfort, and security. Slowing their breathing with nonverbal body language, expressed as outward calmness on the part of the hypnodontist allows patients to relax further.

Dental-phobic patients are given hypnotic suggestions to counteract their previous untoward dental treatment experiences and to set positive expectations for their present treatment. Embedded hypnotic suggestions are intended to set a fresh foundation of trust, security, comfort, and relaxation. In addition, many phobics require a series of formal hypnotic induction appointments to provide optimal imprinting and reinforcement of previous hypnotic suggestions along with ego strengthening and self-hypnosis. Frequently, audio recordings of the sessions or special personalized tapes are created to allow the patient to reexperience the sessions.

One technique recommended by Goodman (2004) for apprehensive children recognizes how quickly induced and disassociated children can be, when necessary. He most often uses a metaphor of enjoying a magic carpet ride to Disneyland. Alternatively, involvement in a cartoon world fantasy is created in hypnosis with a running commentary of hypnotic suggestions.

Correcting Faulty Habits. Thumb sucking in child patients can be inhibited by suggesting to them in hypnosis that the thumb will taste bitter. Another approach is to displace the response to one in which they clench the hands. The two can be combined. The sucking is inhibited by the bitter-suggestion response. The need to suck is then transferred to the hand movement or perhaps to some less-harmful oral activity such as a greater enjoyment of food during mealtimes. The same procedures of inhibition and possible displacement can be successful in reducing tongue thrusting.

Secter (1961) reported the successful employment of behavior therapy reinforcement techniques before behaviorists had fully developed such procedures. A child who was given to tongue thrusting and to nail biting was induced in hypnosis to visualize a very disgusting scene which initiated in her "bad" feelings. This was replaced by a beautiful scene, which caused the bad feelings to dissipate and new, pleasant sensations to be experienced. The first scene was then tied by hypnotic suggestion to the stimulus of tongue thrusting. Every time the patient employed tongue thrusting, she would experience the bad feelings, but as soon as she ceased the activity, the unpleasant sensations would leave and pleasurable ones would emerge. Of course, this procedure employs the principles of punishment and positive reinforcement to extinguish an undesirable response (tongue thrusting) and reinforce a constructive one (the cessation of tongue thrusting). After the linking of the bad feelings with the tongue thrusting and the good feelings with its absence, the procedure was repeated with nail biting and succeeding in eliminating that response, also.

Marcus (1963), in dealing with thumb sucking children, called their attention to the fact that (a) although it was alright to suck when one was little, grown-ups did not suck their thumbs, and (b) that one becomes "prettier" when one does not suck her thumb. Little girls might be asked if their doll sucked *her* thumb. The important point is that children should not be shamed for such behavior because fear and shame are often one of the basic causes of these responses. Rather, a careful consideration of the motivational needs of the child (such as wanting to be grown-up) will enable the practitioner to plan his or her suggestions and images to maximize the child's natural drive and to harness these in the interest of eliminating faulty habits.

Bruxism. Bruxism, or teeth grinding, is one of the most harmful dental habits. The grinding together of teeth, frequently during sleep, is particularly detrimental. Some individuals will completely wear away the tooth enamel and must have their teeth extracted. A number of procedures, some using hypnosis, have been employed in treating this condition.

Clarke (1997) began by having the patient experience hypnosis with a variety of images, phrases, and hypnotic suggestions related to Bruxism therapy. He obtained feedback as to which suggestions are likely to be the most effective on a self-hypnosis audiotape to be made at the next appointment. Clarke pointed out that exploring these experiences with the patient is not a psychological exploration but simply a process intended to discover the patient's strongest areas of hypnotic involvement and image preferences. He collaborated with the patient as to the determination of the most useful suggestions to be included on the forthcoming audiotape.

For nocturnal Bruxism, the tape is usually about 15 minutes in length. Patients are instructed to listen to the tape upon retiring each night. At the end of the tape, hypnotic suggestions are given to go from hypnorelaxation into deep sleep. Some patients begin to fall asleep before the end of the tape, but this is has not been a problem in Clarke's experience. The early stages of sleep are generally a hypnoidal state where the patient remains aware of the suggestions. Daytime clenchers listen once or twice a day in a relaxing place. The suggestions at the end of the tape are to return to the "usual state of awareness, wide awake, refreshed, relaxed, and alert." Daytime tapes are typically no more than 10 minutes long. The hypnotic induction used focuses on relaxed breathing, progressive muscle relaxation and waves of relaxation from head to toes. The images include (a) the jaw hanging like a hammock or sling; (b) muscles soft, smooth, and relaxed; (c) blood vessels dilated and warm; (d) tissues being nourished; (e) hot packs; (f) cold packs; (g) hot tub; (h) sun or skiing; and (i) walking, floating, riding, or drifting. Clarke also used a number of additional positive hypnotic suggestions, including (a) "lips together, teeth apart"; (b) "no problem worth eating yourself over"; (c) "now you can control relaxation rather than stressors controlling you"; (d) "you can take care of yourself"; (e) "approach the world with a sense of humor"; (f) "smile inwardly and outwardly"; and (g) "your body is your most prized possession and you owe it the respect of good health."

The key suggestions for both the waking or the sleep tape are that the patient experience (a) a heightened state of awareness of unnecessary, counterproductive muscle tension; (b) an increased ability to relax; (c) his or her special phrases and images that will trigger jaw muscles relaxation; and (d) that the process will work automatically, whether awake or asleep. These suggestions are stated at the beginning of the tape and repeated at least two or three times throughout the tape. The results of this comprehensive approach typically show sufficient improvement within 4 to 5 weeks, thereby warranting a progress check at that time. To encourage patients to complete the follow-up, the practitioner makes no charge for the follow-up session. This is thought to further encourage compliance with the use of the tape. Psychoanalytically, such an individual is often viewed as having a great deal of repressed anger, which he or she expresses, dreamlike, during sleep. The psychodynamically oriented therapeutic approach would then require that, through abreactions or other analytic techniques, the repressed rage must be released, the origins of it discovered, and a reintegration of the personality achieved. This may be necessary if the previously suggested approaches are unsuccessful. However, such a treatment is a very complicated procedure and normally would require referral to an analytically or hypnoanalytically trained psychotherapist.

Summary

Hypnosis cannot replace the many chemoanesthesias, analgesias, and other dental techniques that have been developed to their present stage of effectiveness, but hypnosis can serve as a valuable adjunct and in some cases will provide the leverage that makes possible successful treatment of previously impossible cases.

Not only will dentists who become experienced with hypnosis have available another modality and additional techniques for the improvement of their practice but in the course of studying the modality they also will learn much about the psychology of human behavior. They are better prepared to deal with the entire patient and his or her reactions to interventions in the oral cavity.

Chapter 16
Hypnosis for Specialized Problems

Irritable Bowel Syndrome

Irritable bowel syndrome (IBS), or spastic colon, is a common disorder accounting for up to half of gastroenterologists' workload. Irregular contractions and distension of the intestines result in disruptive bowel habits. Symptoms include constipation, diarrhea, cramps, bloating, gas, and long-lasting pain. Common extra-colonic symptoms are lethargy, nausea, and backache. IBS patients also have lower perceptual thresholds for pain and discomfort with enhanced sensitivity to visceral stimuli (Naliboff, Munakata, Chang, & Mayer, 1998). They also show increased vigilance toward expected aversive events (Lembo et al., 2000). Symptoms typically fail to respond to medications, and overall treatment by an array of conventional medicine is often unsatisfactory. As a result, IBS patients commonly seek repeated consultations and see their family physicians more frequently for minor ailments (Gonsalkorale, Miller, Afzal, & Whorwell, 2003). The socioeconomic impact is enormous.

In contrast to the failure of conventional medical interventions, gut-directed hypnotherapy has been shown to be extremely effective in the treatment of IBS. Most patients show very substantial improvement in symptoms and quality of life. Several independent studies have consistently confirmed these improvements (Galovski & Blanchard, 1998; Gonsalkorale, Houghton, & Whorwell, 2002; Harvey, Hinton, & Gunary, 1989; Houghton, Heyman, & Whorwell, 1996; Palsson, Turner, & Johnson, 2002; Whorwell, Prior, & Colgan, 1987; Whorwell, Prior, & Faragher, 1984). The

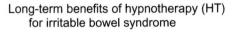

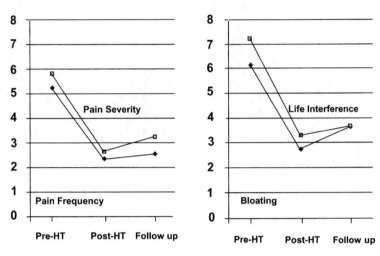

Fig. 16.1 The graphs show reduced irritable bowel symptomology after hypnotherapy and at follow-up. Data adapted by A. Barabasz and J. Roark from Gonsalkorale, Miller, Afzal, and Whorwell (2003).

hypnotherapeutic GUT-directed protocol, developed by Gonsalkorale et al. (2002) involves a course of twelve 1-hour sessions conducted weekly over a 3-month period.

Other than the initial assessment session, each session involves the induction of the hypnotic state and deepening followed by ego-strengthening suggestions tailored to the specific patient. Specific hypnotic suggestions typically involve the induction of warmth in the abdomen using the hands and imagery. Other hypnotic suggestions are directed at the specific control and normalizing of gastrointestinal functions.

The enormous success of this technique, begun by Whorwell et al. (1984), eventually led to the establishment of an IBS treatment unit sponsored by the National Health Service in England, which was exclusively focused on hypnotherapy. The initial 250 patients treated in this unit received extensive follow-up, confirming the beneficial effects of hypnotherapy in the majority of patients (Gonsalkorale et al., 2002).

Perhaps even more impressive has been the follow-up by Gonsalkorale et al. (2003), which involved the follow-up of 200 patients to determine the long-term effects of hypnosis on symptom improvement, consultation rates, and the use or discontinuation of use of various GUT-related medications. Of the 273 patients who were sent questionnaires, an usually high return rate of 204 was found. The returns were also reasonably well distributed among the time since completion of treatment, with between 20% to 30% in each of the categories ranging from 1 to 2 years through 5 years since hypnotherapy had been provided in the special unit.

Of the initial 71% of patients who responded to hypnotherapy for the control of IBS, 81% maintained their improvement over time, whereas the majority of the remaining 19% remarked that the deterioration of symptoms had been only slight. Remarkably, there was no significant difference in the symptoms scores among the patients assessed at 1, 2, 3, 4, or 5-plus years following treatment. Levels of depression and anxiety were likewise significantly improved at follow-up with minimal deterioration. The socioeconomic impact was also apparent in that the majority of patients reported a substantial reduction in consultation rates and significant reduction (or termination) of use of medications following the completion of hypnotherapy that was maintained over the course of the follow-up periods. The finding that the responders continued to improve after finishing hypnotherapy cannot be explained away by their use of other treatments. Only 9.7% (14 patients) had tried other treatments—including dietary changes, alternative medicines, and yoga—and found these helpful. Hypnotherapy was almost universally well-accepted by the patients. Ninety-three percent of the entire patient group considered that the course of hypnotherapy was worthwhile, including all of the responders and more than three quarters of the nonresponders.

Those who wish to construe hypnosis effects as nothing more than placebo might be quick to note the high level of placebo response in IBS patients. However, such placebo response established in IBS patient groups can last up to 3 months. The Gonsalkorale et al., (2003) findings for sustained, long-term effects make placebo response a very unlikely explanation. The improvements lasted at least 1 year and remained at the same level in patients more than 5 years! Furthermore, the nonresponders failed to exhibit significant improvement during the follow-up period, making it extremely unlikely that the improvements observed in the responder group were due to the natural course of the condition. Very similar results have been generated from other clinics using hypnosis for IBS (Barabasz, in press; Galovski & Blanchard, 1998; Gonsalkorale et al., 2002; Palsson et al., 2002). In each of the settings, males were more likely to be nonresponders than females. It seems clear that the beneficial effects of hypnotherapy for IBS are long lasting, and continued improvements after hypnosis is the norm.

Klein and Spiegel (1989) showed that hypnosis could be used to inhibit as well as to stimulate gastric acid secretion. Using the hypnotic state, there was a 39% reduction in basal acid output and an 11% reduction in pentagastrin-stimulated peak acid output. This direct physiological effect of hypnosis on gastric output may account in large part for the ability of hypnotherapy to prevent relapse. Colgan, Faragher, and Whorwell (1988) tested hypnotherapy in relapse prevention duodenal ulcer patients using a carefully controlled design and a 1-year follow-up. Remarkably, 100% of the patients who received medication until their ulcers were healed had relapse, but for patients who also received hypnotherapy, only half had relapse.

Palsson (1998) developed the only standardized hypnosis protocol for IBS. In contrast to the approaches of others, which are focused on the gut, ego-strengthening, and increasing the sense of control over bowels, Palsson's approach was developed from a different paradigm. It is specifically intended to neutralize the symptom-related cognitive processing abnormalities that have been found to be characteristic of IBS patients who uniformally tend toward high somatization (overattention to normal physical sensations and minor symptoms).

Palsson's (1998) approach systematically aims to alter the patient's perception and attentional focus on symptoms and physical sensations and to reduce in a targeted manner the two maladaptive psychological tendencies of catastrophizing and neuroticism in regard to life in general and specifically about bowel sensations. After trance deepening, the hypnotic suggestions that connect to each of the imagery scenes involve a gradual shift to direct hypnotic suggestions about alteration of present experiences. Hypnosis includes suggestions to create a sense of both distance and discontinuity between events in the patients' life and bowel activity. The focus is to enhance nonconscious levels of acceptance of normal sensations. The intervention is both gradual and oblique so that it does not come into conflict with the patient's current cognitive framework and cause resistance. The protocol is written so as to bypass critical-analytical thinking as much as possible, postponing all direct hypnotic suggestions for change to the end of a series of extremely serene scenes. Palsson emphasized that the scenes involve "a kind of double dissociation, for the purposes of maximum suspension of the regular critical frame of mind" (Palsson, personal communication, 2004). The conceptualization of the specific changes in perception and attentional focus are the key to the profound and lasting clinical effects of the protocol.

Unlike other approaches using hypnosis for IBS patients, prior to Palsson's protocol, which involve more general or tailored suggestions, such as those from Gonsalkorale's group, Whorwell's group, or my own (Barabasz, in press), Palsson endeavored to create something that could be reliably delivered to all IBS patients without deviation in procedure. The detailed seven-session protocol is designed for verbatim delivery, thus, to provide scientific documentation of the exact intervention used and to increase the potential for replicability and generalizability among the widest possible range of clinicians. To date, this is the only fully standardized verbatim protocol for IBS that has been tested.

To produce a protocol useful for all patients—or at least all patients with some degree of hypnotizability, regardless of their other personal characteristics—dictated that the protocol involve a rather direct instructional style and rely heavily on direct, detailed descriptions of imagery instead of inviting each person's imagination to fill in most of the details. Palsson recognized that some patients are far better than others in developing their own imagery, so he focused on developing a procedure that would produce clinically meaningful effects for the greatest number of patients.

Palsson (personal communication, 2004) explained, "There have hardly been any patients in my practice who are not able to imagine these scenes in the script, and that this is due the great detail and fixed framework." He emphasized that it is best to help the patient dissociate by bringing him or her deep into hypnosis and into a scene by firmly encouraging the patient to experience the imagery with as many senses as possible; therefore, he uses imagery including sound, touch, colors, textures, temperature, and smells. This is accomplished in the form of permissive hypnotic suggestions and questions such as "Maybe you notice a smell … if you do, what does it smell like?" Despite this open-ended aspect of the protocol, the entire goal remains a word-for-word delivery that can be used for all IBS patients.

The standardized protocol of Palsson (1998) begins by reminding the practitioner to confirm that patient first be diagnosed with IBS by a physician, preferably by a gastroenterologist. Patient's are asked to track their symptoms in a daily symptom log, which produces a summary score for abdominal pain, bloating, and bowel-consistency ratings for 14-day periods, thus providing a quick assessment of improvement in symptoms. It is emphasized with the patient that improvement is frequently not observed until midway through the course of treatment. The patient is treated with a course of seven standardized hypnosis session scripts, scheduled approximately every other week over a 12-week treatment period. The scripts are intended to be followed verbatim except when the induction part of the script needs to be adapted to an individual's specific hypnotic-response rate to ensure some depth.

Following the second hypnosis treatment session, patients are provided with an audiotape recording of a home-hypnosis exercise, which is recorded in the therapist's voice and follows verbatim the audiotape's text script. Patients are instructed to use the recording at home whenever possible, but no less than 5 times a week. Patients are encouraged to continue to use the exercise until after the last of the seven treatment sessions is completed. Patients are also encouraged to try the home exercise once, practiced without the aid of the tape, if they so desire. Once the patient becomes familiar with the language of the recording, it makes it possible to do the exercise anywhere, anytime, without dependence on the tape-recording apparatus.

Smoking

Smoking is a key risk factor in a wide range of serious illnesses. According to the surgeon general's report to the U.S. Department of Health and Human Services (1990), each year, in excess of 400,000 deaths in the United States can be linked directly to tobacco use. Nearly half of those addicted to smoking attempt to break the habit each year, yet at best, only 5% who attempt smoking cessation without professional help are likely to be successful for any significant period of time (Giovino, Henningfield, Tomar, Escobedo, & Slade, 1995). Because of the many addictive agents present in cigarette tobacco, breaking the habit is not easy. Furthermore, smoking is reinforced in many ways as a relaxation agent, for the reduction of anxiety, and for the inhibition of anger. It also is associated as an aid in overcoming social shyness.

Not only does smoking meet many different psychological needs for some people, but the smoker quickly undergoes physiological changes while adjusting to smoking that result in painful withdrawal symptoms when he or she attempts to quit. Helen Crawford and her colleagues have conducted cognitive EEG event-related potential research with smokers and nonsmokers in a collaborative project with biochemists (Crawford, McClain-Furmanski, Castagonli, & Castagonli, 2002). The findings showed that chronic tobacco smokers have substantially less monoamine oxidase in their blood and brains than nonsmokers usually have, and, as they quit smoking, the levels apparently rise again over time. Smokers titrate themselves very closely as to how much they smoke. This raises serious questions about behavioral methods aimed at smokers, such as having them roll their own cigarettes to reduce consumption. Asking them to smoke unknown amounts of tobacco, after rolling them, introduces new problems. The most basic question Crawford raised relates to the ethics of introducing smokers to a new method of smoking.

Many individuals have given up smoking only to find that later, sometimes years and years afterward they find themselves lighting up a cigarette upon the slightest provocation. The therapist who treats smoking is confronted with a patient whose compulsive habit is strongly reinforced and the cessation of which results in tension, anxiety, pain, and initial weight gain as protein lipase metabolism readjusts. The slightest relapse typically results in a full-scale reinstatement of the smoking behavior.

Several approaches have been devised, generally built on the principle of reframing one's commitment to health and living. The literature has become voluminous. Nearly every technique described has been able to report results with varying percentages of success, most often ranging from 20% to claims of more than 90% in terms of curbing the habit (Green, 2004) . However, follow-up studies have shown a great deal of recidivism as a substantial number of the new abstainers, when finding themselves in smoke-filled company and beset with feelings of tension, are seduced into resumption of the habit.

An evaluation of hypnosis as an empirically supported clinical intervention (Lynn, Kirsch, Barabasz, Cardena, & Patterson, 2000) concluded that hypnotic procedures are very cost-effective and have earned a place among entry-level treatments in stepped-care approaches that begin with the least costly and least time-consuming interventions. Studies of hypnosis for smoking cessation intended to demonstrate the specificity of hypnotic procedures and move hypnosis into the arena of empirically supported treatments must make greater efforts to include biochemical measures of abstinence beyond patient self-reports (such as cotinine testing). Nontheless, Green and Lynn (2000) concluded that hypnotic interventions generally yield higher rates of abstinence relative to waiting-list and no-treatment control conditions.

In perhaps one of the most innovative approaches to dealing with the problem of smoking, H. Spiegel (1970) described a single session approach, which offers some patients the opportunity to place their problem in a new perspective. The method has been refined as described by H. Spiegel and D. Spiegel (1978) and more recently by H. Spiegel and D. Spiegel (2004). Once the patient has been assessed for hypnotizability and induced into a hypnotic state using the *Hypnotic Induction Profile* (HIP; discussed in chapter 4) he or she is exposed to deepening techniques and asked to concentrate on three basic points:

1. For your body, smoking is a poison. You are composed of a number of components, the most important of which is your body. Smoking is not so much a poison for you as it is for your body.
2. You cannot live without your body; your body is a precious physical plant through which you experience life.

3. To the extent that you want to live, you owe your body respect and protection. This is your own way of acknowledging the fragile, precious nature of you body and, at the same time, your way of seeing yourself as your body's keeper. You are in truth your body's keeper. When you make this commitment to respect your body, you have within you the power to smoke your last cigarette.

The three suggestions are repeated and elaborated on while the patient remains in hypnosis. Self-hypnosis is then taught so that the points can be reinforced. The patient is instructed to use self-hypnosis typically 3 to 10 times a day. The initial research (H. Spiegel, 1970) reported that, out of a group of 615 patients, 271 returned a questionnaire at a 6-month follow-up. A total of 120 "hard core" smokers had stopped for at least 6 months, and 120 additional smokers had reduced their smoking significantly.

The Spiegels (H. Spiegel & D. Spiegel, 2004) recognized that a more intensive or extensive therapeutic input would result in a higher percentage of responders. They also noted that a more prolonged or involved treatment might better be selected for those patients who are more committed to stopping smoking. The point of their single-session approach is simply maximum therapeutic response with a minimum of time and cost involved. However, subsequent sessions are recognized to be helpful at varying intervals following the initial cognitive restructuring that takes place as a result of the hypnotic suggestions. This is a simple technique requiring minimum time and minimal cost which can be employed widely to help the greatest number of patients. Clearly, others are likely to benefit from more involved treatment, whereas some will remain unresponsive to any approach. The procedure, although outwardly a simple matter of application of the protocol provided, has been shown to be far more efficacious when used by experienced clinicians versus beginners in hypnosis (A. Barabasz, Baer, Sheehan, & M. Barabasz, 1986).

An examination of several studies of hypnosis for smoking cessation reveals that experienced clinicians in an outpatient practice environment (e.g., see Barabasz et al., 1986; Elkins & Hasanrajab, 2004; H. Spiegel &. D. Spiegel, 2004; H. Watkins, 1976) report consistently and relatively higher abstinence rates than those generated from university labs using protocols that are typically administered by inexperienced students or university instructors that have produced far less-startling results. This anomaly in the literature may be responsible, in combination with lack of emphasis on an adequate number of sessions or establishment of an appropriate clinical relationship, for what is reported by some as "mixed results."

Curiously, only one study appears to have addressed these issues directly. A. Barabasz et al. (1986) obtained clinical follow-up data from 307 clients over a 36-month follow-up of hypnosis and restricted environmental stimulation therapy for smoking. Clinician experience level, contact time, and procedural thoroughness varied in six alternative experimental hypnotic intervention conditions for smoking cessation. A seventh intervention combined hypnosis with restricted environmental stimulation therapy where patients spent one to one and half hours in a recliner under sound- and light-free conditions with low-level white noise provided as background before administration of the hypnotic induction protocol.

The major findings of the research showed positive treatment outcomes to be related to greater hypnotizability, as measured by the *Stanford Hypnotic Clinical Scale*, greater absorption, greater therapist experience level, more extensive procedural thoroughness, and greater client-therapist contact time. The least-effective intervention (4% abstinence at only 4 months follow-up) involved predoctoral psychology intern trainees using a single-session approach. Experienced clinicians, with a minimum of 6,000 hypnotic inductions over many years, produced abstinence rates typically in the 30% to 36% range at long-term follow-up (18 months) whether the hypnotic suggestions were administered in a group setting or individually. Typically, the process involved no more than two sessions, an initial evaluation and hypnotizability testing taking approximately 90 minutes followed by a second 90-minute session involving further experience with hypnosis and suggestions for smoking cessation. Given that the inexperienced interns produced a mere 4% abstinence rate at only 4 months, it is remarkable that experienced clinicians who, for one reason or another, only saw their clients for the initial evaluation orientation without hypnosis for smoking, produced a 6% abstinence rate.

Since the A. Barabasz et al. (1986) study, my (A.F.B.) practice has been refined by adding additional tailored hypnotic inductions, deepening, and suggestions tailored to each patient. Patients prepay for a three- to five-session course of treatment (a total of about 5 hours) to be completed within a 10-day period. Psychological evaluation, smoking history, and hypnotizability data as well as an introduction to hypnotic phenomena occur in the first session. The second session emphasizes the client's commitment to protect his or her own body from harm using the H. Spiegel and D. Spiegel (2004) procedure. Hypnotic suggestions, after emphasis on deepening, are carefully tailored to individual clients based on their smoking history and nature of their responsiveness to hypnosis. Subsequent sessions tailor the hypnotic induction to the specific client to achieve maximal hypnotic depth and responsiveness. Considerable effort is made to ensure that the teaching of self-hypnosis, as described by the Spiegels, is not perceived as a ploy to shift the responsibility for treatment success from the doctor to the patient. Telephone follow-ups are conducted frequently between visits, and the information obtained in those follow-ups and in subsequent sessions is used to refine the induction and additional tailored hypnotic suggestions. To verify abstinence reported by patients, therapists have found that one technique that is helpful is the employment of a cotinine saliva test. This has been abandoned in my (A.F.B.) practice in recent years, because fewer than 1% of the clients seen were deceptive in their reports of abstinence from smoking. The typical abstinence from smoking rate, maintained at 12- to 18-month follow-ups, is 45% to 48%.

H. Watkins (1976) described an individualized approach involving 5 weekly sessions. The initial success rate was reported as 78% with 67% still reporting smoking cessation after 6 months. As in the A. Barabasz et al. (1986) approach, an initial smoking history aimed at the client's reason for smoking and for stopping and the feelings derived from smoking is obtained. Hypnosis was tailored on the basis of Barabasz's analysis of the patient's motivations, a series of three suggestions and two visual images were selected from a file of standard protocols. A "concentration-relaxation" induction technique was used, and the patient was presented with a selected suggestion and a visual image during the second and third sessions. An example of a case tailored to the specific patient in question follows:

1. *Relaxation suggestion.* "You tell me that smoking calms your nerves, that it is relaxing and settles you down, but what's so good about a cigarette that shortens your breathe and gives you a dry, cottony feeling in your mouth? A cigarette may seem relaxing because you pause to reach for a cigarette, remove it from the pack, light it, and take a deep inhalation. It gives you a tension-free relaxing moment. But there are other ways to get the same effect, the same relaxing moment. I am going to teach you to substitute a way to get the same effect, by taking a deep breathe in, letting it out slowly, and telling yourself to relax. Do that now—take a deep breath. Breathe in, let it out slowly, and tell yourself to relax."

2. *Victory suggestion.* "You tell me you want to feel a sense of victory over your smoking habit, a sense of willpower and self-control—a feeling of winning over this vice. You can have that a feeling by doing the following: Every time you pick up a pack of cigarettes and put that pack down again, this feeling of victory will come over you. You will feel good and strong. It's like winning one battle

after another. Each time you repeat this behavior of saying 'No' to a cigarette, either in fantasy or in reality, you will be winning one battle after another until the final victory—the victory over your smoking habit."

The good feeling one derives from putting down the pack is the immediate reinforcement. This tends to increase the future probability of actually having put down the pack without smoking.

3. *Anger suggestion.* "You tell me that you smoke to put a damper on your anger and frustration; you can see smoking is one way to handle anger, but you and I know that smoking is no solution to this problem. Smoking ends up hurting you physically, and it cannot discharge or control your feelings. If you are angry with someone, express those feelings in a constructive way. If this is not appropriate, then release that anger energy through exercise, or beating a pillow, or imagine you have a small rubber ball on your hand and knead it as you would dough. Try that now. Just imagine there is a soft rubber ball in your hand and squeeze it; keep working the ball until your hand is tired."

4. *Cost imagery.* "Cigarettes are [insert current cost] a pack. You tell me that you smoke up to two packs a day. That means you must pay at least [insert the dollar amount] a day for cigarettes. Multiply that [insert amount] by 7 and the result is [insert the total for a week] per week. If you multiply [insert number of dollars per day by the number of days in a year], then the total amount you are paying for cigarettes a year is [insert the total amount], and what for? For a habit that makes you miserable, a habit that destroys your health. Wouldn't you like to use the money for something else—for something that would make you happy instead of miserable? If you stop smoking, you deserve to spend the money you save by buying something that wouldn't go up in smoke. Think now of what you would like to buy with the [insert the amount of money for the total year] you would save in a year's time, something, perhaps, that you have always wanted but felt was too much of a luxury. In your imagination right now, buy this item and experience using it. Feel the pleasure while I am silent for a minute."

Using this imagery, Helen Watkins motivated clients by picturing a desirable, long-term goal that they could commit to. She suggested to the clients that, after arousal from hypnosis, the money that is not spent on cigarettes can be saved in a glass jar or a special container and the clients could watch it accumulate daily.

5. *Day of not smoking.* "Imagine that the day has come that you no longer smoke. You are walking across to this building. The air is fresh, the sun is shining, and it is a beautiful day. You woke up this morning feeling good about yourself and your world; you like the way you are handling your life. For one thing, the feeling of being a slave to a cigarette no longer haunts you. You are in control, not the cigarette. You have more energy. Your throat is clear, and you know your lungs are clearing. You feel great, and the more you think about how good you feel, the more energetic your steps become. Continue walking now while I am silent for a minute."

Additional hypnotic suggestions are constructed within a concept of "excuse for a break," then "socialization" (showing that cigarettes interfere with socialization and separate the person from others). Visual images can involve the aversive experience to tobacco smell on clothes. A particularly effective hypnotic image is a "hospital scene," in which the doctor is saying some years later, "I can't do much for you now; I told you years ago you should stop smoking. All I can do now is give you medication for temporary relief before you die of heart and lung failure. I'm sorry, it's all we can do now. If only you had quit when you had the chance."

Next, the patient is taught self-hypnosis to practice the suggestions and visual images alone during the last two weeks between treatment sessions. An important part of this approach is the therapist's insistence at the end of the second session that the patient phone each day for one week and report success or failure. No scolding or praise is administered, simply an acceptance of the report; but if the patient fails to call, the therapist calls the patient on that same day. H. Watkins (1976) noted that the greatest difficulty in smoking cessation is for those individuals who use smoking to dampen feelings of anger to quit.

Given Holroyd's (1980) conclusion that the likelihood of success for hypnosis in the treatment of tobacco dependency is when four criteria are met (more than one session, tailored hypnotic suggestions, adjunctive treatment and follow-up, and an intense interpersonal relationship), the excellent success reported by H. Watkins is understandable.

Perhaps recognizing the success rates obtained with H. Spiegel and D. Spiegel's (1978) approach and the advantages of adding at least one additional separate session (A. Barabasz et al., 1986) in terms of cost-effectiveness versus H. Watkins's (1976) 5-week treatment program, Elkins and Hasanrajab (2004) developed a cost-conscious three-session intervention. Their preliminary data is based on a sample of 30 smokers enrolled in a health maintenance organization who are referred by their primary care physician for smoking cessation. The sample, with an average age of 47 years and an average number of 26 years smoking approximates the "hard-core" smokers treated in the studies by the Spiegel's and A. Barabasz et al. This contrasts with the less-developed habit characteristic of the university-community population treated by Helen Watkins.

The Elkins and Hasanrajab (2004) treatment protocol of three sessions begins with an initial evaluation without hypnosis. Sessions 2 and 3 involve tailored (individually adapted) hypnotic suggestions and emphasis on individualizing the therapeutic relationship with each patient, as is characteristic of the work of the H. Watkins protocol. To reinforce the face-to-face sessions therapists provide patients with a cassette tape recording of the hypnotic induction, which includes the direct hypnotic suggestions for relaxation and feelings of comfort. The three sessions were scheduled biweekly.

The first session included a history of the patient's smoking and previous attempts to quit and a mental status and psychopathology assessment. The session also included a discussion of the addictive aspects of nicotine and the relationship between stress and cigarette smoking. Patients were also asked to select a date to stop smoking, to discard all tobacco products, and to return for hypnosis treatment on the stop-smoking date. An assessment was made of the patient's social support and the patient was introduced to hypnosis, emphasizing a debunking of myths and misconceptions. The primary purpose of this session is to develop rapport and a positive relationship before completing a hypnotic induction for smoking cessation.

In the second session, patients participated in the 25-minute hypnotic session with hypnotic suggestions aimed at relaxation and comfort as well as deepening, absorption, a commitment to stop smoking, decreased craving for nicotine, tailored posthypnotic suggestions, and practice of self-hypnosis. Patients were also asked to visualize positive benefits of smoking cessation. All inductions include emphasis on a dissociation from potential cravings and using a floating image. Posthypnotic suggestions also emphasized to the patient to not eating excessively and that the patient would find an appropriate amount of food to be satisfying. This procedure must be regarded as in its infancy, but the results are encouraging. Eighty-one percent of patients reported they had stopped smoking, and 48% reported abstinence at 12-months posttreatment. Furthermore, nearly all the patients (95%) indicated they were satisfied with the treatment they received.

Shirley Sanders (1977), another highly experienced clinician, described an approach that is perhaps as intriguing as that of the Spiegels'. Her patients were hypnotized as a group after first brainstorming to produce as many reasons as possible for becoming a nonsmoker. Then, after induction of hypnosis and deepening, patients were "time progressed" into the future to picture themselves as nonsmokers. Imagery and hypnotic dreams tailored from the brainstorming sessions were used to develop the hypnotic suggestions. This was followed by relaxation practice through self-hypnosis. Sanders reported that 84% were nonsmokers by the fourth session and 68% remained so after 10 months.

Nail Biting

Some individuals acquire and maintain the oral habit of nail biting. In one of the most thorough analytically oriented reviews of literature, Gruenewald (1965, pp. 210–215) noted that different writers have attributed nail biting to "an ego-integrative search for homeostatic equilibrium through motor channels," "a substitute activity for the release of hostile conflict libidinal needs," "a discharge of oral-aggressive impulses," "a self-mutilation including both indulgence and punishment," "a depression equivalent in the form of a partial attenuated suicide," "a guilt expiating device with an element of restitution (i.e., nails grow back)," and "a hysterical conversion symptom and a masturbation equivalent."

Regardless of its etiology, patients seldom seek long, intensive, psychoanalytic treatments for it, because it is not usually regarded as seriously incapacitating. The case discussed by Gruenewald (1965) reveals that the patient's symptoms were tied to a deep-seated impairment of self-concept and was psychodynamically related to very early childhood conflicts, perhaps stemming from a disruption of developmental attachments. The patient did eventually resolve her nail-biting habit, but the hypnotic suggestions for its cessation were only effective after resolution of inner conflicts using complex hypnoanalytic techniques.

Crasilneck and Hall (1985) explored the dynamic meaning of nail biting with the child. He or she is simply asked to comment on which fingernail needs biting most. "How much? At what time of day? How much blood is needed to taste it, just a little or a lot?" Using their psychodynamic orientation, the hypnotic intervention is intended to simply to draw attention to the habit as follows: "You will no longer wish, nor desire, to continue this outgrown, unwanted habit that injures your hands and embarrasses you before your family and friends. As you begin to discontinue the habit of biting your nails, you will feel a sense of well-being and self approval." (Younger children are instead told, "You'll just feel good inside about yourself.")

My (A.F.B.) approach is based on Erickson (1958), where, in hypnosis, the child is told how useful it would be to have just one nail not bitten off. Hypnotic encouragement to bite the others even more to make up for it is provided. Once one nail has been allowed to grow, I describe using light hypnosis, "How lonely that nail must be. Could you let it have a friend?" This procedure is carried out gradually over several sessions and is, therefore, suitable only for severe cases after other brief methods have failed.

Weight Reduction and Obesity

In the early 1970s, doctors Ken Cooper (1970) and Covert Bailey (1991) started the fitness booms with their respective famous books *New Aerobics* and *Fit or Fat*. The fitness boom lasted from the 1970s to about the 1980s. Today, many Americans suffer from obesity. According to the Centers for Disease Control and Prevention more than 60% of Americans are obese. Adult-onset Type 2 diabetes is up 39% from 1990 to 1999. Currently, 25% of Americans get no exercise at all, and this increases to 34% for those ages 50 and older. Few Americans consume even the basic minimum of recommended healthy foods. The resultant harm to our biological systems and the cost of disease care is now pandemic (Hatfield, 2000).

It seems that the majority of American adults have nearly all at one time or another been involved in some form of dieting. The inevitable has been a resumption of old eating habits and a loss of lean body mass. Diet without exercise is physiologically disastrous in the long run. For example, let us take a hypothetical person, Mr. Smith, who is 200 pounds, with 30% body fat; that equates to 140 pounds of lean body mass (water, bone, muscle). He may be a relatively healthy fat man. He sees his family physician who looks at a chart and says, "Mr. Smith, you have to lose weight." So Mr. Smith involves himself in a dieting program, either one he has read about or perhaps a costly program such as Weight Watchers, Nutra-Sytems, or Physician's Fat Loss Clinic. Religiously following the diet program, Mr. Smith manages to reduce his weight to 160 pounds. He, is however, still 30% body fat, meaning he now has only 112 pounds of lean body mass. Mr. Smith is now a small, sick fat man, so he eats and eats. Now, once he has returned to his 200 pounds or perhaps more, which is the norm, he now is 35% body fat; that is, 130 pounds of lean body mass.

What does this mean? It means that he must eat less, just to maintain the weight that he had before all that dieting. The yo-yo cycle goes on and on and this is why some people who are enormously fat are actually telling the truth when they say they eat very little. The more a person diets without proper exercise, the more the yo-yo cycle goes on.

For the reasons we discussed previously, to be ethical and responsible in our use of hypnosis for weight loss, we must focus on creating a new philosophy of life, a new commitment toward one's body and health. Hypnosis that focuses on diet plus cardiovascular training such as walking or using a treadmill or perhaps even jogging, plus resistance training (ideally with weights) allows a person to eat more at a reduced body weight. The point is that the person, by gaining muscle, which is normally lost because of the aging process, is able to maintain a higher level of health and a higher caloric intake, without becoming obese.

Muscle mass is absolutely critical to maintaining quality-of-life youthfulness and vigor. People who lose a lot of muscle mass during standard diet weight loss programs lose fitness. They cannot do much physically so their performance declines whether it be skiing, playing golf, gardening, or even just carrying the groceries. Muscle mass is also critical to bone health. Women in particular lose bone mass with age (osteoporosis). Muscle mass is also critical to body temperature control because muscle holds a lot of water it is essential for temperature regulation. Loss of muscle robs the body of precious water stores. Therefore, a person has more trouble regulating heat and suffers a decrease in blood volume, which decreases endurance. When using hypnosis to reduce a persons weight and increase their fitness level, we must recognize that one lowers their metabolic rate when they lose weight. Muscle mass maintenance helps a great deal but it is still not enough in the short term. In the long term, the natural link between muscle mass and metabolic rate reestablishes itself. Once a client increases lean mass by building muscle, metabolism also increases. That means they can eat more.

Vigorous resistance training, which can be facilitated when encouraged with a hypnotic protocol, increases lean body mass. Fat-loss efforts are considerably enhanced and longer lasting and this is why dieting alone or dieting with only aerobic exercise is simply not the answer. It is essential that the client understand that the more muscle he or she has the greater their metabolic rate. Muscle is the best way to stroke the metabolic fire and to keep tissue active. Hypnosis should also be aimed at teaching the person to eat five to seven small meals per day rather than the usual three squares. This keeps one from going into fat storage mode, which begins to occur for most people at about 3 hours after their last meal.

Weight loss clients should be taught that they need to outsmart their evolutionary control center. That is, if they satisfy their liver approximately every 3 hours with a small meal they should never get hungry. They should never allow themselves to get thirsty. The quickest way to develop a bloated look is to restrict your water intake. Your body simply thinks it has been placed in the desert and tries to hold on to every bit of water it can. It is also essential that clients understand that before exercise they should eat. Clients should be encouraged, in hypnosis, to "keep your tanks full, without adding fat." But to remember that if they overfill on carbohydrates, the carbs are stored as fat. Increased carbohydrate diets simply become high-fat diets. The popular "food pyramid" is a license for overfilling on carbs. The food pyramid is a wonderful way to fatten up cattle in the feedlot and one of the reasons behind the creation of obesity in the United States. The problem is that high-fat storage is associated with increased insulin response and even more fat storage. If our carbo- hydrate stores run out, we then must rely on protein and fat for energy, which is simply not efficient for high-intensity work or even for keeping one's mind active while attempting to study or do other sedentary brain- intensive tasks.

Loss of lean body mass also decreases metabolic rate. When blood- sugar levels drop, we crave high-energy foods and then tend to overfill, thus creating a very vicious cycle. These factors should be borne in mind when therapists construct tailored hypnotic inductions for their patients.

Hypnosis has considerable scientific support for its effectiveness with weight loss. The review of hypnosis as clinical intervention (Lynn et al., 2000) presented evidence that hypnotic procedures have received a great deal of empirical attention in many areas, comparable to, if not exceed- ing, the attention lavished on some of the most rigorously researched psychotherapies.

The powerful meta-analysis statistical technique permits a direct com- parison of treatment outcomes that span diverse methodological approaches and interventions. Perhaps producing one of the most fre- quently cited meta-analyses, Kirsch, Montgomery, and Sapirstein (1995) evaluated hypnosis as an adjunct to cognitive-behavioral psychotherapy. The results indicated that hypnosis can be a useful adjunct to cognitive- behavior therapy for a wide variety of problems but is particularly so (Kirsch, 1996) in the treatment of obesity. Most important is the finding across many studies showing that hypnosis helps sustain long-term weight loss. This is important, given that nearly all obese individuals who lose weight in nonhypnotic treatments quickly regain it (Stunkard, 1972). The findings of the meta-analyses were so strong as to suggest that training in hypnosis should be included routinely as part of clinical training in cogni- tive-behavioral therapy. The average patient receiving hypnosis was better off at the end of treatment and in the long term than 75% of clients receiv- ing the identical therapy without hypnosis.

M. Barabasz and D. Spiegel (1989) tested the effects of hypnosis for weight control. Hypnotizability was assessed with the *Stanford Hypnotic Susceptibility Scale,* Form C. Forty-five participants completed the study with experimenters who were masked with respect to hypnotizability scores. Participants exposed to a simple self-management technique and to the H. Spiegel and D. Spiegel (1978) hypnosis intervention modified to include specific food aversion, lost significantly more weight at a 3-month follow-up than did participants exposed only to the self-management treatment or control condition. The specificity of hypnosis in the program was supported by a significant correlation between weight loss and hypnotizability scores. Participants perceived all treatment groups as active interventions.

H. Watkins (personal communication to J. Watkins in 1979; see J. Watkins, 1987) emphasized the use of hypnosis in groups. After ensuring that each participant was in a hypnotic state, she suggested that they visualize two tables of food. On the first table are all the rich foods that are high in calories, high fats, and carbohydrates. As they see these foods, she asked the participants to recognize that they could feel a complete lack of interest and a desire to turn away. They then look at another table, filled with salads, cottage cheese, high protein items, fresh vegetables, and low-calorie foods, and at once, they feel very hungry. Their mouths begin to water, and they begin to see and think about how good it is to eat these foods. In this approach, aversive factors are minimized and positive images of enjoyable eating are suggested.

H. Spiegel and D. Spiegel (2004) adapted the procedure they use for smoking in their treatment of eating disorders. The intervention generally takes place in one or two sessions if patients exceed their normal weight by less than 15% percent. Regular therapy sessions are scheduled for patients who weigh in excess of this limit. After taking a brief psychological history, the hypnotic induction profile is explained to the patient and administered. The patient is also taught an exercise in self-hypnosis, which emphasizes the concept of eating with respect for his or her body. Once the hypnotic state is ensured, the patient is instructed to choose a varied diet, which can include a high-vegetable day, or a high-protein day, or even a liquid day. They emphasized that the major issue is that of the total calories taken in in relation to physical activity, rather than blindly following some specific formulated diet plan. Their point is to get the person to change the relationship to his or her body and realize that fighting calories is simply too narrow a focus. They also emphasized that the patient accept responsibility for his or her own eating behavior. They pointed out that far too many people blame their eating on their parents, boyfriend, girlfriend, the mayor, or even the phase of the moon. While in hypnosis, the absurdity of this notion is emphasized, and the patient is told that there is nothing for which one is more clearly 100% responsible for than one's own eating behavior.

The final major point is that as people prepare for normal weight while losing weight, it is mandatory that they reacquaint themselves with the body so that they can prepare to meet the new body at a normal weight and realize that this will be like meeting a long-lost friend. Preparing patients to meet their bodies at a normal weight prevents creating the feeling of being a "stranger" in the body, which is thought to make it more likely for patients to resume the previous self-destructive overeating behavior.

Patients are encouraged to eat like a gourmet who pays full attention to every swallow. In this way, there is total involvement and much more fulfillment with each swallow. They note that gourmets are typically of normal weight or underweight. The same basic self-hypnosis procedure used for smoking cessation is employed for overeating: (a) "For my body, overeating is a poison," (b) "I need my body to live," and (c) "I owe my body this respect and protection."

The procedure developed by Arreed Barabasz is more holistic and comprehensive. It involves training and education in exercise science as well as nutrition to produce a lifelong fitness and ideal body fat-muscle mass ratios. Patients are taught in hypnosis to reverse the normal muscle loss that occurs with aging to "stoke the metabolic fire, keep tissue active, and make it possible to eat substantial amounts of food while maintaining extremely low body fat levels and high levels of fitness in both strength and endurance." Alert and active alert hypnotic inductions are used to ease fitness-training perceptions of excursion while aiding the levels of excursion that are necessary to create muscle hypertrophy. The additional specific hypnotic suggestions administered after assessment and induction of the hypnotic state were inspired by the work of the Spiegels. Both moderate and light levels of hypnotic depth are employed before the following suggestions are administered:

1. When you choose a lifestyle of true fitness and fat loss, you have made the choice of a lifelong commitment to health and the happiness it makes possible.
2. Your body is a precious physical plant that you need to live. You wouldn't think of putting kerosene into the gas tank of your car or for that matter even using regular gas in an engine designed for high test; these are the same choices you make every day in fueling your precious body.
3. If you accept yourself, you will always feel good about yourself when fueling your body properly.
4. This lifelong commitment is a special agreement you have with your body to love and protect it from harm and thus at the same time counteract many symptoms of aging which are actually signs of illness. These are preventable in a large part by your own commitment to fitness and proper body fueling.

The hypnotic suggestions are repeated by clients in a self-hypnosis protocol tailored to their hypnotic talents before each of the five to seven small meals that they have each day. In the office sessions, patients learn about the issues that must be considered when making eating and fitness choices each day. Once a light to moderate state of hypnosis has been induced the patient is instructed:

> As the ancient Greek philosopher Aristotle recognized, a virtuous person is one who recognizes that excellence is destroyed by deficiency or excess. Moderation is the key to achieving the highest human potential or areté. Modern science relating to nutrition and exercise makes it possible today for almost any normal person to build a body worthy of comparison to the ancient Greek gods. The key is simply a moderate and continuous approach to energy intake. Always satisfy your liver every 2 and a half to 3 and a half hours. A typical male's liver holds 400 calories, while a female holds about 300 calories. The maximum number of calories to be taken at any one time then should not exceed 800 for males or 600 females to avoid fat storage. By eating at those frequent intervals, you will never run out of liver stores of energy. In so doing your body continues at its ideal metabolic rate rather than believing it has been sent off to some land of famine where every calorie must be held to stay alive. (This weight-loss program is being taught to physicians and psychologists worldwide by the first author (A.F.B.)

The general ineffectiveness of cognitive explanations and reasoning to patients is quite well-known by therapists. Usually such explanations are brushed off, rapidly forgotten, and prove quite ineffective in the face of a patient's strong emotional needs and unconscious motivations. However, the inculcating of such material in a hypnotic state can have more effect than simple conscious, intellectual arguments no matter how well reasoned they maybe. A person's maladaptive resistances are usually lowered in hypnosis, and the possibility of significantly imprinting new and more constructive attitudes in patients appears better. I (J.G.W.) have done much with "dynamic education" of patients in hypnosis regarding their underlying motivations and conflicts, and I consistently noted that the results were more significant than when the same material was presented to the fully conscious, alert participant. This is precisely why Barabasz' program is so effective when combined with fitness training.

Substance Abuse

Despite intense counseling, education programs such as Just Say No, D.A.R.E., and law enforcement efforts, the core of sensation seekers continues to use drugs (Meddis, 1994). Decades ago, attempts were made to use hypnosis to recreate the cognitive-affective characteristics of drug-induced states (Barber, 1970; Bauman, 1970; Tart, 1969; Ulett, Akpainar, Itil, & Fakuda, 1971). These pioneering efforts relied only on self-report and failed to measure hypnotizability and provide accepted experimental control conditions. As A. Barabasz and M. Barabasz (1992) noted, little can be said about the specificity of hypnosis in a clinical intervention if hypnotizability is not measured. Research conducted at Washington State University brought experimental controls to this area of study to shed light on the potential utility of hypnosis as a safe drug-state alternative that might be useful for clinicians involved in treating sensation-seeking patients.

Nishith, A. Barabasz, M. Barabasz, and Warner (1999) stringently selected individuals for high and low hypnotizability based on testing by the *Harvard Group Scale of Hypnotic Susceptibility*, Form A (Shor & Orne, 1962) and the *Stanford Hypnotic Susceptibility Scale*, Form C (Weitzenhoffer & Hilgard, 1962). The 20 high-hypnotizable participants and 20 low-hypnotizable participants were also matched for age and gender.

The study first compared the effects of alparazolam (Xanax) and a placebo identical in appearance on mood state and EEG brain activity. Participants who experienced the true alparazolam condition were invited to participate in the second research stage, which investigated the effects of hypnosis with a suggestion to recreate the alparazolam effect on mood state and EEG. The hypnotic suggestion used to recreate the alparazolam effects was derived from participant-reported experiences of alparazolam in the first part of the study. Participants were also exposed to a hypnosis-only condition to determine if the effects of suggestion with hypnosis were greater than the relaxation effects of hypnosis alone. Our aim was to determine whether a simple hypnotic induction with an alparazolam experience derived suggestion would recreate the subjective effects of alparazolam and determine whether the effects of alparazolam are greater than the effects of hypnosis plus the suggestion, and whether the effects of hypnosis plus the suggestion were greater than the relaxation effects produced by hypnosis alone. We also tested the EEG correlates of alparazolam, placebo, waking, and hypnotic conditions. After induction and deepening, the hypnotic suggestion was as follows:

> All right then ... your state of hypnosis makes it possible to fully recreate the pleasant state you experienced the other day with

Xanax. Now imagine you are taking a large dose of Xanax, twice as much as you took in the previous experiment. This is the best possible dose you can take. You can feel its effects spread throughout your body. You will have a nice and light feeling, like you floating and looking down on yourself ... you will feel a warm glow inside of you, and it feels really nice ... really good. ... Now go ahead and experience these warm and pleasant sensations until I speak to you again in a few minutes. You will feel just as you did the other day when you took the pills but even more so. (Pause about one minute, confirm the effect of the hypnotic suggestion by asking, "Do you feel it?" The patient will say yes or nod. Then say, "It will get even better.")

Participants exposed to the hypnosis-plus–hypnotic-suggestion condition demonstrated significantly greater levels of relaxation as measured by the tension-anxiety scale of the profile of mood states (Eichman & Umstead, 1971) than in the alparazolam condition or the hypnosis-only condition. The high-hypnotizable participants showed significantly greater levels of relaxation than the low-hypnotizable participants in all three conditions (hypnosis plus suggestion, hypnosis only, alparazolam only). The EEG findings showed frontal and occipital areas of the brain were specifically involved in both the alparazolam and the hypnotic suggestion conditions. This controlled study suggests that hypnosis can be useful as a substitute for at least sedative (benzodiazopines) drug use.

Cocaine addiction is generally considered to be far more serious than addiction to benzodiazopines as in the study we discussed previously. Page and Handley (1993) presented an unusual case in which hypnosis was completely successful in overcoming a $500.00 (5 grams) per day cocaine addiction. The patient was in her mid-20s and had been heavily addicted for 6 months before acquiring a commercial hypnotic weight-control tape that she used successfully to stop smoking by mentally substituting the word *smoking* for *eating*. She also used the tape to bring her down from her cocaine high to allow her to fall asleep. Eight months into her cocaine addiction, she decided to use the tape in an attempt to overcome cocaine use. For a period of 4 months she listened to the tape 3 times a day, mentally substituting the word *coke* for *eating*. Her addiction was completely broken and she established a drug-free history for a follow-up period of 9 years. The authors noted that this was quite an extraordinary recovery because hypnosis was the only intervention and there was no support network of any kind beyond the hypnosis tape available to her.

Ludwig, Lyle, and Miller (1964) at the U.S. Public Health Service Hospital in Lexington, Kentucky, used a teaching in hypnosis method for groups of 6 to 10 patients. Hypnosis was induced by "the method of high eye-fixation while making continual suggestions for tiredness, relaxation, drowsiness, and sleep." While in hypnosis, patients were then given "educational talks" in which drug addiction was explained to them, and inspirational hypnotic suggestions designed to enhance self-confidence, and encouragement to live up to their potentialities were also provided. The evils of taking that first shot of drugs were emphasized. Hypnotic suggestions were also provided to increase group cohesiveness. The procedure was exceptionally successful. However, attempts to use hypnosis to have patients mentally return to a time in their lives when they were leading a happy drug-free existences were unsuccessful with all but a few patients.

One technique was viewed by Ludwig et al. (1964) as particularly potent. Patients were told that they would feel a branding iron that "was becoming red hot" and they would soon be branding their brains with words, "I must never take the first shot of drugs." The concept is that of planting a very vivid and powerful hypnotic suggestion under what must have been an emotional experience for the patient. The branding-iron technique was also reported to have a great deal of appeal to drug-addicted patients. Perhaps the strong, authoritative approach was much more effective than a permissive, analytic one because of the kind of dependant personalities typical of drug addicts.

Ludwig et al. (1964) also tested the ability of hypnosis to influence drug symptoms and withdrawal symptoms. They reported success with 11 participants who were patient-prisoners. They did this by regressing these patients in hypnosis to times when they had been thrown in jail and had to quit cold turkey. The patients reported painful symptoms as a result of this hypnotic suggestion but not as severe as from using an actual drug. Of most interest to therapists is that, in part of their study in which they removed the behavioral and painful symptoms during an actual administration of drugs and subsequent withdrawal, the physiological symptoms remained but the psychological components were either eliminated or substantially mitigated. Obviously, these effects are similar to those established to be obtained by hypnotic anesthesia as discussed in previous chapters.

The use of hypnosis in drug dependence and drug addiction has received little controlled experimental research focus. Further investigation is needed to determine the best methods to achieve the greatest possible success rates. The difficulties that adhere in hypnotically treating alcoholism generally should be thought to apply even more so when treating drug addicts.

Insomnia

There are several theories of insomnia. The most prominent suggest either excessive physical arousal or excessive cognitive activity. Simple nonhypnotic solutions to getting to sleep when it is time to do so is to begin to quite the atmosphere down around the patient. Loud music and bright lights or excessive noise are all contraindicated if one is to settle down into a deep, sound sleep.

A sleep-facilitating self-hypnotic induction I (A.F.B.) have found useful in my practice begins in the office with an induction technique tailored to the particular patient followed by the hypnotic suggestions:

> You can transport yourself to a tropical island, all alone on a tropical island beside a jungle pool, which is fed by a waterfall. The pool is so inviting and clear that you have decided to remove your clothing and to go for a swim. As you grasp this image in your mind and are able to focus on it, let me know by raising a finger on this hand [the nondominant hand is touched]. Now soon you will be able to experience the pool on the island just as if really being there. [Once the patient has lifted a finger, continue.]

> Now the water in this crystal-clear pool is gently heated by volcanic rocks, and rifts of steam lift from the surface of this clear, pure water. You can see all the way to the bottom; it's just the perfect temperature for bathing. You decide to wade into this beautiful pool's warm, gentle massaging water. ... Now just enjoy the warmth of the water, moving up your feet into the calves of your legs, up above your knees into your thighs. This gentle, calming, soothing, warmth, water is relaxing your entire body. Now immerse yourself completely and take a relaxing short swim to a large flat rock that makes a little island almost in the middle of this pool [for nonswimmers, indicate they can wade to this flat rock]. Now that you are up on the rock you can stretch out on it. It's shaped perfectly for your body from years of being worn by the tropical waters and rains. Stretch out on the rock. You can hear the jungle birds and you might even be able to hear the ocean waves as they come rolling on the beach because it's less than half a mile away. At the same time you hear the sounds and feel the comfort of the warm, shaped rock, you may be able to smell the beautiful, tropical flowers surrounding your pool. The sun filters through the palm trees. Just enjoy. [Substantial hypnotic depth is not required for this image; even those who respond minimally to hypnosis can

benefit from it.] Now as you enjoy your experience, the warmth, the sound of the water, the tropical island sounds, tropical island flower smells and earth smells, you notice that you can hear a waterfall, and there it was all the time, at one end of this large pool, and you decide to swim [or wade] over to this waterfall. You can sit or stand underneath the waterfall. The warm water rushes down over your head, massaging your body and washing away any worries, cares, ruminations. Just savor the experience and feel the infinite sensations of peace, calm, tranquility. Enjoy the relaxation that this brings to every muscle in your body. As you move away from the waterfall you can again choose to go back to the sunny rock for a nap, or rest by the side of the pool. The relaxation takes over all by itself—the fresh air, the sunshine, the warm rock, the safety—that you experience, and the soft jungle sounds are so pleasant, so soothing, so peaceful, so calm, your whole body relaxed, calm as you're able to turn on the sleep switch and let yourself go deep asleep, sleep.

Now you know that you can recapture these feelings anytime you wish to. At night when you wish to sleep, simply practice this experience again in your mind, and whenever you do, you will go to sleep promptly, perfectly, with ease, feeling the calm tranquility flowing into every muscle fiber in your body, deep asleep.

Stentorian Snoring

Cotecha and Shneerson (2003) reviewed 10 surgical procedures or devices currently available including sleep apneas. Objective evidence of the benefit of these interventions is at best sparse, noting that the long-term success of any surgical procedure "is likely to be no more than fifty percent."

Ewin (2004) reported on a technique to deal with Stentorian snoring. The patient, a woman in her late 50s, snored so loudly that when her family went on vacation she had to stay in a separate hotel room. At home, she had a separate bedroom in the back of the house. An eyes-closed eye-roll induction was used accompanied by deep inspiration and the instruction to hold for 5 seconds, then progressive muscle relaxation for deepening (Ewin, 1992). The patient reportedly went into a deep trance within 3 to 5 minutes of progressive muscle relaxation deepening. She was then told, "From now on you will find that you can let it be impossible to make that sound no matter how hard you try. Try to do it … try again." She took several breaths through her nose and with her mouth open, and then with it closed, with no snoring sound. After alerting, she was asked to try again, and there was no sound.

She completely stopped snoring and moved back into the bedroom with her husband. A year later, she returned, noting she had started snoring again the previous month. Upon questioning, she first insisted that nothing of significance had occurred at that time frame but then revealed she had strained her back and had received a muscle relaxant from her orthopedist. The snoring returned upon her taking the medicine. The previous hypnotic session that had been successful was repeated and for the 4 remaining years of her life, her daughter who lived at home reported that the snoring had never returned.

The concept as explained by Ewin (2004) is that a positive hypnotic suggestion "let it be impossible" is better than a negative "won't be able to," and that the verb "try" implies failure, so Ewin uses it only when he does not want something to happen. He also believes that it introduces confusion because the patient had been "trying" not to snore and that it had never occurred to her to actually try to do it.

Oropharyngeal muscle relaxation occurring in sleep is related to snoring. Obviously, these patients do not snore while awake and in conscious control of their musculature. Hypnosis can be used to consciously create the symptom to bring it under voluntary control. In the present case, it may be that the muscle relaxant medication precipitated the reoccurrence of the symptom as a significant cue. This is consistent with literature showing that hypnosis can be highly successful in treating a variety of muscular disorders such as dystonia (Prussack, 2002).

Academic Performance

College students often come to their counseling centers complaining of inability to concentrate, anxieties about examinations, and reading-speed concerns. This is usually a result of poor study habits. Correction of such faulty habits is assigned to counseling psychologists who may employ a variety of directive, nondirective, or cognitive-behavioral procedures intended to teach the student how to establish regular hours of study and how to banish distracting thoughts during those periods. Hypnosis can be very helpful.

Stanton (1993) used hypnotherapy to overcome examination anxiety with 11 medical practitioners who had previously failed their fellowship examinations and who sought assistance for combating the anxiety they felt was responsible for the lack of success. They were seen individually for only two 50-minute sessions of hypnotherapeutic training aimed at engendering increased confidence in their ability to overcome examination anxiety.

In the first session, hypnotizability was assessed, and rapport was built before inducing hypnosis with a relaxation technique, which focused on attention to the breath. Participants were encouraged to develop an attached attitude as if they were watching someone else breathing. Mental calmness was encouraged with images of the mind as a pond, the surface of which was completely still, like a mirror that thoughts could be watched in a detached way, being allowed to drift above the water. They were instructed that they were "able to dispose of rubbish by dumping mental obstacles such as fears, doubts and anxieties down a shoot from which nothing can return." Hypnotic suggestions included "removal of a barrier representing everything that is negative" in the lives of the participants. Embodied in this barrier are self-destructive thoughts, doubts, fears, forces of failure and defeat, mental obstacles, and self-imposed limitations.

In the second session, the hypnotic state was again induced with the relaxation induction. Participants were then asked to "recall a positive past situation in which they experienced feelings of calmness, confidence, or decisiveness." As they mentally recreated these feelings, they were asked to clench the fist of their dominant hand. It was then suggested that in the future whenever they close this hand into a tight fist they would reexperience the desired feelings. Additional practice was afforded with two further positive past experiences to increase confidence in their ability to evoke the desired emotional state. Attention was also focused on the unpleasant emotional state experienced in the examination room, such a state usually including anxiety, indecision, or self-doubt. As the participants mentally recreated this scene, it was hypnotically suggested to them that the unpleasant feelings could be funneled down through the shoulder and the arm into the nondominant fist where they would be locked up tightly. The concept was to link the two parts of the procedure by simultaneously squeezing their dominant hands into strong, confident, happy fists, and opening their nondominant hands to allow the unpleasant feelings to wash away and evaporate into the abyss. In this way, they were able to exchange negative emotional states with pleasurable positive ones. Two objective outcome measures were used to access the effectiveness of hypnosis; the actual examination result and an attitude scale. After hypnosis, 10 of the 11 practitioners successfully passed their examinations; 9 of the 11 indicated an attitude change toward lower levels of test anxiety.

Wark (1996) focused on teaching college students better learning skills with self-hypnosis. This is one of the few studies in the area to employ an alert hypnotic induction (A. Barabasz & M. Barabasz, 1994a). Participants learned to deepen the trance, to give themselves a suggestion for study

improvement, to open their eyes and begin to study while remaining hypnotized. The induction developed by Wark is as follows:

> This is a practical technique to quickly bring your mind to a state of
> focused attention and your body to a state of efficient relaxed calm-
> ness. The technique is called the Lever, because you lever your
> mind to a state of sharp focus and relax your body while holding
> your mind's tension. Then you lever up your mental focus a bit
> higher, and again relax your body. And then a third time you raise
> your mental focus and relax your body. In that state, you give your-
> self suggestions to affect your body. Sit comfortably in your chair.
> Pick a spot to focus on, and attend to it alertly. Take a deep breath,
> sit up in your chair and extend your spine right up to the sky. Focus
> your attention on the target and begin to exhale. As you do, keep
> your spine straight, but allow your shoulders to relax like a cape
> falling over your back. Take another deep breath while focusing on
> your target. Tense all of the muscles below your waist; your hips,
> and thighs, and calves, and feet. Increase your alert attention on the
> target, and slowly relax your lower body as you exhale. Take a third
> deep breath. Tense your whole body and even more alertly observe
> your target as you keep your spine erect, but exhale and relax your
> whole body. Notice that your mind is alert and your gaze is fixed on
> the target while your body relaxes. When you're ready, give yourself
> your suggestion to study.

After learning to use the alert hypnotic procedure, the students all
employed self-hypnosis to a variety of learning skills. They learned to generate their own hypnotic suggestions to overview assignments before starting to study, to listen, and to take notes more attentively in class.

Grades were collected the quarter before the course, during the course,
and the quarter after the course. Satisfaction and depth data indicated that
students were involved all through the course. Students who scored highest on the creative imagination scale (a scale that correlates with hypnotizability) and had the lowest grade point average before hypnosis, improved
the most during the course. They also significantly increased their grade
point average in the quarter thereafter.

Koe and Oldridge (1988) tested the effects of hypnotically induced suggestions on reading performance in 52 volunteer university students. The
students met for four 1-hour hypnotic sessions over a 1-month period
with hypnotic induction relaxation followed by administration of the
Stanford Hypnotic Susceptibility Scale, Form A. Deepening procedures were
also used involving visualizations of a scene developed by the authors.

Hypnotic depth was assessed with the *Long Stanford Scale of Hypnotic Depth* (Tart, 1972), a 1- to 10-participant self-rating scale. Ego-strengthening hypnotic suggestions were administered using Hartland's (1971) approach modified for reading. Suggestions were reinforced in the four treatment sessions. The wording of the suggestions was modified for the other-esteem groups so that the suggestions influenced perceptions of the opinions of significant others such as "others will feel you read better." A combined-esteem group was administered a combination of self-and-other-esteem suggestions such as "you and others will feel you read better." The Nelson-Denny reading test (Nelson & Denny, 1960) showed that hypnotizable participants scored higher than nonhypnotizable participants, and the other-esteem suggestions were found to improve reading performance significantly.

A. Barabasz and M. Barabasz (1994a) used active alert hypnosis with direct suggestions for increased reading speed, confidence, and comprehension with the control and experimental groups. Both high- and low-hypnotizable groups significantly increased readings speeds, but only the high-hypnotizable participants were able to demonstrate significantly improved comprehension scores on the Nelson-Denny test.

In one of the more unusual approaches to examination anxiety, Erickson (1965) induced hypnosis and suggested to the student that he was to pass this examination but only with the "lowest possible passing grade." Erickson's point was that these problems could stem from self-defeating needs. By using such a suggestion, his intent was to provide for their satisfaction while still keeping the student above the passing level. He also suggested that each question would "seem to make a little sense," "a little information will trickle into your conscious mind. When the time is up, you will have answered all the questions."

In an unpublished study, I (J.G.W.) suggested to a 19-year-old college sophomore that she was now 29 years of age, had a doctoral degree from a famous university, and could read with enormous speed and comprehension, whereupon she increased her speed 50% and her comprehension 10% on an ophthalmograph reading machine, during which her eye movements were photographed. Although one would not normally distort self-perception to this extent in treating study problems, it was established that hypnosis could very significantly influence reading behavior, at least for a short time. This clinical experiment lends weight to the idea of improving study habits and reading speed by a hypnotic enhancement of the participant's self-concept.

As we have shown in this chapter, many new and innovative approaches using hypnotic procedures are now being developed and employed. The early pioneers, such as Lieblault, Bernheim, Janet, and Freud would be amazed.

Chapter 17
Hypnosis With Children

Hypnotic Responsiveness

Unique treatment approaches are called for when treating the problems of childhood. Sophisticated verbal psychotherapies can be of little use when dealing with the immature cognitive processes and emotions of the developing child. The use of hypnosis for the treatment of many problems in children is especially indicated because hypnotizability increases from the age of 3 years and peaks at about the age of 11 years, declines slightly from that point to about the age of 16 years, and remains fairly stable throughout the rest of adulthood (A. Morgan & Hilgard, 1978-1979).

Children are much more likely than adults to pass nearly every one of the items on standardized measures of age-appropriate hypnotizability scales. Such remarkable developmental variations point to the special potential of hypnosis as an even more potent intervention than when used with adults (Milling & Costantino, 2000). However, the literature on hypnotherapy with children is meager compared with the more than 7,000 publications on hypnosis in 150 different general medical, psychological, and interdisciplinary adult categories (Nash, 2000). Olness and Kohen (1996) authored the most comprehensive text devoted only to hypnosis with children.

Hypnosis represents a kind of regression, thereby making its use for the treatment of the many problems of childhood especially appropriate. Children also think more concretely than adults and are more suggestible, even outside of the hypnotic context. Other than a small group of nonresponders, children are, more easily hypnotized than adults. Failures in treating them often stem from the fact that the therapist does not reason like the child does. Therapists who work with children, whether or not hypnosis is used, must be able to gear their thinking and feeling modalities to the level of the little patients if success is to be achieved. Unfortunately, by the time many of us reach adulthood we have forgotten or repressed our own childhood states so that they can no longer be brought to conscious levels to relate to children in their own frame of reference. Such therapists simply should not be treating children, and their mentors should guide them to work in other areas of psychology.

The induction of hypnosis with children is best conducted by some form of fantasy or play (J. Smith, A. Barabasz, & M. Barabasz, 1996). The child may be asked to look carefully at her doll: "Dolly [use the child's name for the doll] is getting very tired. Do you see how her eyes want to close? If you closed your eyes like she wants to do, maybe you could still see her, as she is relaxing. She feels so good, so nice and warm, and you can go to sleep right beside her."

The last thing most children would be interested in doing is closing their eyes, particularly if some sort of medical procedure is about to be performed. In those cases, it may be better to talk to them about how they can use their imaginations to do or feel different kinds of things. Instead of using the word imagination, you may choose to ask what it's like to "pretend things," to "make-believe." Then simply ask, "Do you ever pretend things or make-believe that you are someone else? It's when you can do anything you want to do. What is it you like to do more than anything else?" Then, as recommended by A. Morgan and J. Hilgard (1978-1979), use the interest selected by the child to develop a scene. Then go on to say something like, "Okay. We can do that right now. Let's pretend we are on a picnic, and there is a big picnic basket right in front of us. What does the basket look like? How big is it? I'm going to spread a bright yellow table cloth on the grass here. Why don't you take something out of the basket. Tell me about it. What else is in the basket?" Then simply indicate, "You know you can do lots of interesting things by thinking about it this way. It's like pretending something so strongly that it seems almost real. How real did it seem to you?" The child indicates it was quite real. This can be used as the avenue to the hypnotic induction required for the procedure at hand. The concept comes from the *Stanford Hypnotic Clinical Scale for Children* modified form for ages 4 to 8 years (A. Morgan & Hilgard, 1978-1979).

The use of television imagery is also very effective. Children are asked to say what their favorite TV program is and then asked to imagine watching that favorite program. The therapist draws an imaginary screen in space with a finger and then asks the little patient to watch until they see whoever represents a screen character that they particularly enjoy. If a therapist is familiar with the show, as many child therapists are, it is better to substitute a specific character from that program to further improve rapport: "Can you see Scooby-Doo, Spider-Man, Superman, Strawberry Shortcake?" Children can then be told to watch the whole program, that it is funny, and that they are to tell the therapist about it when their eyes open after it is all over.

Another technique that has empirical support (J. Smith et al., 1996), asks the child to take the part of a character in a favorite storybook. This technique is most effective when children have been afforded the opportunity of using homework assignments as regular practice with the parent of their choice under the guidance of the therapist. Once the child is imaginatively involved in either the story or the television program, the physician can go about the painful medical procedure as needed.

Magic is another avenue particularly appropriate for children (Zarren & Eimer, 2001). They can be told that if the doctor strokes their finger it will become magic. It can go all numb and has no feeling. They can transfer the numbness to any part of their body: arm, gums, face. Children greatly enjoy the feeling of power that they have and thus rapidly develop the ability to achieve this type of anesthesia. Such hypnotic procedures give them mastery and control over situations where they were previously frightened and helpless and forced by physical restraint to undergo a painful procedure.

Rational thinking is the marker of adulthood. Psychological adjustment, success, and happiness are dependent on reacting to realistic external cues with a view to the future rather than on internal fantasies. Yet it is precisely this ability to fantasize that is characteristic of more hypnotizable adults (J. Hilgard, 1979; Rhue, Lynn, & Kirsch, 1993). Josephine Hilgard (see A. Barabasz, 1982) found that individuals reared in homes using strict discipline tended to be more hypnotizable. This finding has been misunderstood by some as a form of conditioning of the child to not question response to authority, but Hilgard's findings indicated that children who are treated very strictly and punished frequently develop their fantasy resources as an escape from an external situation that they cannot master. Similarly below-average hypnotizable adults developed imaginary capacity, in an effort to cope with 6 hours of restricted environmental stimulation (A. Barabasz, 1982). They were then able to achieve double their previous hypnotizability scores on the *Stanford Hypnotic Clinical Scale* and to very significantly increase their ability to achieve anesthesia to painful stimuli.

As children become older, their levels of hypnotizablity become more stable (Cooper & London, 1971) and begin to decline slightly with the advent of adolescence. Therefore, as children grow and mature, alternative approaches to hypnotic induction should be used. Gardner and Olness (1981) recommended for very young tots (the first 2 years) stroking, patting, rocking, music, whirring sounds, visual objects, or holding a doll or stuffed animal. Between the ages of 2 and 4 years, the telling of stories becomes more effective. Describing the child's favorite activity; speaking to the child through a doll, teddy bear, or puppet; and watching an induction by video might be quite effective. For children ages 4 to 6 years, the therapist will find that storytelling, television fantasies, and describing the child's favorite place is frequently the most useful. Eye fixation, involving staring at a coin, can be effective at these ages also as this extends into the middle childhood range of 7 to 11 years. More traditional approaches can be employed in adolescents.

One of the most important motivations is their drive for mastery and independence, considering that the world of children is filled with big people to whom they must defer and adults are giants who tell them what to do and how to behave. It is no wonder that opportunities to show independence and to master events in one's world would be attractive.

Interestingly, many of these same needs appear when child ego states are activated spontaneously (or through hypnotic regression in adults) (Emmerson, 2003; J. Watkins & Watkins, 1997). When a child ego state that was fearful of "monsters" became spontaneously executive in a multiple-personality case (dissociative identity disorder) (J. Watkins & Johnson, 1982), H. Watkins taught the individual to control the fear by shouting "MONSTER, go away!" The hallucinated monsters would then disappear and the child ego state was reassured by being able to master the situation. It would seem that many child therapy techniques can be used with adults when they are hypnotically regressed to such states.

Practicing social situations under hypnotic visualization or imagery is like going to school by one's self, dealing with a bully, or approaching the other sex as a teenager, and can do much to build ego strength and minimize traumatization. This is not unlike dealing with repressed material in hypnoanalysis prior to fully egotizing it in the conscious state.

Numerous general medical conditions such as asthma, dermatitis, and gastrointestinal disorders occur in children just as they do in adults. The hypnotherapeutic techniques described in our earlier chapters were designed primarily for adults. However, by considering the differences in children's modes of communication, many of these can be adapted for use with younger patients. The hypnotherapist who would treat children will need to modify the hypnotic suggestions to coincide with the specific child's more limited attentional abilities. The need for independence from adult control and for self-mastery of situations as well as their proclivity for nonverbal communication, concrete thinking, and imaginative abilities must also be carefully evaluated in formulating hypnotic suggestions. The creative child therapist will consider these factors in general when applying hypnotherapy to younger patients. Deep hypnoanalysis is seldom indicated, but some general knowledge of personality dynamics is of great value, as is understanding the potential difficulties of attempting to curtail a symptom that might well have been generated in response to an unconscious need or a subtle parent-child conflict.

Parent-Child Problems

Working hypnotically with children can be imbued with the attitudes of parents. In general, the public still secures so many concepts about hypnosis from movies and television that parents often refuse to allow the use of hypnosis on their children, believing either that it is ineffective or that it is a diabolical instrument of control. Unless parents understand to some degree what hypnosis can and cannot do and are willing to cooperate, it becomes virtually impossible to use the modality with their children. The lack of information plus prejudice displayed by many parents is frequently supported by misinformation and prejudices voiced by the few uninformed physicians remaining in practice, the teachings of some religions, and other healing arts personnel who deprecate the procedure to both the child and the parents. Dealing with such attitudes in a constructive manner can be effective and make it possible to apply hypnosis successfully in the treatment of childhood problems.

Cooperation of the parents is particularly well-assured when the protocol allows for the parents to be involved in the hypnotic intervention with the child (J. Smith et al., 1996). Alternatively, educating parents about the possibilities and limitations of hypnosis can be effective. It is important to reassure parents about their fears as well as to mitigate unrealistic expectations. Invariably, the most cooperative parents are those who have experienced hypnosis. For this reason, I (A.F.B.) invite parents to participate in the early sessions with their children and to involve themselves with the imaginative experiences discussed earlier.

It is important to recognize that symptoms such as enuresis and soiling are frequently signs of child-parent conflict and struggles for control. Unconsciously, the child, through such actions, is securing positive gratification in frustrating the parent, and at the same time is receiving much more attention, even though unfavorable. School teachers are quite aware that children are often satisfied with unfavorable attention as an alternative to being ignored. Surprisingly, a number of parents seem unaware of this.

Children's Hypnotizability Scales

Hypnotizabilty in children has not had as intensive or exhaustive study as that in adults. However, the clinician or the researcher in the area of child hypnosis does have access to standardized measures of hypnotic responsiveness including the *Children's Hypnotic Susceptibility Scale* (London, 1963) and the *Stanford Hypnotic Clinical Scale for Children* (SHCS:C) (Morgan & Hilgard, 1978–1979). The SHCS:C has also received major revision and updating (Zeltzer & LeBaron, 1984). The scale items and their wordings are far more suitable for children than those in the adult scales that we described in chapter 4.

Effectiveness of Hypnosis for Childhood Conditions

The number of childhood conditions reported in the literature as being successfully treated with hypnosis is so vast as to be legend. However, Milling and Costantino (2000) pointed out that only 15 clinical hypnosis outcome studies were fully controlled to the point of utilizing a between-subjects design in which the hypnotic intervention was compared against at least one alternative hypnotic or nonhypnotic intervention or a placebo, attention, or no-treatment control condition. Applying this criteria, hypnosis for children has been found to be effective for the following conditions: acute pain (Liossi & Hatira, 2003); test anxiety (Stanton, 1993); academic performance and self-esteem of learning disabled children (L. Johnson, Johnson, Olsen & Newman, 1981); peripheral temperature control (Dikle & Olness, 1980); control of salivary immunoglobulin (Olness, Culbert, & Uden, 1989); cystic fibrosis (Belsky & Khanna, 1994); nocturnal enuresis (Banerjee, Srivastav, & Palan, 1993; Edwards & Van der Spuy 1985); nausea and emesis (Jacknow, Tschann, Link, & Boyce, 1994; Zeltzer, Dolgin, LeBaron, & LeBaron, 1991); cold pressor pain (Zelter, Fanurik, & LeBaron, 1989); bone marrow aspiration (Katz, Kellerman, & Ellenburg, 1987); lumbar puncture with bone marrow aspiration (Kuttner, Bowman, & Teasdale, 1988; Zeltzer & LeBaron, 1982); venipucture and bone marrow aspiration (J. Smith et al., 1996). All of these studies showed significant effects of hypnosis versus control or standard treatment conditions. Some studies showed hypnosis to be equivalent to a focused distraction condition, whereas others found hypnosis to be significantly more effective than distraction. In studies where hypnosis was found to be more effective than distraction, the researchers endeavored to ensure sufficient hypnotic depth. This suggests that, as with adults, children can achieve greater control when the clinician strives to assure sufficient depth as well as sufficient hypnotizablity. Adequate hypnotic depth seems essential if true hypnotic effects beyond those that could be wrought by distinction are to be obtained.

After the Milling and Costantino (2000) review, new controlled research also demonstrated the efficacy of hypnosis for attention-deficit/hyperactivity disorder. Alert hypnosis (A. Barabasz, 1994) in combination with neuro-therapy has been effective for children with attention deficit disorder with or without hyperactivity (Anderson, Barabasz, Barabasz, & Warner, 2000; A. Barabasz & Barabasz, 2000; Warner, Barabasz, & Barabasz, 2000).

Induction Techniques for Children

Adults and children respond rather differently to hypnotic induction procedures. Accordingly, techniques must be modified when dealing with young people. Children are usually so easily hypnotized and so close to spontaneous hypnosis much of the time that they may be in a hypnotic state and yet, at a superficial glance, appear to be acting quite normally. Like hypnotized adults, children can become focused and highly concentrated in concrete situations. They can often be entirely absorbed to the exclusion of hearing communications addressed to them or other distractions. This narrowing of the field of attention is also typical of the hypnotized adult (H. Spiegel & D. Spiegel, 2004).

Transient fears are more salient in children than in adults. Children who are subjected to a heavy diet of television, movie, and computer game violence are more likely to manifest such fears. If they do not show such fear overtly, attempts to hypnotize them can result in failure simply because the therapist has failed to recognize that they are fearful and distrusting. Accordingly, time spent in the early contacts with children, establishing rapport and building confidence, is essential for success in treating children.

Relating to children calls for a unique set of traits. Children resent being talked down to. More likely than not, children are more sensitive than adults in identifying phony overtures. One needs to be genuine and authentic, and at the same time able to think and feel like a child. One lets one's own child ego-state emerge and resonate with the little patient. If therapists are able to accomplish this, they will be successful in working with children. As important as the therapeutic relationship is with adults, it is considerably more significant when working with children.

The lives of children are embedded within the context of the total environmental situation in which they exist. It is, therefore, essential to evaluate the home environment, insofar as possible, to infer the nature of the relationship patterns that exist within the total environment if one is to plan a therapeutic program successfully. Children cannot be treated in a vacuum. They must be treated with an awareness of the circumstances and pressures that surround them. This is probably true of most individuals but even more so with children.

Even children with attention deficit disorder can become absorbed in certain tasks for hours at a time (A. Barabasz & M. Barabasz, 1996). Accordingly, reinforcements, to be effective, should be administered immediately following successfully achieved target behaviors. Inductions will need to be accomplished as quickly as feasible. Eye-fixation objects that are moving are generally considerably more effective than motionless points. This technique can be used as a direct bridge to increasing hypnotic depth sufficient for the task at hand.

Given that children's thinking is more concrete than that of adults, they tend to fixate on some aspect of a situation to the exclusion of its general meaning. Remarkably, this latter characteristic seems to be carried forward into early adulthood by otherwise intelligent and successful university students. But unlike anyone in adulthood, children may ask why dead people do not open their eyes.

There is a great love of fantasy. What the world does not immediately supply in the form of desired stimulation, most children can create in their own play. This means that fantasy becomes a valuable way of reaching them. "Let's pretend," can be effective yet simple. But therapists who attempt to foist their own fantasies on children, instead of those secured from the little patients' associations, will find a frequent breakdown in communication. Given these issues, stories created by the children can be more effective than those made up by the therapist.

A 9-year-old who had suffered a severe burn on the upper-back region is one example. Each time the dressing required changing, he would scream loudly and had to be restrained by several nurses. The experience was becoming a real trauma. He was referred to me (J.G.W.) with the hope that hypnosis might mitigate his severe pain to the point that he would become more cooperative. Together we made up a story about a boy playing in a field, a scene that was very pleasant to him. He was told that whenever he had to have his dressing changed he would go back to the field and spend the entire time playing in the field, and that while so playing he would not experience any discomfort. The attending physician reported that from that time on the boy ceased to scream, that he lay quietly during the changing of dressings, and that he did not complain of further pain.

In another comparison of imagination-focused hypnosis against distraction, Zeltzer, LeBaron, and Zeltzer (1984) employed 19 children from

6 to 17 years of age who had a history of distress from chemotherapy. Again, hypnosis was found to be an effective treatment. Jacknow et al. (1994) focused on testing the effects of hypnosis versus the effects of standard antiemetic medications that were available on an as-needed basis for chemotherapy distress. Twenty children between ages of 6 and 18 years participated. The hypnosis condition consisted of two to three sessions of practice learning self-hypnosis, which emphasized imagination of favorite activities and favorite places. Progressive muscle relaxation also served as part of the induction. Specific hypnotic suggestions for emesis control focused on "locating the brain's vomiting control center and turning it off." Controls conversed with the therapist for an equivalent amount of time and received antiemetic medication as they requested it. Both groups experienced significant reductions in episodes of nausea and vomiting that were equivalent between standard medical treatment and hypnosis. Perhaps even more important was the finding that 1 and 2 months later the patients in the hypnosis group experienced significantly less anticipatory nausea than did children in the control group who received the antiemetic medication.

Enuresis

A common medical intervention of enuresis is use of Imipramine, a tricyclic antidepressant, which has a side effect of urinary retention. Banerjee et al. (1993) studied 50 nocturnally enuritic children between the ages of 5 and 16 years testing hypnosis versus Imipramine interventions. Hypnotic suggestions were administered for specific use of the toilet at night. Children were encouraged to practice self-hypnosis before going to sleep each night. The Imipramine condition involved the simple administration of 25 mg every night. The first week of treatment doses increased an additional 25 mg each week as necessary to produce dry nights. After 3 months, both treatments were discontinued and both hypnosis and Imipramine were found to be effective in significantly reducing bed-wetting nights. There was no significant difference between hypnosis and Imipramine groups at 3 months. However, 6 months after treatments had been discontinued a significant difference between the two treatments emerged that was accounted for by a substantial relapse in the medication group. The children in the hypnosis condition had maintained their dry nights.

Understanding and cooperative parents can become valuable auxiliary therapists in assisting their child to develop hypnotic mastery over the child's symptoms. However, the emphasis should be on "assisting," not controlling. Practice in sessions with parent and child will make it obvious to the therapist as to whether an overanxious parent is resorting to pressure the child to achieve hypnotic phenomena if the child resists and therapeutic efforts are blocked. Authoritative hypnotherapists can easily be identified with authoritative parents in the minds of children and be reacted too similarly.

Acute Pain

A recent controlled investigation of the efficacy of clinical hypnosis in alleviating pain (Liossi & Hatira, 2003) involved comprehensive manualized therapy with 80 pediatric cancer patients ages 6 to 16 years. All were undergoing routine lumbar punctures and were randomly assigned to direct hypnosis with standard medical treatment, indirect hypnosis with standard medical treatment, attention control with standard medical treatment, or standard medical treatment alone. The six-phase study included (a) assessment of the degree of the pain in pain-related anxiety during three consecutive lumbar punctures, (b) interventions, (c) assessment of the degree of pain and pain-related anxiety during the first two consecutive lumbar punctures in which interventions were used, (d) training in which self-hypnosis was taught to patients in the hypnosis direct and hypnosis indirect groups, (e) assessment of the degree of pain and related anxiety during the first, third, and sixth lumbar punctures in which self-hypnosis was used, and (f) measurement of hypnotizabilty using the *Stanford Hypnotic Clinical Scale for Children*. The direct-hypnosis group received hypnotic suggestions such as:

> "We will do some strong magic now. First you'll have to make your lower back go to sleep for a few minutes — I'll show you how to do it. I'll just put my hand up on your back to help it become numb ... sleepy and numb ... soft and sleepy." For topical anesthesia, the group received suggestions such as "Just imagine painting numbing medication on to your back." For local anesthesia, the group received suggestions such as "Imagine injecting anesthetic into your lower back ... feel it flow into your body ... notice the change in feeling as the area becomes numb." Glove anesthesia with a direct suggestion to "pay attention to your hand ... notice how you can feel tingling feelings in the hand ... let it become numb ... when it is very numb, touch that hand to your lower back ... let the numb feeling transfer from the hand to the back." The routine hypnotic switch-box technique of being able to "flip the switch off" to turn off pain to various parts of the body was also employed.

The indirect hypnosis group received a setting-sun fantasy adapted from Levitan (1990):

> "See yourself sitting on a beautiful Greek beach at sunset ... notice the bright sun as it descends on the far horizon ... see the sun gradually sink into the sea ... see the colors change red to purple and then to blue ... enjoy the tranquility ... tranquility is available to you whenever you need it, merely by giving yourself your own signal to relax! Maybe you enjoy letting your finger and thumb come together to make a magic OK sign ... that is your signal to enjoy immediate relaxation and calmness whenever you like."

Patients in the hypnosis groups reported significantly less pain and anxiety and were rated as demonstrating less behavioral distress than those in the control groups. Both direct and indirect suggestions were equally effective, and were consistent with the J. Smith et al. (1996) study. Hypnotizability was significantly associated with treatment benefit in both hypnosis groups. Therapeutic benefit degraded when participants were asked to use only self-hypnosis (Liossi & Hatira, 2003).

Imagination-focused hypnosis was compared with distraction for alleviating the excruciating pain of bone marrow aspirations and lumbar punctures for 33 oncology patients ages 6 to 17 years (Zeltzer & LeBaron, 1982). The hypnosis condition involved imagination of fun activities, play, and child-interest fantasies. Distraction involved coaching using deep breathing and diversion to external cues. Hypnosis was found to be significantly more effective than distraction in reducing both pain and anxiety. The superiority of imagination-focused hypnosis over distraction was particularly marked in reducing self-reported distress of the invasive medical procedure.

J. Smith et al. (1996) compared hypnosis and distraction in twenty-seven, 3- to 8-year-old oncology patients. Children and their parents were randomly assigned to one of two balanced sequences of treatment. Parents were taught to help their children involve themselves into hypnotic fantasy by taking a journey with the child to a favorite place developed from one of the child's favorite stories. Parents were also involved in the distraction condition and were taught how to engage their children in pop-up toy play activities and the hospital's normal breathing ("blowing") and counting technique. The training sessions for the parents and practice sessions for the children were monitored to ensure compliance.

Rather than involve the therapist at the time of the medical intervention, the parents served as therapists for invasive medical procedures such as a bone marrow aspiration. Parents then crossed over to the alternative intervention for a third procedure. The study obtained a wide range of pain and distress measures including parent report, child report, and blind observational measures of pain and anxiety with independent videotape raters, as well as nurses assessments of the patient's response. Data were collected at baseline, hypnosis, and distraction phases. Unlike many other studies, this study also measured hypnotizability using the *Stanford Hypnotic Clinical Scale for Children* to determine whether hypnotizabilty accounted for the results of the study.

The majority of children were moderate to highly hypnotizable and all showed highly significant reductions in pain perceptions and observed pain or distress by independent raters to the medical procedures. Consistent with E. Hilgard's (1992) neodissociation theory, these children also showed significantly lower pain, anxiety, and distress scores in response to hypnosis in contrast to low-hypnotizable children. Distraction produced significant positive effects in observer rated distress for the low-hypnotizable children. The value of measuring hypnotizability in children seems apparent in that the few children that are of low hypnotizability are more likely to benefit from distraction techniques, whereas those who have hypnotic capacities (the vast majority) are likely to respond to a hypnosis intervention.

Kuttner et al. (1988) tested hypnosis against distraction and control conditions for 48 boys and girls between the ages of 3 and 10 years who were receiving bone marrow aspirations. Hypnosis involved several interventions, including imaginative fantasy, direct suggestions for analgesia, and the special "pain-switch" metaphor in which it was hypnotically suggested to children that they could switch off pain messages to various parts of the body. Despite only 5 to 20 minutes of preparation before the bone marrow aspiration procedure, hypnosis was found to be more successful than standard medical practice. It was noted that the older children in the hypnosis and distraction conditions achieved significantly greater reductions in observer rated pain and anxiety compared to the control condition, whereas the younger children in the hypnosis condition achieved significantly greater reductions in distress then those in all other conditions. Younger children responded better to hypnosis than distraction.

Kohen (1986) focused on pediatric emergency situations and produced similar results. Self-hypnosis was used emphasizing relaxation and mental imagery as an adjunct for rapid reduction of anxiety and discomfort. Fear was diminished, self-control improved, and self-perception of discomfort was altered.

As addressed in previous chapters, the literature supporting the use of hypnosis for acute pain conditions shows enormous effectiveness. There is far less controlled research available on children but the research extant is extremely promising. It is noteworthy that in contrast to the frequently equivalent effects between hypnosis and distraction conditions for chemo-therapy symptoms, a very different picture emerges with the use of hypnosis for acute pain.

Academic Performance

A number of studies have focused on academic performance and self-efficacy with college student's (Rather, Barabasz, & Barabasz, 1993) and reading speed and comprehension performance (A. Barabasz & Barabasz, 1994b). Hypnosis for academic performance improvement has also been used to help children with learning disabilities (A. Barabasz, 1973; Crasilneck & Hall, 1985; Krippner, 1966)

In one of the most frequently cited studies, L. Johnson et al. (1981) focused of the effects of group self-hypnosis on self-esteem and academic performance of children with learning disabilities. The study involved 33 boys and girls, ages 7 to 13 years, and their parents and teachers. The hypnosis condition involved three group-training sessions where the children listened to a hypnotic induction with suggestions for imagery emphasizing improved academic performance and enhanced self-esteem. The children were also instructed in self-hypnosis to experience similar imagery that they could create on their own. Parents and teachers participated in the same sessions. Unfortunately, hypnotizability was not assessed and hypnotic depth was not considered, thereby mitigating against significant effects. The findings were intriguing in that they suggest that self-hypnosis has promised for test anxiety in children similar to that demonstrated for adults (A. Barabasz & Barabasz, 1981; Stanton, 1993). Before the present author's (A.F.B.) formal training in hypnosis, an earlier study (A. Barabasz, 1973) unwittingly employed hypnosis in the group-desensitization of test anxiety with 87 fifth and sixth graders. High and low test-anxious students were determined by obtaining physiological anxiety arousal measures during guided imagery. The lengthy progressive muscle relaxation procedure of Wolpe and Lazarus (1966) was repeatedly used to train participants to create a state antagonistic to test anxiety. Years later, this was recognized as serving to induce hypnosis for what was in all likelihood the majority of children over the 5-day training program.

Unreported in the published study (A. Barabasz, 1973) were the qualitative reports from children. Dozens of children reported their own images of dealing with test anxiety beyond the prescribed desensitization protocol. One student explained that, after the relaxation, he imaged, "unzipping the top of my skull, taking out my brain, and putting it on the desk, then taking a fire hose to wash away all the bad worries about the test." Another child went into great detail about "an army in the head, attacking, blowing up, bombing, annihilating, and destroying the bad [test-anxiety producing army in the brain] guys that made me forget stuff I knew before the test." Such self-generated imagery was typical of student reports among those that bettered their pre- to posttreatment Lorge-Thordike (LT) test scores. Overall, findings showed the treatment produced significantly higher LT scores for the high test-anxious students. The findings were corroborated by significant effects on physiological measures. Unfortunately, hypnotizability test data and depth measures were lacking as in the L. Johnson et al. (1981) study.

Further research in this area is warranted. Attention should be paid to the measurement of hypnotizability and to one-on-one therapist-child interactions, perhaps involving hypnotic suggestions tailored to the specific difficulties or needs of the child.

Medical Problems

Trichotillomania

Trichotillomania, or chronic hair pulling resulting in alopecia, is predominately a habit disorder exhibited by children and young adults. The scalp is most often the depilated, but often eyebrows, eyelashes, pubic hair, and axillary hair can be the target of hair-pulling behavior. The disorder is widespread, with an estimate of more than 8 million people chronically pulling their hair out (Azrin & Nunn, 1978). Behavioral formulations view the disorder as an isolated habit. Applied behavioral analysis (Wolf, 1978 points to the anxiety-reducing function served by this behavior that is maintained by endogenous or exogenous antecedents with consequences of varying complexity. A wide range of behavioral techniques with both children and young adults frequently fail because of noncompliance.

A serious problem with behavior-therapy interventions is that they are universally highly dependant on client and parental cooperation. It is not surprising, therefore, that treatment failures and relapses have been blamed on compliance problems.

Hypnosis has a long history of success in the treatment of habit disorders without the complexity of most of the behavioral interventions focused on trichotillomania. Furthermore, hypnosis does not seem to foster such problems with client compliance. Given the promise shown by the work of H. Spiegel and D. Spiegel (1978) in the treatment of two highly hypnotizable adults for trichotillomania, a procedure was developed for testing with children.

Approaching the problem differently from the Spiegels, I (A.F.B.) tested a technique involving awareness and control with 4 teenage boys and girls, each with at least 2 years history of severe hair pulling. After introducing hypnosis by means of an imagination exercise that included the "favorite television program" procedure, the *Stanford Hypnotic Clinical Scale for Children* form was administered. All 4 participants had scores between 3 and 5 showing above-average to high hypnotizability. Hypnosis was induced using a variation of the eyes-rolled-up alert induction technique (A. Barabasz, 1985). After hypnotic suggestions for deepening, the following posthypnotic suggestion was given: "You will be very aware whenever you put your hand to your head. Then it's entirely up to you, you have the power, you have the control, no one else, and no habit controls you. You can pull your hair out if you want to or you can choose to control the habit." All 4 children had ceased hair pulling within 3 to 5 days of the single application of the hypnotic induction. All 4 also reported that they had looked regularly at the 3" × 5"card with the suggestion on it that had been provided to them and that they had continued to practice the eyes-rolled-up hypnotic induction and enjoyed the experience very much.

Shortly thereafter, M. Barabasz (1987) tested a more sophisticated form of the hypnotic suggestion with four females ages 19, 21, 24, and 34 years with histories of two to eight years of trichotillomania. She also added a relaxation induction instruction from the *Stanford Hypnotic Clinical Scale* to the rolled-eyes induction. Three of the 4 patients ceased hair-pulling following treatment, whereas one patient who had been seeing her psychiatrist for psychoanalytically oriented therapy once a week for the past 30 months made an "emergency" telephone call in the late evening complaining that she could not pull her hair out and that the "tension" was unbearable. She was reminded of the posthypnotic suggestions emphasizing awareness of the habit and the choice involved. She reported feeling "more relaxed and in control" and "having no particular concerns about touching my hair." Unlike the other 3 patients, this patient's hair-pulling behavior returned to the pretreatment baseline and remained so at 6- and 9-month follow-ups.

Peripheral Temperature Regulation

Peripheral temperature regulation is important and efficacious in the treatment of a variety of disorders including Raynaud's disease and migraine headache. Patients who learn how the increase peripheral blood circulation, warming the extremities, also report feelings of relaxation and calm, which can be useful in a number of therapeutic endeavors. Thermal biofeedback with temperature sensors attached to a person's fingers for example, was once thought to be the most efficient method of training patients to direct blood flow to the extremities. However, within a short period of time the subgroup of patients who were able to actually respond to the auditory or visual feedback relating to the amount of warming going on in a finger rapidly would learn only to warm the specific extremity upon which the sensor was attached. This was a less than an ideal situation for the treatment of the disorders in question!

Clinical trials (A. Barabasz, 1977; A. Barabasz & Wright, 1975) suggested that hypnosis could be a more generalizable alternative method of increasing peripheral circulation. A controlled experiment was conducted to determine whether biofeedback with or without hypnotic suggestion is effective in training the vasodilatation response as contrasted to mediated biofeedback in hypnosis (A. Barabasz & McGeorge, 1978). Experimental conditions included a standard auditory feedback protocol, a false feedback condition, relaxation training instructions, and an experimental group, which received hypnosis in which the hypnotic suggestions for hand-warming were mediated on the basis of participants' continuously monitored hand temperature with the feedback data provided to the therapist rather than to the patient. There were no statistically significant differences among the first three groups, but the hypnosis group showed significant hand-warming effects. Seventy-three individuals participated in this initial study, which was subsequently replicated in a number of clinical situations.

Shortly thereafter, Dikle and Olness (1980) investigated the potential of hypnosis for children by testing biofeedback against self-hypnosis as well as a combination of self-hypnosis and biofeedback. Using a sample of 48 boys and girls ages 5 to 15 years of age with previous training in self-hypnosis, emphasis was placed on relaxation effects with imagery of the child's favorite activities. Participants were also asked to imagine their hands becoming warmer or cooler depending on the specific condition. Again, hypnosis was found to be effective in providing peripheral temperature control for children.

Immune-System Modulation

Early investigations of psychoneuroimmunology produced findings supporting the use of hypnosis as facilitating voluntary alteration of immune activity (Hall, Minnes, Tosi, & Olness, 1992; Kiecolt-Glaser et al., 1985; Olness et al., 1989; Smith, McKenzie, Marmer, & Steele, 1985). Unfortunately, none of these studies controlled for hypnotizability, making it difficult to determine the specificity of hypnosis in the positive outcomes of the investigations. Zachariae and Bjerring (1992) did show that immunoreactivity to dinitrochlorobenzene and diphenylcyclopropenone could be modulated by direct hypnotic suggestion using guided imagery in children as an induction deepening procedure. Unfortunately, there was no control for relaxation effects that could have accounted for the results without hypnosis.

Our laboratory at Washington State University tested the effects of hypnosis on immune response with 65 high- and low-hypnotizable university student volunteers exposed to hypnosis, relaxation, or control conditions (Ruzyla-Smith, Barabasz, Barabasz, & Warner, 1995). Blood samples were obtained before treatment and twice thereafter and subjected to flow cytometry analysis. Significant alteration of the immune response as measured by B cells and helper T cells was shown only for the highly hypnotizable participants exposed to the hypnotic induction. This study demonstrated the specificity of hypnosis in alterating the immune system in a positive direction.

The key application of immunomodulation with children is that of Olness et al. (1980), who employed 57 healthy volunteer youngsters age 6 to 12 years. One group listened to a self-hypnosis audiotape with instructions for relaxation and imagery, a self-hypnosis and hypnotic suggestion group heard a similar audiotape that contained specific instructions to increase the number of immune proteins in the saliva, while children in the control group were engaged in an attention condition involving conversation for the same amount of time. Only the relaxation plus hypnotic suggestion group showed a significant increase in IgA levels, an antibody that protects the upper respiratory tract from infection and plays a role in fighting dental cavities.

Cystic Fibrosis

Cystic fibrosis causes severe respiratory distress as a result of major effects on the lungs. Twelve children, 7 to 18 years old, were taught self-hypnosis to enhance pulmonary function and psychological adjustment (Belsky & Khanna, 1994). The self-hypnosis individuals participated in three training session where they listened to a hypnotic induction with imagery to enhance relaxation and specific hypnotic suggestions related to clear lungs, healthy feelings, and comfortable breathing. They were asked to listen to the tape at home on a daily basis. The findings indicated that the hypnosis group achieved significantly greater improvements in lung function, self-esteem, state anxiety, and health compared with a matched control group.

Nausea and Vomiting (Emesis) from Chemotherapy

These are a routine side effect in the treatment of childhood cancers. Noncompliance with treatment protocols frequently exceeds 50% because children view chemotherapy as worse than that of the cancer itself. J. Hilgard and LeBaron (1984) explored the use of an imagination-focused form of hypnosis for pediatric cancer patients. They hypothesized that imaginative activities could be particularly helpful because children can become involved and interested in the process as opposed to simple distraction techniques such as deep breathing or diversion to external objects.

First, children were interviewed about their favorite television programs, movies, games, activities and foods, and favorite activities. This information was then used to develop fantasy stories that they could experience during hypnosis when used with the symptom or medical procedure at hand. The hypnotic intervention was designed to heighten multisensory involvement. Imagination-focused hypnotic procedure was first developed to help counteract the adverse effects of chemotherapy, but has been used in later studies to ease to pain of medical procedures as well.

Zeltzer et al. (1991) tested the effects of imagination-focused hypnosis on 54 children between the ages of 5 and 17 who were undergoing distress from chemotherapy. The three experimental conditions included a hypnosis condition where the therapist trained children to use imagination-focused hypnosis for use during the next administration of chemotherapy. The therapist then involved the child in imaginative fantasy development during training. Children in a distraction condition were trained to use attention diversion techniques such as deep breathing or counting objects in the room. During the next chemotherapy session, these children were helped by their therapist to use the distraction techniques. A third group was an attention placebo group, which met with the therapist for an equivalent amount of time in conversation. Results of the study showed that both hypnosis and distraction or relaxation conditions produced shorter durations of nausea and vomiting.

LaClave and Blix (1989) treated a 6-year-old girl with malignant astrocytoma of the left-brain hemisphere. During the course of the child's chemotherapy, severe vomiting developed to the degree that on several occasions she became dehydrated. The symptom was so severe as to warrant the consideration of discontinuation of chemotherapy when she was referred for hypnotherapy. Despite severe neurological impairments, which excluded many traditional techniques, hypnosis was successful in eliminating emesis. Hypnosis was also used to decrease pain and to improve sleep patterns.

The child came to her first hypnosis session understanding that she was going to learn something called hypnosis to help her decrease the incidence of vomiting. She had already been told she had a brain tumor and that it was serious and sometimes people died from them. Hypnosis was described to her, and it was explained the there are two parts of each of us: there is a body and there is a mind. She was told the mind could do all sorts of different things: "Sometimes it's awake, sometimes it's asleep, and sometimes the mind is in hypnosis. When in hypnosis the mind has more control over how the body feels." Therapists had low expectation that hypnotherapy could help the child given her severe neurological impairments. She had little control over her right arm, and walking was laborious. Speech was extremely difficult and receptive language slowed.

Despite these problems, trance induction was attempted using eye fixation, which was a complete failure and the child became frustrated and anxious. Progressive relaxation was also not possible because of the loss of muscle groups on the right side of her body. Guided imagery was used, and although she was attentive, she was unable to achieve a trance state. The family was advised to give the matter some thought before continuing, but the child's mother persisted saying, "Hypnotherapy was their last hope." Neither she nor her husband nor the child was psychologically ready to give up the hope that chemotherapy could offer.

The child was seen twice weekly in preparation for her next course of chemotherapy. Difficulties in entering trance were frustrating. Despite the difficulties, she tenaciously persisted in engaging in therapy. The child nearly always came close to the therapist's chair, which was interpreted as an attempt to identify with the therapist. She delighted in the fact they both shared the same middle name. There was no overt evidence that she was in trance during the first four or five attempts to experience hypnosis. Together the patient and the therapist designed an audiotape for practice at home using a multiple-induction technique described by Gardner and Olness (1981). She became highly motivated and practiced more frequently than recommended. Gradually, rhythmic breathing, evidence of catalepsy, and general relaxation during the office sessions was observed. Her parents also reported that she appeared to be getting some pain relief from the practice sessions at home. Seven more sessions were held before the course of chemotherapy was scheduled, during which time the child was hospitalized. It was recommended that the child use the hypnosis tape every 4 hours with suggestions for stomach comfort and each half hour without vomiting would be acknowledged with a sticker. The child's parents happily reported that she had not vomited once.

Attention-Deficit/Hyperactivity Disorder

Once most widely known as MBD (minimal brain dysfunction) or MCD (minimal cerebral dysfunction) the term *attention-deficit/hyperactivity dis-*

order (AD/HD) has been adopted. The disorder, characterized by the inability to self-regulate focused attention, is a biologically based developmentally disabling condition that has a pervasive negative impact on adaptive functioning. It is one of the most frequently diagnosed disorders among school children (A. Barabasz & M. Barabasz, 2000).

Until recently, treatment had been limited to management of symptoms by the use of powerful stimulate drugs, such as methylphenidate (Ritalin) or traditional behavioral modification. Trafficking and abuse of methylphenidate have fostered the search for more suitable treatments. Furthermore, concerns about the long-term use of psychostimulant drugs have been raised due to side effects of unmanageable high blood pressure and heart failure. Behavior modification programs, while effective in the short run, remain highly dependent over the long term on compliance and cooperation between parents and teachers. Both treatment programs are by their very nature, at best, palliative (Feussner, 1998; Gaddes & Edgell, 1994, p. 279). Cessation of either treatment results in the rapid return of symptoms to their pretreatment levels and dysfunction. Feussner (1998) noted that school-age boys in the United States now consume nearly 9 tons of Ritalin a year, making it obvious that treatments that go beyond symptom management are urgently needed. Neurotherapy (brainwave biofeedback) provides a habilitative alternative to traditional approaches, but typically takes 40 sessions or more to achieve lasting effects. However, instant alert hypnosis (A. Barabasz, 1985, 1994), used as an adjunct to neurotherapy, may make it possible to reduce treatment time by half, while potentiating the efficacy of behavioral neurotherapy (A. Barabasz and M. Barabasz, 2000).

Neurotherapy (also known as EEG feedback, neurofeedback). Neurotherapy is a relatively new habilitative approach to the treatment of AD/HD. The goal is permanent normalization without dependence on drugs or continuous behavioral management. Consistent with its neurological basis, children with attention deficit disorder (ADD) produce greater EEG slow wave (theta) activity (4 to 8 Hz) and less beta (14 to 32 Hz) activity compared with normal controls (Sterman, 2000). Logically, the most appropriate treatment for the disorder should be derived from and focused on the underlying problem.

Neurotherapy is intended to teach patients to normalize their brainwave responses to stimuli (A. Barabasz & M. Barabasz, 1995, 1996; A. Barabasz, Crawford, & M. Barabasz, 1993; Mann, Lubar, Zimmerman, Miller, & Muenchen, 1992).

When people without AD/HD are presented with attentional task, such as reading, doing simple arithmetic, or listening to a story, their EEGs normally shift to the faster beta frequency. Lubar (1991) observed that persons with AD/HD do just the opposite. Instead, they shift down to the lower theta frequency band. Slow activity, remaining in the lower alpha range or dropping down to theta is characteristic of the wandering mind, nonvigilance, and unfocused thought. Perhaps the only adaptive aspect of ADD and AD/HD is possible enhancement of creativity (Low, 1999).

In neurotherapy, EEG responses to stimuli are analyzed and displayed on a computer screen. The computer provides feedback information, in the form of visual displays and auditory tones showing how well the individual is responding to the feedback. Candidates for neurotherapy include stimulant medication nonresponders, persons with a suspected stimulant-use disorder, and children of parents who are skeptical about the unknown deleterious effects of long-term stimulant drug use.

Instant alert hypnosis. Instant alert hypnosis is conducted in two distinct phases (A. Barabasz, 1994; A. Barabasz & Barabasz, 1994a, 1994b, 1996). In the training phase, patients are instructed to roll eyes up, as if trying to look at their foreheads. The eyes are also led to this position by instructions to focus on the therapist's thumb. The thumb is then moved slowly from 10 to 15 centimeters in front of the patients' noses to the approximate center of their foreheads. The speed of movement should be carefully coordinated with the patient's ability to follow without swimming eyes or obvious loss of focus. When eyes dart or focus seems to be lost, the procedure should be reinitiated. Normal adults seldom have a problem, but clinical experience may need to be brought to bear in the treatment of hyperactive children to get their eyes as rolled up as possible and then kept steadily rolled up as required for successful instant alert hypnosis effects. It is important to allow ample therapy time for practice trials using verbal reinforcement as the child successfully approximates the appropriate response, such as "Good, that's it," or "Good job" (to maintain an eyes-steady, rolled-up position).

Once the eyes are fully and steadily rolled up, instructions are then given to take notice of breathing, relaxation, calm, confidence, and the special calm alertness felt at this point. Direct hypnotic suggestions can also be given as the patient progresses in therapy, which are aimed directly at the computer-displayed feedback, such as, "It's easier and easier to produce more beta and less theta, more beta and less theta, focused, concentrated, relaxed yet focused; it's easy to focus and concentrate, more beta and less theta."

Once subjective signs of hypnosis are observed by the experienced clinician, the patient can be asked to raise a finger upon perception of the suggested responses: "Just lift a finger on this hand [for right-handed patients the clinician touches the patient's left hand] when you feel the comfortable, relaxed, special calm alertness." Upon observation of the patient's signal, which should occur with in 5 to 10 seconds, the patient is given the attentional process specific suggestions such as "In this special state of alertness you will be able to focus your attention any way you like; you can concentrate as completely as you desire." Upon completion of the suggestion, the patient is told to let the eyes roll down and enjoy the calm alert feelings. Then the specific attentional task is begun. Once the child begins to learn exactly what each of the graphic video feedback displays represent, hypnotic suggestions can be tailored to specific levels of understanding that emphasize "more and better beta, less theta." As progress is made over the course of several sessions, patients are encouraged to use instant alert hypnosis on their own (self-hypnosis). If the clinician has been executing the procedure correctly, and the patients do their part, the effects of enhanced beta with inhibition of theta are usually so dramatic as to be immediately obvious on the computer-screen feedback representation. This sometimes profound response can greatly enhance neurotherapy effects and patient motivation.

The first tests of instant alert hypnosis as an adjunct to neurotherapy were case studies (A. Barabasz & M. Barabasz, 1995, 1996; M. Barabasz & A. Barabasz, 1996). Patients were all boys diagnosed with AD/HD who had prior treatment with psychostimulants and behavior modification. Instant alert hypnosis accelerated the response to neurotherapy so that half the usual sessions required to achieve results similar to neurofeedback were required. Three quarters of the cases responded with greatly reduced overactivity, improved attentiveness, and significantly improved school grades and deportment ratings.

Progress beyond the case-study level has been made involving independent researchers outside of my (A.F.B.) practice. Anderson et al. (2000) randomly drew 16 EEG data files from patients with AD/HD treated in a previous year. The *Stanford Hypnotic Clinical Scale for Children* form scores showed all the patients were above-average to highly hypnotizable, which is not usual for this population. Anderson et al. found that instant alert hypnosis neurofeedback trials produced significantly greater beta-theta ratios than neurofeedback alone. Because theta is associated with poor attention concentration, the significant augmentation of beta with instant alert hypnosis contrasted with neurofeedback alone provides rationale for the hypothesis that instant alert hypnosis potentiates the effect of neurotherapy in the treatment of AD/HD.

In another test of instant alert hypnosis as an adjunct to neurotherapy, Warner et al. (2000) randomly selected 19 of my (A.F.B.) child patient files that had been terminated. All had met *DSM–IV* criteria for the disorder with histories of 4 to 10 years, and all had previous largely ineffective responses to psychostimulant drugs and behavior modification treatments. Parents described the prior treatments as "problematic and ineffective." Parents completed the *Attention Deficit Disorder Evaluation Scale–Home Version* (McCarney, 1989) at the beginning of treatment and again at the end of treatment. Posttest scores showed that all indications of AD/HD were significantly lower than pretreatment scores. Patients had markedly decreased inattentiveness, decreased impulsivity, and decreased hyperactivity.

The instant alert hypnosis and neurotherapy findings showed rather remarkable improvements in AD/HD symptomology (Warner, Barabasz, & Barabasz, 2000) and significant changes in the beta-theta ratios criteria data (Anderson et al., 2000). Furthermore, the elimination of dependence on psychostimulants by all but 4 patients in the studies and the marked reduction of intake for those remaining 4 lend further credibility to the efficacy of hypnosis as a potentiater of neurotherapy effects in the treatment of AD/HD. Positive and substantial clinical changes were obtained in an average of 23.2 sessions (3 to 14 weeks of treatment, mean = 11.2 weeks), a number well below the usual 40 to 80 sessions for neurotherapy alone typically reported in the literature. These outcomes were achieved despite the fact that all the patients had long disorder histories and previous treatment with traditional psychostimulants and behavior modification without receiving significant beneficial effects.

Although the problem that always arises in the study of the effectiveness of therapy is to find out what aspects of the interventions are contributing most to the outcome — the therapist or the procedure — we have no reasonable reason to believe that already-discouraged parents would be more likely to rate this approach more favorably than previous treatments without valid reasons for doing so. This procedure is still in its infancy, and it is hoped that other practitioners and researchers trained in hypnosis will further test the use of instant alert hypnosis in this treatment area to shed additional light on what appears to be a very promising treatment combination.

Summary

Even more so than adults, children have a greater facility to engage fantasy. Most children also demonstrate greater responsiveness to hypnosis. The range of disorders that hypnosis has been empirically supported as effective for children is enormous. It seems clear that these findings warrant better understanding by clinicians and hypnosis far greater use as the treatment of choice.

Chapter 18
Hypnosis and Sports Performance[*]

Considerations and Techniques for Using Hypnosis in Sport

As we know, hypnosis has proved to be effective in a wide variety of health fields, but its use as a performance enhancement tool in the area of sport continues to remain negligible (Liggett, 2000b). Pates, Maynard, and Westbury (2001) believed that sport psychologists fail to employ hypnosis as a performance-enhancing strategy because of the lack of training and supervised experiences in hypnosis, as well as confusion over the multitude of methods, strategies, and orientations. They also pointed to the scarcity of methodologically sound research in the sport domain, and "perceived difficulties involved in controlling a spontaneous abreaction" (p. 85). Despite the roadblocks, the use of hypnosis and the use of hypnosis in combination with other techniques that have some research support such as imagery and restricted environmental stimulation therapy has increased over the years and has been employed as a means of enhancing physical, motor, and athletic performance for some time (A. Barabasz, M. Barabasz, & Bauman, 1993; Garver, 1977; Jacobs & Gotthelf, 1986; Liggett, 2000a, 2000b; McAleney, A. Barabasz, & M. Barabasz, 1990; Nideffer, 1981; Orlick, 1980; Pressman, 1979; Pulos, 1979; Wagaman, A. Barabasz, & M. Barabasz, 1991).

[*]This chapter was contributed by Erik Dunlap, Ph.D. Dr. Dunlap completed his Ph.D in physical education and sport psychology from the University of Idaho in 2004. His training includes introductory and advanced hypnosis courses and experience in A.F.B.'s attentional processes and hypnosis laboratory at Washington State University. His undergraduate degree in chemistry and psychology is from Duke University, where he was an offensive lineman on the football team.

Hypnosis and Athletic Performance

Imagery and relaxation are two of the most popular intervention techniques used by sport psychologists to enhance athlete's performance (Cornelius, 2002a). Most sport psychologists and researchers agree that imagery and relaxation have greater effects on performance when combined (Kendall, Hrycaiko, Martin, & Kendall, 1990; Weinberg, Seabourne & Jackson, 1981). When imagery and relaxation are used simultaneously in an intervention, it is essentially a form of hypnosis. Unfortunately, it is lacking in controls for hypnotizability and is without efforts to achieve depth of trance that may be required for the purpose for which it is intended. Nevertheless, the connection between hypnosis and sport interventions seems natural. However, researchers examining the physiological processes that occur in the brain and the self-reports of specific instances in sport have indicated that athletes actually experience "hypnotic-like" experience during peak performances. It is not surprising then that the theoretical explanations describing the characteristics of peak performance are very similar to popular theories explaining hypnotic phenomena (Pates, Maynard, et al., 2001).

Altered States in Sport

There is a great deal of theoretical and empirical support in the literature in sport psychology describing the use of hypnosis as a performance enhancement tool. It has been suggested that such an optimal performance is dependent on the intensity and experience of a specific state of mind, which is very similar to that described by Ernest Hilgard's (1992) neo-dissociation theory and Erika Fromm's (1992) altered state theory, in which each describes a special state that differs from the waking state and involves the reorganization of cognitive structures including alterations in arousal, perception, attention, cognition, and memory. Within sport psychology, this special state of mind has been dubbed various names, such as the "ideal performance state" (Unestahl, 1979, 1981, 1983, 1986), "flow" (Csikszentmihalyi, 1990), and "peak performance" (Cohn, 1991). According to the description of each of these states (see Csikszentmihalyi, 1990), athletes who enter flow essentially are entering hypnosis. Peak performance, flow, and the ideal performance state essentially represent the same dissociated altered state described by E. Hilgard (1992) and Fromm (1979, 1992) and have similar characteristics, which include high levels of self-confidence while being relatively relaxed. Actions happen almost automatically, the actions are perceived as effortless concentration on the task at hand. There is a sense of control, and there is a dissociation from everything but the task at hand. In addition, the other constructs that are integral components of sport and athletic performance (imagery, arousal regulation, attentional focus) are also integral to "of the experience of hypnosis.

Theoretical Bases

The rationale for using hypnosis in sport interventions stems from several theories in sport that discuss or allude to creating these "special states" through which maximal performances can occur. Some of the more commonly discussed theories are those put forth by Csikszentmihalyi (1990), Hanin (1978, 1999), Unestahl (1979, 1981, 1986), and Gorton (1959). Although each of these theories espouses unique philosophies, all suggest that hypnosis can be an extremely useful intervention tool with the athletic population.

Csikszentmihalyi (1990) coined the term "flow" to describe "the state in which people are so involved in an activity that nothing else seems to matter" (p. 4). There are eight characteristics that have been used to describe the experience when flow occurs. These characteristics include a challenging activity that requires skill, the merging of action and awareness, clear goals and feedback, concentration on the task at hand, paradox of control, the loss of ego and self-consciousness, the transformation of time, and an autotelic experience.

Hanin (1978, 1999) suggested that each athlete possesses an individual optimal zone of functioning at which a maximal performance can occur. Hanin empirically demonstrated that athletes will perform their best when they fall within this zone of functioning. Athletes who achieve this state also have a high probability of experiencing flow. Hanin's theory incorporates retrospective recall of precompetitive state anxiety levels (ego state), first identified by A. Barabasz et al. (1993). Hanin believed such states can be obtained in the nonhypnotic state but this phenomenon can represent spontaneous hypnosis as suggested by Barabasz (A. Barabasz et al., 1993). Morgan (1996, p. 108) pointed out that although there is "no mention of hypnotic procedures in his theoretical formulation, the potential for hypnotic intervention is obvious."

Unestahl's (1981) theoretical views are similar to Hanin's (1978) with respect to the affective state the athlete achieves during peak performance. Both agree that a peak performance occurs when the athlete's affective state (anxiety or arousal level) is optimum. The major difference in Unestahl's theory is that he suggested athletes experience amnesia after experiencing a peak performance, "whereas Hanin believes that these states can be accurately recalled" (W. Morgan, 1996, p. 109), a conceptualization introduced as a recall of a specific sport-performing ego state (A. Barabasz et al., 1993). Unestahl related the ideal state performance to a hypnotic trance because of this hypothosized amnesia. The ideal performance state is similar characteristically to flow in that it also includes dissociation and transformation of time; characteristics similar to the hypnotic phenomena.

Gorton (1959) believed that physical performance is limited by inhibitory mechanisms. He believed that there exist reserves of muscular power that are inaccessible under normal conditions (W. Morgan & Brown, 1983), which is in part because of a tendency to protect oneself from injury or overexertion. Gorton believed that if people or athletes could disinhibit their inhibitions, theoretically, they could transcend normal performances and achieve peak performances. According to Ikali and Steinhaus (1961), alcohol, drugs, loud noise, and hypnosis are means through which disinhibition of inhibitory mechanisms can facilitate maximal muscular performance. Hypnosis could potentially allow for the "disinhibition of inhibitory mechanisms" allowing the individual to access those reserves of muscular power, transcend these limits, and perform at their peak levels (Gorton, 1959; W. Morgan & Brown, 1983). Gorton's (1959) conceptualization of using hypnosis as a disinhibiting mechanism to enhance performance supports its use as a performance-enhancement technique.

Arreed Barabasz (personal communication to Erik Dunlap, 2003) focused on self-hypnosis to specifically inhibit the Golgi tendon organ. (This organ causes reciprocal inhibition within the musculotendon unit overriding the stretch reflex that occurs in the muscle spindle causing the muscle to relax thus, preventing injury. The mechanism also serves to attenuate the athlete's ability to produce the maximum benefit from training to muscular failure.) In two cases, Barabasz included himself as a participant (A.F.B. is a nationally certified fitness trainer, who trained to a plateau in weight lifting) and used alert hypnosis to inhibit the Golgi to reliably increase maximum one-repetition lifts by an astounding average of 16% over the previously plateaued maximum. The intention was to produce the required micro tearing of muscle to enhance rebuilding. Barabasz suffered a macro tear (sports injury), which suggests the potential power and risk of hypnosis. He recommends experimental research to explore the potential of this hypnotic intervention.

Empirical Support

Several reviews dating back to 1933 have been published regarding the relationship between hypnosis and motor performance (R. Cox, 2002; Taylor, Horevitz, & Balague, 1993). Unfortunately, the results of research in this area are mixed, and, too frequently, the results are equivocal (Gordin, 1995; Jacobs & Salzberg, 1987; Pratt & Korn, 1986; Taylor et al., 1993). W. Morgan and Brown (1983) suggested that determining the effectiveness of hypnosis based on these studies is difficult given numerous concerns about experimental controls. They concluded that "hypnosis can facilitate the physical performance of selected individuals under certain circumstances" (p. 246). As in previous reviews, they questioned methodological problems regarding hypnosis as an ergogenic aid. They also explained that the mixed results found in earlier reviews can be accounted for. Some studies incorrectly generalized the results from nonathlete participants in a laboratory setting to the dynamic environment of sport where athletes perform more complex skills. According to Morgan (1972), it is easier to enhance the physical performance of nonathletes than trained athletes performing near their maximal levels. This is precisely why A. Barabasz (personal communication, 2003) used two individuals who were trained to plateau over a 3-year period in the Golgi tendon disinhibition pilot experiment. Second, the traditional research paradigm "has been characterized by the confounding of state of hypnosis with simple suggestion. This is why Barabasz carefully established adequate hypnotic depth as well. With very few exceptions (the Barabasz case study is one), it has been difficult to delineate the effects due to hypnosis per se versus those due to simple suggestion, because hypnosis with suggestion typically were contrasted with nonhypnotic interventions without suggestion" (W. Morgan, 1996, p. 109).

Third, the tasks used in these experiments often differ significantly, making comparison across studies difficult. Comparison is also difficult given the poor descriptions of the tasks employed in the studies. Finally, the type of induction has not always been specified in the previous literature. As we have learned in previous chapters, the nature of the induction can have a profound effect on outcome (A. Barabasz, 2000; A. Barabasz, Christensen, & Barabasz, 2004). For example, "inductions that are primarily 'relaxing' in nature would theoretically have a different effect on physical performance than those that are primarily alerting in nature" (W. Morgan & Brown, 1983, p. 232). Although previous studies have made determining the effectiveness of hypnosis on athletic performance difficult, studies within the past few of years have found hypnosis to positively affect athletic performance and help athletes achieve flowlike states (Liggett; 2000a, 2000b; Pates et al., 2000, 2001; Taylor & Gerson, 1992).

Considerations for Using Hypnosis With Athletes

Athletes, like most people, are likely to have misconceptions regarding hypnosis. Before any hypnosis intervention is used with this population, it is imperative that these misconceptions are addressed, including what level of change or experience can be expected. One approach that has been helpful has been to introduce hypnosis as a combination of relaxation and imagery; two techniques familiar to every athlete. Determining the appropriate induction protocol and suggestions can have a significant impact. As we discussed earlier, most inductions that have been used in sport have involved some form of muscular relaxation (e.g., Jacobsen's progressive muscle relaxation). Yet it must be made clear that muscular relaxation may benefit only some athletes. For those athletes involved in ballistic (football or hockey) or explosive sports (track and field), a relaxing induction might be detrimental to an athlete's performance. It is doubtful that middle-aged Frederick Hatfield, a psychologist who accomplished the world record for a hard bell squat (1,040 pounds), used muscular relaxation. Alternative hypnotic suggestions can involve the idea of a calm mind but also a primed body or images of an animal or machine.

As we explained in the chapter on hypnosis for childbirth, the consultant should be aware of the requirements of the client's task and adapt the induction to meet those needs. It is helpful to have a good understanding of the environment the athlete performs in. It is important for the therapist to get specific feedback from the athletes and then to incorporate those characteristics into the hypnotic protocol. For example, most athletes watch tapes of themselves or their opponents performing. Thus, it makes sense that after the initial induction and deepening, the therapist may find that having athletes picture themselves sitting in front of a large television is helpful in creating images. Using this format, the therapist can have the athlete imagine performing specific skills successfully, during a competition, facing an opponent. Because of their familiarity and use of videotape in competition preparation, using suggestions for viewing themselves from a third-person perspective, rewinding, pausing, performing in slow motion, make visualizing a TV or screen an ideal tool in such hypnotic protocols.

Finally, several reviews of previous research reveal consistent considerations clinicians should take into account (see W. Johnson, 1961b; W. Morgan, 1972, 1980, 1985, 1993; W. Morgan & Brown, 1983), which include the following: (a) The deeper the hypnotic trance, the more likely it is that the hypnotic suggestions will provide the intended results; (b) general arousal techniques might be more useful in enhancing muscular strength and endurance than hypnotic suggestions alone; (c) hypnosis can help a successful athlete, but it cannot make a good performer out of a poor one — mastery requires practicing hypnosis as one would any other physical skill; (d) inappropriate use of hypnosis can do more harm than good — persons providing hypnosis should have the necessary training; (e) autohypnosis (self-hypnosis) as opposed to heterohypnosis is recommended to avoid the problems associated with dependency on a therapist; (f) the evidence that hypnosis can affect muscular strength endurance is unclear; (g) hypnotic suggestions designed to enhance performance generally have not, as of yet, been effective, whereas suggestions designed to impair muscular strength and endurance have consistently been successful; (h) individuals who are not accustomed to performing at their maximal levels usually experience gains in muscular strength and endurance when administered "involving" suggestions in the hypnotic state; however, suggestions of a "noninvolving" nature are not effective when administered to individuals who are accustomed to performing at maximal levels; (i) efforts to modify performance on various psychomotor tasks have effects similar to those observed in research involving muscular strength and endurance; for example, efforts to slow reaction time are usually effective, whereas attempts to improve reaction time are not; (j) case studies involving efforts to enhance performance in athletes by means of hypnosis appear to be universally successful; (k) hypnotic suggestion of exercise in the nonexercise state is associated with increased heart rate, respiratory rate, ventilatory minute volume, oxygen uptake, carbon dioxide production, forearm blood flow, and cardiac output (these metabolic changes often approximate responses noted during actual exercise conditions); and (l) perception of effort during exercise can be systematically increased and decreased with hypnotic suggestion even though the actual physical workload is maintained at a constant level.

Techniques for Sport Hypnosis

The application of hypnosis in the sporting realm is not new and has been used for years in sport and exercise psychology to investigate and influence the underlying mechanism of athletic performance. However, most of the clinical applications of hypnosis in sport are anecdotal in nature (Gordin, 1995, p. 193). In sport, hypnosis has been used to improve and develop a variety of issues, including pain management (Ryde, 1964), aggression issues (W. Johnson, 1961a), anxiety (Naruse, 1965), arousal control (Garver, 1977), and performance analysis (W. Morgan, 1980). Hypnosis also has been applied to resolve consistency issues, fear of reinjury, and performance and technique evaluation (W. Morgan, 1996). Despite a growing body of literature on hypnosis and sports, few authors have specifically discussed the "how-to" aspect of using hypnosis to enhance athletic performance beyond anxiety reduction and attention (Liggett, personal communication, March 11, 2000, to Erik Dunlap). In this chapter, we describe how to use hypnosis to address some of the commonly identified areas that concern athletes. We break down the techniques by various aspects within athletic performance. However, it should be noted that because psychological constructs (confidence, motivation, imagery, etc.) overlap, many of the techniques can be used for a variety of issues.

Relaxation

Most athletes have been exposed to various relaxation techniques, whether formally or informally. Two of the most adapted techniques used in performance enhancement interventions are E. Jacobson's (1938) progressive muscle relaxation and Suinn's (1980) visual motor-behavior rehearsal. Jacobsen's progressive muscle relaxation involves tensing and flexing various muscle groups in a specific order. Suinn's visual motor-behavior rehearsal technique combines relaxation with covert behavior (technique) rehearsal, which is essentially hypnosis. Visual motor-behavior rehearsal comprises two phases. During the first phase the athlete becomes totally relaxed using a modified version of Jacobson's progressive muscle relaxation. During the second phase the athlete uses imagery (and suggestion) to rehearse various skills or movements. For those athletes with some hypnotic capability, these relaxation and imagery techniques are in essence hypnotic inductions and are likely to induce at least a light trance. Support for the use of hypnosis to aid in relaxation and performance enhancement has been noted in previous literature (see Jacobs & Gotthelf, 1986; Taylor et al., 1993). "Hypnosis aimed at increasing relaxation and alleviating psychological anxiety may have a positive and enhancing effect on the performance on athletes" (Jacobs & Gotthelf, 1986). Although most hypnotic inductions (except those asking alert and active-alert models) will suffice to induce a relaxed state, adding posthypnotic suggestions using verbal or tactile cues can add to the effectiveness of relaxation training.

Following Deepening of Hypnosis. [Athlete's name] you are so deeply relaxed ... so comfortable ... that your mind is completely open ... and completely receptive ... to everything that I have to say ... it will be easy for you to experience all that I ask you to experience. You are now deeply hypnotized and completely relaxed ... nothing will disturb you. Pay attention ... to the complete relaxation that has now come over you. It is easy ... just to sit [lie] there ... and feel completely relaxed ... notice how pleasant it feels ... how nothing can disturb you ... it is easy ... to sink deeply into the chair and let it support you. Feel the heaviness ... in your limbs ... how the tension has melted away. Your mind is so calm ... so focused on this complete state of relaxation that has come over you. Take a moment ... enjoy how this feels ... when you are done indicate by raising your right index finger [pause]. Good. [Athlete's name] you can achieve this state whenever you need to. ... Whenever you wish to return to this deep state of complete relaxation ... all you to do is ... take a deep breath and think or say to yourself [cue word] ... and then ... your body will begin to relax and your mind will become clearer ... and more alert. ... With each deep breath the tension will melt away ... and you will become more relaxed. your mind will remain clear and alert ... your body will feel heavy and warm as it becomes ... more and more relaxed ... just by taking a deep breath and thinking or saying to yourself [cue word]. You will always be able to return to this state of complete relaxation when-ever you choose to. [Bring athlete out of hypnosis and then rehyp-notize and practice the technique several times with the athlete.]

[Athlete's name] Stay completely relaxed, but continue to listen care-fully to what I tell you next. In a moment I will count backwards from 10 to 1. You will gradually come out of hypnosis, but you will be the way you are now for most of the count. When I reach "1" you will be awake and alert as you usually are. You will be able to recall all the things I have said to you and the things you did. You will find it easy to return to this complete state of relaxation whenever you need to ... just by taking deep breaths and saying to yourself [cue word]. It will become easier to recall this state of complete relaxation each time you say to yourself [cue word]. After you wake up you will feel refreshed. I shall now count backwards from 10 to 1. At "1" you will be fully awake. A little later I shall ask you to take a deep breath and say to yourself [cue word] like this. [Demonstrate with a deep breath and cue word.] When I do, you will feel a sudden wave of relaxation come over you. And then you will be completely relaxed ... but always keenly alert to all that you need to perform well. You will always be able to return to this state whenever you choose to. All right, ready — 10, 9, 8, 7, 6, 5, 4, 3, 2, 1.

Imagery and Visualization

Athletes invariably use imagery, intentionally or not. Athletes are thinking of plays, movements, parts of or whole games, or performance possible outcomes, which makes it a valuable skill to take advantage of to enhance their performance. Imagery and relaxation have become the foundation of most performance-enhancement interventions (Cornelius, 2002a; Weinberg & Gould, 2003). One possible explanation for its effectiveness is that hypnotically induced imagery can "enhance skill development at the motor-learning level through low-level neuromuscular innervations in those muscles associated with a particular motor skill" (Taylor et al., 1993, p. 70). Williamson et al. (2002) found that hypnotically induced imagery can influence cardiovascular response and perceived exertion (through activation of the anterior cigulate and insular cortices) in highly susceptible individuals. That means highly hypnotizable athletes will be able to "experience" the images more realistically, thus increasing their familiarity, confidence, and reaction time with the imaged skill or task.

There are several theories that attempt to explain how imagery works to enhance performance, but one thing is clear; it works (Cornelius, 2002a). Because hypnosis frequently incorporates an imagery component, it seems only natural to use hypnosis in the same way one would use imagery to address an athlete's performance concerns. In fact, Taylor and colleagues (1993) suggested that hypnotically enhanced imagery can be used in a variety of ways, including (a) increasing self-confidence by creating success or positive imagery, (b) improving kinesthetic awareness, and (c) addressing the origins to performance inconsistencies.

The possibilities are limitless for using hypnotically induced imagery; some of which we present shortly. In an example of a sprinter, Liggett (2000b, p. 53) had the athlete observe the attributes of a large predatory cat. He then had the athlete image assuming that feline's characteristics, visualizing his muscles exploding like the great cat's and then running smooth and controlled during a race. In another imagery case, the athlete imaged himself as a machine (a locomotive), not getting tired and churning out consistent performances (Liggett, 2000b, p. 54). According to Taylor et al. (1993), "There is a growing body of evidence that hypnosis may enhance the quality of mental imagery."

Imagery is a polysensory experience. When working with an athlete, the therapist must gather as much information as possible from the athlete prior to beginning and to incorporate as many of the senses as possible in the imagery. The key to the use of hypnosis-based imagery is to ask the athlete to image, see, or picture, rather than to imagine.

Following Deepening of Hypnosis.

Say:

> [Athlete's name] You are deeply relaxed ... deeply hypnotized ... nothing will disturb you. It is easy just to listen to all that I say. ...

As you sit [lie] in that chair [bed], picture a large TV, or maybe screen, whichever you choose, in front of you. ... You have now become so deeply relaxed ... so hypnotized ... that you will be able to visualize everything that I ask you to. The images will be so familiar that it will be easy just to see whatever it is that I ask ... in just a moment you will see yourself running [one of the plays the athlete will be performing in the next competition]. See yourself in the huddle ... the QB [quarterback] calling out [play]. You break and run to the line. ... Picture in your mind getting into your stance, smell the sweat rolling down your face, feel the wet ground up turf beneath your fingers. You have practiced this play all week ... you know what to do. Feel the tightening ... tensing of your fingers as they grip the ground. Feel your leg muscles tightening ... tensing ... ready to propel you forward ... you are so confident. ... You know the count ... everything else is automatic ... your moves, where to place your head and hands ... you are ready. Just before the ball is snapped, your mind is focused, and your body is primed ... you are powerful ... strong ... and pre-pared. The ball is snapped ... you explode forward ... powerfully ... gracefully ... your hands shoot the inside of the defender's pads ... he is jolted back ... you grab fast ... you have him ... your feet driving into the ground ... you begin to move him back ... he struggles ... but ... you are in control. As you move forward you extend your arms and pull him out of his hips ... you have him ... you keep driving ... see yourself ... powerful ... strong ... driving him into the dirt ... as the back runs off your back for a first down. You did your job.

[Athlete's name] Stay completely relaxed, but continue to listen carefully to what I tell you next. In a moment, I will count back-wards from 10 to 1. You will gradually come out of hypnosis, but you will be the way you are now for most of the count. When I reach "1" you will be awake and alert as you usually are. You will be able to recall all the things I have said to you and the things you did. You will find it easy to return to this state of complete concentration ... and confidence whenever you need to ... when-ever the QB says "down." It will become easier to recall this state of concentration ... and confidence each time the QB says "down." You will remain in that state until the referee blows the whistle for the play to end ... but ... you will be able to return ... when the QB says "down." After you wake up you will feel refreshed. I shall now count backwards from 10 to 1. At "1" you will be fully awake. A little later today I shall ask you to practice becoming more confident and more focused at practice whenever you hear the QB say "down." When you do, you will feel a sudden wave of awareness ... confidence ... and concentration come over you. And then you will be completely confident and keenly alert to all that you need to perform well. You will always be able to return to this state whenever you choose to. All right, ready — 10, 9, 8, 7, 6, 5, 4, 3, 2, 1 — wide awake and ready.

Goal Setting

Almost all athletes set goals in one way or another, whether they are vague "do-your-best" goals or specific goals, such as having a "hang time" of 4.3 seconds and downing the ball between the 5- and 10-yard line. Goals help us focus our energies toward a specific objective, keep us motivated and focused on that objective, and help reduce confusion on what needs to be done to accomplish that goal. Although setting goals in sport is very common, many athletes have difficulty following through with the changes necessary to achieve their goals. Falling short of reaching a goal may be a result of not knowing how to incorporate the changes. Usng hypnosis, athletes can image the various stages and changes that are necessary to achieve the goal. Athletes can even image what it will be like to achieve that goal, which can help increase their enjoyment and motivation for competing.

Goals should be discussed in terms of long-term (dream goals [terminal objectives]) and short-terms goals (enabling objectives). Usually, achieving these intermediate goals moves athletes closer to achieving their long-term or dream goal. For example, most athletes tend to focus on outcome goals (placing first, winning the championship, etc.) but frequently ignore the small steps that will make it possible to achieve these goals. Keep it simple. When discussing goal achievement with an athlete, the therapist should ask the athlete to think of a staircase; the top being the long-term goal (i.e., championship) and the steps being the short-term goals that lead to the long-term goal (out scoring opponent, recovering from mistakes, fitness level, etc.). Once specific goals are established and a time line is set, hypnosis can be used to help athlete sees (image) themselves at each stage in the process. Caution should be taken not to suggest visualizing changes that are too drastic or too far ahead compared to the athletes' current ability level. It would be difficult to visualize being at a particular level of goal attainment if the athletes have never come close to such a level. In doing so, the consultant (hypnotherapist) increases the probability of failure and reduces the athletes' self-confidence and the probability of future success.

Following Deepening of Hypnosis.

Say:

[Athlete's name] You are deeply relaxed ... deeply hypnotized ... nothing will disturb you. It is easy just to listen to all that I say. ... As you sit [lie] in that chair [bed], picture a large TV, or maybe screen ... whichever you choose, in front of you. ... You have now become so deeply relaxed ... so hypnotized ... that you will be able to visualize everything that I ask you to. The images will be so familiar that it will be easy just to see whatever it is that I ask ... in just a moment you will see yourself backing into the blocks ... working on your takeoff ... and when you master your takeoff ... you'll come closer to the 6.87 mark ... Now ... see yourself on the track prior to your start ... going through your normal warm-up routine ... prior to your race ... placing your right hand down ... then your left ... kicking out your right leg ... then the left ... shaking it out [pause]. you are now in your blocks, head down ... waiting for the command ..."runners take your mark" ... ass up and coiled ... you are primed to explode ... the gun goes off ... you drive with your left foot and pull with your right. ... You remain low ... as you power for the first 10 steps ... then you pop up. See yourself improving ... how each time you get into your blocks ... you Feel more confident ... more powerful ... becoming better at driving out low and hard ... each time you come out of the blocks. ... The more you practice exploding out and driving into your step ... the faster you will become ... it will become so natural ... so fluid ... that it will just happen on its own ... so natural that it becomes automatic ... getting better ... more fluid ... and smoother each time. See yourself ... making progress at coming out of the blocks ... becoming stronger ... faster with each attempt ... feeling more confident ... more in control ... becoming more graceful ... more fluid ... with each start ... with each start ... your form ... will improve ... you will be more in control of your body ... driving low for the first 10 steps before popping up ... with each successful start ... you move closer to achieving your goal. with each successful start ... you will move closer ... to your goal ... your confidence in your ability to achieve your goals will increase ... each time you visualize coming out of the blocks ...

each time ... it will be easier to take what you have learned ... and do it ... on the track. ... You will feel yourself ... just as you did here ... exploding out ... driving low ... for the first 10 steps ... and when you are able to do this ... you will get closer to your goal of 6.87. You will get closer to your goal ... closer ... with each step ... with each successful start ... you will get closer ... because you have all the skills in you ... now ... you can begin right away ... with that first step ... and it will feel good ... to do it. [After visualizing several successful starts, assess the athlete for successful attempts using an ideomotor signal.]

Now [athlete's name] ... allow yourself to experience the success, the feeling of achieving your goal ... of exploding low out of the blocks ... the confidence ... the power. You are now closer to your goal ... you feel good. ... Take a moment ... Enjoy these feelings ... the sense of accomplishment. As you take each step toward your goal ... you will feel more ... and more comfortable ... you will be able to recall what it feels like to accomplish your goal. When you awaken ... in just a few moments ... you will be able to recall the process of achieving your goal ... the steps you will take ... and how it will feel along the way. You will look forward to working toward your goal. [Bring the athlete out of hypnosis and debrief.]

Skill Development and Technique Enhancement

Technical development is another area in which hypnosis has been found to be beneficial (Liggett, 2000a, 2000b; Liggett & Hamada, 1993; Taylor et al., 1993). Hypnosis can help the athlete learn new skills or perfect current ones by "assisting the athlete in attending to relevant cues in the sequencing and timing of complex responses" (Taylor et al., 1993, p. 68). Taylor et al. (1993) stated that hypnosis "appears to facilitate conscious access to subtle neuromuscular processes and mechanisms that would otherwise seem to be beyond direct conscious control," allowing the athlete to develop skill mastery by improving kinesthetic awareness and control (p. 70). In hypnosis, athletes are able to practice new strategies, identify and work on skills needing improvement, and make quick and accurate decisions during competition.

Researchers have used hypnosis to enhance technical performance and facilitate skill development of gymnasts (Liggett, 2000a, 2000b; Liggett & Hamada, 1993), basketball players (Pates, Oliver, & Maynard, 2001; Schreiber, 1991), volleyball players (Baer, 1980); golfers (Pates & Maynard, 2000), and tennis players (Taylor et al., 1993). Liggett and Hamada (1993) described using imagery to help gymnasts perfect their performance. Using hypnotically based imagery, a gymnast was asked while in trance to picture himself performing a double backflip with a full twist. He reported being able to see himself performing the movements in slow motion to understand timing and body placement throughout the moves. Slowly, the athlete began to increase the speed of the movements until he reached real-time speed. Hypnosis can also help an athlete tap into first-person imagery (looking through the athlete's eyes) allowing the athlete to incorporate kinesthetic feelings, smell, touch, sounds, and images more vividly in a hypnotic state (Liggett, 2000b; Taylor et al., 1993). The more vivid the imagery, the easier it is for athletes to generalize their success to the real world. The athletes are able to practice new skills mentally several times until they feel comfortable doing it on their own, without expending too much energy or getting injured because of overtraining.

For example, let us examine a scenario of a long jumper whose long-term goal is to increase his jumping distance by 4 to 5 inches over the next 5 weeks. After establishing this as a realistic yet challenging goal, we gather more information regarding what the athlete needs to improve to reach this goal (usually such information comes from a coach). There are several technical issues that he needs to improve, including perfecting footwork, maintaining proper form in the air, and leaning into the landing. On the basis of this information, we can begin to help the athlete move closer to his long-term goal by becoming more technically sound in these areas. Using hypnotically induced imagery, the athlete can practice his movements first in slow motion to get the coordination down, then in real-time speed to get the feel of hitting the mark and jumping at full speed.

Following Deepening of Hypnosis.

Say:

> [Athlete's name] You are deeply relaxed ... deeply hypnotized ... nothing will disturb you. It is easy just to listen to all that I say. ... As you sit [lie] in that chair [bed], picture a large TV, or maybe screen, whichever you choose, in front of you. ... You have now become so deeply relaxed ... so hypnotized ... that you will be able to visualize everything that I ask you to. The images will be so familiar ... that it will be easy just to see whatever it is that I ask ... in just a moment you will see yourself at the starting mark ... maybe a little vague at first, but soon you will see yourself very clearly ... [pause] ... can you see yourself ... [ideomotor signal]? Good. ... See yourself in slow motion ... rocking back on your

right heel ... feel the weight shift from left to right as you rock ... feel the rhythm build in that rock ... so smooth ... so naturally ... it feels ... to shift from one leg to the next. ... see yourself now ... as you shift and explode ... off of that left foot ... and drive into the next step ... powerfully ... feel the natural rhythm of shifting power as you explode off the balls of your feet. See yourself stride down the strip ... feel how each leg turns over ... so fluid ... so graceful ... you approach the mark with good form ... you hit the mark in stride ... and explode ... into the air ... extend forward ... reaching for your toes ... you landing feet first ... and roll out ... you are pleased with your jump ... you look over to the measure ... a new personal record!

There are several key points that will make this more effective. First, the more information and detail the therapist includes in the script, the better. This script is more of a skeleton that would be built on following feedback. Using the athlete's language makes it the imagery more effective. One suggestion is to have the athlete come up with a description of his jump process using his words and then adapt that into a script. Following the first run through, it is important to get feedback about what worked and what did not. After adjustments to the script are made, go through the process several more times, each time having the image get faster and faster. Finally, add suggestions for self-confidence, control, power, and gracefulness to maximize effectiveness.

Achieving Optimal Arousal

Arousal is an innate part of sport performance. Arousal alone is not usually sufficient to achieve the desired goal. There is a small window or zone in which the athlete's level of arousal is optimal for achieving peak performance. It is the optimal zone of functioning (Hanin, 1999). Arousal levels outside this window, too little or too much, can have a detrimental impact on performance. Csikszentmihalyi (1990) revealed that a psychological state he termed "flow" was strongly associated with peak performance. Where this window or zone occurs on the continuum depends on a variety of factors: the task, sport, position, personal preference, and so on. For example, a golfer putting requires a different level of arousal than a football player preparing to tackle someone or a hockey player checking an opponent into the boards. Athletes who can activate their zone of optimum functioning increase the probability of experiencing flow. Unfortunately, it is difficult for many top athletes to get into this zone on a consistent basis. However, in hypnosis it is possible to have athletes recall successful performances and reexperience the feelings (self-confidence, arousal level, thoughts, etc.) and movements that accompanied that performance. Once the athlete is able to recall at various sensory levels these experiences vividly, the therapist can associate the athlete with a cue word or trigger. The athlete can reexperience when needed to increase the chance of experiencing flow. Pates, Oliver, et al. (2001) (see also Pates, Cummings, & Maynard, 2002) showed that hypnosis could be used to facilitate flow and improve performance by improving confidence, focus, and control. Repeated practice in hypnosis can then help strengthen the use of the posthypnotic suggestions using the cue word or trigger.

Following Deepening of Hypnosis.
Say:

> [Athlete's name] You have now become so deeply relaxed ... so deeply hypnotized ... that your mind has become so clear ... and so focused ... on everything that I am about to say ... that you will be able to experience all that I ask you to. Continue to go deeper ... and deeper into this hypnotic state that you are currently experiencing. I will now count from 5 to 1. ... At the count of 1 you are going back to a time when you were in the "zone" ... when everything seemed to click ... a time when you felt extremely confident in your abilities ... when the game seemed to play out in slow motion ... a time when you knew what was going to happen ... before it happened. Just allow yourself to go back to that pleasant experience ... and feel those positive feelings again. ... When you are there, allow your right index finger to float up from the arm of the chair [following the ideomotor response]. Good. ... As you enjoy that moment ... once again ... you will be able to sense those feelings of being extremely confident ... relaxed ... and in control. And when you begin to have those feelings again, allow your right index finger to float up off of the arm of the chair to let me know [wait for signal]. Good. Feel those emotions getting stronger ... as you continue to immerse yourself in that previous experience [pause]. And now as you are experiencing these feelings, I'd like you to [suggest a trigger such as touch your right knee or elbow, close your dominant hand into a tight fist, squeeze the ball twice, etc.], and as you do so, these positive feelings will become even stronger. That's right, just [trigger], as a sign and symbol of confidence and control. And as you [trigger], feel the feelings of confidence ... and control ... flowing back over you ... energizing you. Whenever you want to experience these feelings again, all you

need to do is [trigger], and this same kind of memory and feelings, will come back into your experience ... becoming more relaxed ... more focused ... more alert ... and more confident. ... Each time you practice recalling these feelings ... they will return more rapidly ... more clearly than before [pause].

[Athlete's name] Stay completely relaxed, but continue to listen carefully to what I tell you next. In a moment ... I will begin counting backward from 10 to 1. And ... as I do ... you will gradually come out of hypnosis. When I reach "1" you will be as awake and alert as you were when your first came here today. You will be able to recall everything I have said to you and the things you did. ... you will find it easy to recall these feelings of confidence ... control ... and relaxation ... whenever you need to ... just by [trigger]. It will become easier to recall this state of confidence ... control ... and relaxation ... each time you [trigger]. I shall now count backward from 10 to 1. At "1" you will be fully awake. A little later I shall ask you to take a deep breath and [trigger]. When I do ... you will feel a sudden wave of confidence ... control ... and relaxation come over you. ... And then ... you will be completely confident ... and keenly alert ... to all that you need to perform well. You will always be able to return to this state whenever you choose to. All right, ready — 10, 9, 8, 7, 6, 5, 4, 3, 2, 1 — wide awake and ready.

Arousal Management

Arreed Barabasz, winner of more than a dozen Formula Atlantic race car championships by 1995, was once asked by a TV sports reporter why the word *calm* appeared above the tachometer in his cramped-cockpit, open-wheel car, which he took through turns at 150 plus miles per hour. Without mentioning hypnosis, Barabasz replied, "Oh, it's just a reminder of what I must do to win."

Athletes frequently experience increased levels of anxiety, stress, and arousal preceding and during competition (Jones & Hardy, 1990). Because of this, many sport psychologists involve some form of physiological management as part of the athlete's skills training. Most athletes are concerned with decreasing their levels of precompetitive anxiety, or heightened arousal, but some athletes struggle to "get up" for their performances. Outside of competition, the previous arousal script and relaxation script can be used to help regulate arousal. However, there are times when athletes are in "crisis," when they are out of their zone during competition. In these situations athletes must be able to quickly reduce their levels of arousal to focus, or performance will suffer. We offer here are a few rapid hypnotic inductions that can be used in the competition setting. Previous hypnosis practice will enhance the effectiveness of these techniques.

Hands moving together to decrease arousal.
Say:

> [Athlete's arms are stretched out, palms facing each other approximately 6 to 8 inches apart.] Watch your arms as they come together on their own. As the distance between your hands grows small, the rest of your body becomes more and more relaxed. Soon your hands will touch each other while you are watching, and you will become more and more relaxed. The closer your hands move together the less tense you will become. Closer and closer ... more and more relaxed. ... Good, that's it. ... wonder how much tension you want to keep for today's performance. And when you feel your level of arousal is where it needs to be, you will be ready to enter the zone.

Eye roll to increase arousal (derived from A. Barabasz, 2000).
Say:

> [Athlete's eyes are rolled to center of forehead.] Allow yourself to become comfortable. Stand [sit] with your feet slightly apart and flat on the floor ... place your hands by your side [or on your lap]. Drop your head slightly and roll your eyes upward so that they are looking at a point though your forehead to where my finger is [place finger on top-middle of forehead]. It may feel a little uncomfortable, but try to focus on that point. Take a deep breath and let it out slowly. Listen carefully to what I say. ... As your eyes become more and more tired, your body will become more and more energized. You will become more alert as your eyes become heavier ... more and more alert and more ready to play. And when your eyes finally decide to close, you will have reached an optimum state of arousal. [Repeat several times. Following an indication of trance, the therapist slowly brings finger down past nose; athlete's eyes should follow and close.]

Focus and Concentration

Motivation and arousal can greatly influence an athlete's ability to remain focused and make quick, accurate decisions in the heat of competition.

There are numerous obstacles on and off the field that can distract athletes from being able to perform at their best. Worrying about what others (coaches, teammates, etc.) think, the previous play that did not go well, plans after the game, and various other thoughts are just a few examples of distractions athletes face. The very nature of some sports may lead to a decrease of concentration over time because of complacency. The dilemma these athletes face of not being focused could cost them the game. However, staying constantly vigilant for nine innings, for example, could lead to mental fatigue resulting in slowed reaction time and poor decision making. In situations like these, attending to specific cues can help athletes maximize the time they need to pay attention and when they can mentally relax. In trance, the athlete can be asked to image specific cues that would signal them to increase their level of focus. In our baseball example, when the pitcher steps on the rubber, it is a cue (for the other players) that play is about to begin. When the pitcher is off the mound, it is a cue to the outfielders to decrease their level of arousal and concentration. Suggestions can be given, for example, that when the outfielder slaps his glove, players will be optimally alert and aroused. When a play is over (batter strikes out or steps out of the batter's box, or pitcher is off the mound), the outfielder can be given the suggestion to adjust his hat as an indication to the players to momentarily relax their focus. Repetition of these cues with the suggestions of focus or alertness in trance can strengthen these techniques and sharpen the athlete's ability to adjust his or her concentration. The athlete's level of concentration can then be recalled using a quick induction (e.g., eye roll), cue word, or trigger. Alternatively, some athletes respond more reliably to posthypnotic suggestions to execute the suggestions.

Following Deepening of Hypnosis.

Say:

> You have now become so deeply relaxed ... so comfortable ... so deeply hypnotized ... that your mind has become so open ... so receptive to all that I say ... everything that I say ... will sink so deeply into your unconscious mind ... and everything I say to you will make so deep and lasting an impression ... nothing will change it. ... Your mind is so receptive that it will be easy to not think ... or understand ... the things that I am saying. in fact, it isn't even necessary to listen very closely to the things that I am saying, because your unconscious mind will be able to hear ... and understand ... everything ... that I say to you. Just allow your conscious mind ... to enjoy the pleasant state ... of complete

relaxation ... that has come over you ... and let your unconscious mind take over. As these things I say, begin to sink deeply into your unconscious mind ... they will soon begin to exert a greater influence over the way you think ... over the way you feel ... over the way you play. And ... because these things will sink so deeply ... into your mind ... they will continue to influence ... the way you think ... the way you feel ... and the way you play. ... [athlete's name] You are deeply relaxed ... deeply hypnotized ... nothing will disturb you. ... As you sit [lie] in that chair [bed], picture a large TV, or maybe screen, whichever you choose, in front of you. ... You have now become so deeply relaxed ... so hypnotized ... that you will be able to visualize everything that I ask you to. ... It will be easy just to listen to all that I say. ... The images will be so familiar ... that it will be easy just to see whatever it is that I ask ... and maybe even experience it as well ... in just a moment you will see yourself on the screen ... at bat ... there are many distractions all around you ... the crowd ... the lights ... the catcher behind you ... and the players in the field ... it is difficult to focus [pause]. ... When you step into the batter's box, you are stepping into a special zone. In the box you will find that you are able to concentrate on the ball's rotation ... because the distractions are muted inside the box ... everything else begins to fade ... you will begin to feel more confident ... more in control ... and ... more alert in every way. When your step into the box ... you will become so focused ... so aware ... and so alert ... that it will be easier to pick up the rotation of the ball as it leaves the pitcher's hand ... you will become so deeply focused in the box that the ball will seem bigger ... and move slower ... you will no longer think nearly so much about yourself ... about your opponent ... or the crowd ... you will become much less aware of what you are doing ... and how you feel. ... You will recognize the rotation of the ball ... without thinking ... without doubt ... and without fear of striking out. ... You will be able to make the right decision ... the right move ... automatically ... without thought ... because you will become more confident ... and more focused ... when you step into the box. it will become easier day by day to feel more and more Focused ... when you step into the box ... every day. When it is time to perform ... in practice ... or in a game ... you will be able to think more clearly ... be more focused ... when you step into the box. It will be so easy to just play the game you have so much passion for ... that it will just happen without you knowing it. every day ... you will become less anxious ... less concerned about the crowd ... and less concerned about your opponents. you will become ... and you will remain ... more and more completely focused at bat ... just by stepping into the box on the field. now ... [athlete's name] ... I want you to practice stepping into the box ... notice the noise begin to fade when you are in the box ... becoming more confident and more aware ... take a moment and practice stepping in and out of the box ... and notice ... how you can become more focused by stepping into the box. ... When you feel comfortable stepping into the box and feeling more alert ... allow your right index finger to float up from the arm of the chair [following the ideomotor response]. good ... the more you practice stepping into the box ... the sooner you will become more focused and alert on the field. ... This thing that I put into the unconscious part of your mind ... stepping into the box ... after you have left here ... when you are no longer with me ... will continue to enhance your ability to become confident ... focused ... and be alert ... just as strongly ... just as clearly ... just as powerfully ... when you are back home ... or at work ... as when you are actually with me in this room.

[Athlete's name] Stay completely relaxed, but continue to listen carefully to what I tell you next. In a moment I will count backward from 10 to 1. You will gradually come out of hypnosis, but you will be the way you are now for most of the count. When I reach "1" you will be as awake and alert as you usually are. You will be able to recall all the things I have said to you and the things you did. You will find it easy to return to this state of complete concentration whenever you need to ... just by saying stepping into the box. It will become easier to recall this state of complete concentration each time you step into the box. After you wake up you will feel refreshed. I shall now count backward from 10 to 1. At "1" you will be fully awake. When you go to practice later today, I shall ask you to practice stepping into the box. when you do, you will feel a sudden wave of awareness and concentration come over you. and then you will be completely focused and keenly alert to all that you need to perform well. You will always be able to return to this state whenever you choose to. All right, ready — 10, 9, 8, 7, 6, 5, 4, 3, 2, 1 — wide awake and ready.

Self-Confidence and Motivation

Athletes frequently find it difficult to maintain a consistent level of self-confidence and motivation. It is one of the most frequent issues mentioned by athletes (Weinberg & Gould, 1995). Athletes have a tendency to allow their most recent performances in competition and practice determine how they will perform in future situations. In the 1990s Arreed Barabasz faced Lynn St. James, an experimented Indy car driver, in a Formula Atlantic national championship race in Portland, Oregon. His confidence running against a professional team that even arrived with a spare race car came from his setting the track record there just weeks before. Barabasz went on to win that race after a tight battle. St. James went on to qualify in the second row for the Indianapolis 500, just ahead of the reigning Formula 1 world champion Nigel Mansell. St. James had run that race before and Mansell had not. Confidence can make a huge difference.

Alternatively, beginning the season with a few losses can create a snowball effect of negative thinking and loss of self-confidence for the rest of the season. Slumps can also lead to a decreased sense of competence and self-doubt. Russell (1980) suggested using positive self-suggestions combined with hypnotically induced imagery to increase the athlete's confidence and coordination. Gardner and Olness (1981) described a case of an 11-year-old girl who was anxiety ridden over an upcoming ice skating competition. When she was regressed to the earlier ages of 8, 9, and 10, she recalled an unpleasant incident. After being rehypnotized, she was asked to "send it off" by pony express (an image that had meaning to her). Her anxiety about the ice skating competition subsided and she competed very well in the event.

Ego-strengthening (self-confidence) hypnotherapy does just what its name suggests. Supportive ego-strengthening hypnotherapy is a strategy used to facilitate self-esteem and self-confidence by supporting the client and emphasizing the client's strengths (Hammond, 1990; Taylor et al., 1993). Ego-strengthening protocols can be used to help athletes "reprogram" their internal dialogues by using suggestions for confidence and self-esteem.

Richard Morris, a friend and former student of John Watkins (1982), described hypnotic techniques he has used successfully in improving the skill of wrestlers and in combating batting slumps as a consultant to the New York Mets baseball team. He reported that he often found destructive ego states that emerged temporarily to impair players at these times. Morris employed a hypnoanalytic ego-state approach to resolve the conflicts, which seemed to resolve the slumps. The technique was especially effective for pitcher's slump (see our volume II, *Hypnoanalytic Techniques* to learn the procedure). Examples of the suggestions used in this method of performance enhancement include "You will feel stronger with each step; more alert and interested in what you are doing"; suggestions for arousal include "You will experience a sense of pleasure and calmness as you drive forward with each step." Tying these feelings to a trigger such as squeezing the dominant hand can further facilitate the athlete's ability to recall feelings of confidence. Practicing this script multiple times can increase the effectiveness of the trigger (e.g., squeezing the fist).

Following Deepening of Hypnosis.

> You have now become so deeply relaxed ... so comfortable ... and so deeply hypnotized ... that your mind is completely open ... and completely receptive ... to all that I say ... everything that I say ... will sink so deeply into your unconscious mind ... and everything I say to you ... will make so deep and lasting an impression ... nothing will change it. ... your mind is so receptive that it will be easy to not think ... or understand ... the things that I am saying. in fact, it isn't even necessary to listen very closely to the things that I am saying, because your unconscious mind will be able to hear ... and understand ... everything ... that I say to you. Just allow your conscious mind ... to enjoy the pleasant state ... of complete relaxation ... that has come over you ... and let your unconscious mind take over. as these words begin to embed themselves ... deeply into your unconscious mind ... they will soon begin to exert a greater influence over the way you think ... over the way you feel ... over the way you play on the field. And ... because these things will become ... so permanently embedded ... into your mind ... they will continue to influence ... the way you think ... the way you feel ... and the way you play ... even after you have left this office ... they will continue to influence the way you think ... and feel ... just as powerfully ... just as clearly ... on the field ... at practice ... and in your everyday life ... as they do right when you are here with me. These thoughts will have become so engrained ... so entrenched ... into the unconscious part of your mind ... after you have left here ... when you are no longer with me ... they will continue to exercise that same great influence ... over your thoughts ... your feelings ... and your actions ... just as strongly ... just as clearly ... just as powerfully ... when you are at practice ... when you play ... or when you are back home ... as when you are actually with me today. With each practice and competition ... you will begin to feel more confident ... physically stronger and fitter in every way. You will become more focused ... more aware ... more energized. ... You will become much less easily tired ... much less easily fatigued ... and much less easily discouraged ... everyday ...

you will become so motivated to do your best ... that everything else will fade ... you will no longer think nearly so much about yourself ... about your opponent ... or the crowd ... you will become much less aware of how you are doing ... and how you feel ... you will begin to make decisions on the field ... without thinking ... without worrying about the consequences ... and without fear of failing. ... You will be able to make the right decision ... the right move ... automatically ... without thought ... because you will become more confident ... and sure of yourself ... every day. when it is time to perform ... in practice ... or in a game ... you will be able to think more clearly ... be more focused ... because you are more confident in your abilities. it will be so easy to just play the game you have so much passion for ... that it will just happen without you knowing it. every day ... you will become less anxious ... less concerned about the crowd ... and less concerned about your opponents. you will become ... and you will remain ... more and more completely relaxed on the field ... and less concerned about what you have to do ... because you will know ... what to do ... more quickly ... and more accurately ... every day. With each passing day ... you will feel more confident ... more in control ... and more powerful on the field ... than you have ever felt before. Every day ... these things will begin to happen ... exactly as I tell you. ... You will play with more vigor ... more effort ... and more passion.

In just a moment, I will count backward from 10 to 1. You will gradually come out of hypnosis, but you will be the way you are now for most of the count. When I reach "1" you will be completely awake and alert as you usually are. Everything that you accomplished today will stay with you. DAY by DAY ... you will grow more and more confident in yourself as a person ... and as an athlete. ... After you wake up you will feel refreshed ... beginning today ... when you leave my office, you will FEEL good about yourself and about your ability to perform well. I will now count backward from 10 to 1. At "1" you will be fully awake and comfortable ... and maybe more confident. All right, ready — 10, 9, 8, 7, 6, 5, 4, 3, 2, 1 — wide awake and ready.

Performance Evaluation and Reconstructing

In a hypnotic state, the athlete is more receptive to the suggestions and recollection. Russell noted that the individual is able to remember minute details of an occasion almost as though they were reliving the event in its entirety. As we have discussed earlier in this volume, hypnosis can help one reexperience auditory, olfactory, tactile, and sensory-kinesthetic sensations. Because of this introspective effect of hypnosis, athletes can reexamine past performance to better recognize mistakes or errors in performances. Athletes can use the hypnotic state to help correct movements and enhance skills. In hypnosis, they can regress back to the moment they began to notice having difficulty. The affect bridge (J. Watkins, 1971) is one ideal method to accomplish this regression that Arreed Barabasz and Jack Watkins will discuss in volume II, *Hypnoanalytic Techniques.* After deepening, it is possible to discuss the athlete's experiences as they are happening. The information can later be used in a skill development.

Following Deepening of Hypnosis.

[Athlete's name] You have now become so deeply relaxed ... so deeply hypnotized ... that your mind has become so clear ... and so focused ... on everything that I am about to say ... that you will be able to experience all that I ask you to. Continue to go deeper ... and deeper into this hypnotic state that you are currently experiencing. I will now count from 5 to 1. At the count of 1 you are going back to the first time you began to struggle at [issue]. Five ... you are going back into the past. It is no longer 2004 or 2003 or 2002, but much earlier. Four ... you are going back to the first time you began to experience trouble at [issue] ... it is now coming back to you ... with each moment, that performance is becoming clearer ... more vivid ... presently you will be back in that game, the game that you began to notice something different with [issue]. Three ... almost there ... getting clearer and clearer. soon ... you will be back in that game ... you will feel the experience exactly as you did once before on that day that things began to be different with [issue]. Two ... very soon you will be there ... once again in that game ... when you first noticed [issue]. You are nearly there now. ... In a few moments you will be right back there. One! You are now back in that game ... when things seemed different with [issue] (adapted from the *Stanford Hypnotic Susceptibilty Scale,* Form C; Weitzenhoffer & Hilgard, 1962).

At this point, the therapist can gather information regarding events that took place, specific thoughts, and so on that may have been inconsistent with previous performances or that the athlete notes as different. Following information gathering, the therapist will then bring the athlete back to the present and continue with positive and corrective hypnotic suggestions to correct the errors the athlete was experiencing in the performance. The suggestions are reviewed again after the athlete is brought out of hypnosis. Using hypnotically induced imagery, athletes can use images of completing the skill correctly to help regain confidence and enhance their performance.

Injury and Pain Management

As we discussed in the chapters devoted to pain management, hypnosis is widely recognized as a complementary means of treating a variety of conditions in which pain is prominent. It is also useful in rehabilitation after surgery (Taylor et al., 1993). Ryde (1964) reported its use to treat 35 individual cases for a variety of injuries, including tennis elbow, shin splints, chronic Achilles tendon sprain, bruised heels, arch sprains, and other common ailments involving minor trauma. Hypnosis was so effective in the treatment of minor trauma resulting from injuries in sport that Ryde opted "to treat these disabilities initially by hypnosis and only proceed with conventional methods, should hypnosis fail or be refused" (p. 244; as cited in Morgan, 1996, p. 115).

It is not uncommon for athletes to heal completely on the physical level, but they remain psychologically injured. Whether the pain is real or exaggerated, the feelings of discomfort or pain prohibit athletes from reengaging in their sport with the same intensity and confidence they had prior to the injury. In some cases the team physician has cleared the athlete to begin participating again, but performing timidly can increase the athlete's chances of reinjury. Controlling the pain can restore the athlete's self-confidence and motivation to return to the sport. Earlier in this volume techniques addressing surgical, acute, and chronic pain management were elucidated. The following script represents one approach to helping the athlete recover from injury and pain.

Following Deepening of Hypnosis.

Say:

> [Athlete's name] You have now become So deeply relaxed ... so deeply hypnotized ... that you mind has become ready ... and open ... to all that I have to say. everything that I ask you to experience ... you will experience ... maybe not all at once ... but ... gradually the pain in your [location] will slowly begin to diminish. ... With each passing day, the feeling will begin to decrease. ... Before you know it, it will be so vague. So much you

won't recognize anymore with each passing day. You will feel stronger ... healthier each day. ... The more you focus on [the athletic task], the more the feelings diminish and these feelings will continue to increase or decrease... every day. ... You will be so deeply interested in [specific task] that your mind will be completely distracted away from the feeling in your [add the painful part of the athlete's body] you will no longer be aware of it. ... With each passing day healthier and stronger ... even when you are no longer with me ... more confident ... more interested in [the task] ... that the pain will grow smaller ... and smaller ... so small that you will not recognize it ... it will be so hard ... to recognize that it will be easy to ... let it go ... with each passing day ... it will continue to shrink ... until it is gone ... and you will have so much difficulty remembering the feeling ... it will disappear. [Awaken the athlete with suggestions for feeling more comfortable and confident.]

Rehabilitation Hypnosis

At least once in athletes' careers, they will experience some type of injury and therefore miss competition or practice. Recovering from surgery or serious injury is difficult. There is not only the discomfort associated with healing but also the painful experience of weekly rehabilitation. Facing months of pain and discomfort, athletes not surprisingly feel a negative impact on their motivation, self-confidence, and self-worth. Injury is likely to have a serious psychological impact on the athletes. They experience emotions and ruminations that can hamper the recovery process. "Education about the injury, rehabilitation process, goal setting, relaxation, imagery," and other cognitive strategies are among the many techniques that sport psychologists use to help move the athlete along in the recovery process (Cornelius, 2002b, p. 243). Hypnosis can be an effective alternative to help speed the athlete along the course to recovery by aiding in pain management and in actually healing of the tissue.

Following Deepening of Hypnosis.

Say:

Pain is your body's way of letting you know something is wrong ... a warning system ... your body's way of protecting itself from harming itself ... Pain is a natural part of healing ... it is often necessary ... but not all pain is necessary ... the more you begin to understand your own body, the more you will begin to know how much pain is useful to you ... continue to sink deeply into this complete state of relaxation ... deeper ... completely relaxed ... nothing will disturb you ... you will always be able to hear me very clearly ... very distinctly ... with each passing moment ... you will become more deeply relaxed ... more deeply comfortable ... so relaxed ... so deeply comfortable. ... In fact, it isn't even necessary to listen very closely to the things that I am saying, because your unconscious mind will be able to hear ... and understand ... everything ... that I say to you. Just allow your conscious mind ... to enjoy the pleasant state ... of complete relaxation ... that has come over you ... and let your unconscious mind take over. As these things I say begin to sink deeply into your unconscious mind ... you will soon begin experience all that I ask you to ... now ... begin to focus on your left hamstring ... become aware of the pain in your left hamstring ... recognize how intense ... and maybe ... uncomfortable it feels ... focus all your attention on it ... allow those feelings to be present in your mind and body. ... Now ... see it begin to heal ... feel a surge of warm healing energy flow from your core into that hamstring ... allow the energy to heal that hamstring ... notice a warmth beginning to build ... that warmth is your body healing itself ... new tissue is replacing the old and your body is healing ... each day ... picture more healing energy flowing into that left leg [pause]. That is good, your body is beginning to heal ... now ... getting stronger ... with each passing day ... day by day ... you will become healthier ... stronger ... than the day before. ... You may even notice the discomfort beginning to ... fade into the background ... each day ... your hamstring will get stronger ... heal ... and feel comfortable again ... feel the tissue getting stronger as it grows ... as new cells replace old ones ... the warmth is the circulation of blood removing the part that is not healthy ... away. [Awaken the athlete with suggestions for feeling greater comfort; the only sensory feeling needed is that which serves to protect from further injury.]

Summary

Hypnosis has been shown to be a useful technique in various other professions, including medicine, dentistry, and psychotherapy. Given further research, the potential uses of hypnosis to enhance performance seem limitless. We are at the frontier of its use in sports. In this chapter, successful hypnotic techniques to enhance athletic performance were provided to address many common problems confronting athletes. Its appropriateness seems natural, given the similarities between performing at a peak level and the hypnotic state. Unfortunately, within the field of sport psychology, hypnosis remains a virtually untapped tool for enhancing athletic performance. Although it has limitless potential in the field of sport medicine and sport psychology, it has not been employed on a systematic basis by researchers or clinicians (W. Morgan & Brown, 1983). This is surprising, given its well-documented efficacy in the management of pain (E. Hilgard & J. Hilgard, 1994) and in psychosomatic medicine in general (Burrows & Dennerstein, 1980; W. Morgan & Brown, 1983, p. 234). As more research is conducted on the effects of hypnosis on muscular and athletic performance, hypnosis might eventually become a technique of first choice to aid athletes in achieving the athletic performance.

Appendix
Societies and Journals

This list is intended to provide a flavor of the scientific-professional societies and journals in the field of hypnosis. It is by no means exhaustive.

Major International Scientific and Professional Societies of Hypnosis and Their Publications

Society for Clinical and Experimental Hypnosis (SCEH)
Massachusetts School of Professional Psychology
221 Rivermoor Street
Boston, MA 02132
USA
Phone: (617) 469-1981
Toll free number: (888) 664-6777, extension 203
Fax: (617) 469-1889
E-mail: sceh@mspp.edu
Web site: www.sceh.us or http://ijceh.educ.wsu.edu
Publications:
International Journal of Clinical and Experimental Hypnosis (IJCEH)
The major citation impact journal in the field
Focus: The quarterly bulletin of SCEH
Editor: Arreed Franz Barabasz, EdD, PhD, ABPP
Official Journal of the Society for Clinical and Experimental Hypnosis
Washington State University
P.O. Box 642136

Pullman, WA 99164-2136
Phone: (509) 335-8166
E-mail: ijceh@pullman.com
Web site: http://ijceh.educ.wsu.edu

International Society of Hypnosis (ISH)

Austin & Repatriation Medical Centre
Repatriation Campus, 300 Waterdale Road
Heidelberg Heights VIC 3081
Australia
Phone: +61 3 9496 4105
Fax: +61 3 9496 4107
E-mail: ish-central.office@medicine.unimelb.edu.au
Web site: http://www.ish.unimelb.edu.au/ish.html
Publication:
International Journal of Clinical and Experimental Hypnosis
Official journal of the International Society of Hypnosis

National Societies of Hypnosis and Their Publications

American Psychological Association Division 30—The Society of Psychological Hypnosis
750 First Street, NE
Washington, DC 20002-4242
USA
Phone: (800) 374-2721, (202) 336-5500, (202) 336-6013
TDD: (202) 336-6123
Fax: (202) 218-3599
Publications:
International Journal of Clinical and Experimental Hypnosis
Official journal of the society of psychological hypnosis
Psychological Hypnosis
The quarterly newsletter of the society

American Society of Clinical Hypnosis (ASCH)

140 N. Bloomingdale Rd.
Bloomingdale, IL 60108-1017
USA
Phone: (630) 980-4740
Fax: (630) 351-8490
E mail: info@asch.net

Web site: http://www.asch.net/
Publications:
American Journal of Clinical Hypnosis (AJCH)
(See information for the American Society of Clinical Hypnosis)
Editor: Thurman Mott, MD
Newsletter of the American Society of Clinical Hypnosis (quarterly)

Association Francaise d'Hypnotherapie

74, Rue Lamarck
75018 Paris
France
E-mail: dfayolet@noos.fr
Web site: www.afhyp.org

Associazionne medica Italiana per lo Studio dell Ipnosi (AMISI)

E-mail: amisi@mw.itline.it

Australian Society of Hypnosis (ASH)

Victoria Branch, ASH
P.O. Box 5114,
Alphington VIC 3078
Australia
Phone: +61 3 9458 5133
Fax: +61 3 9458 5399
E-mail: hypnosis@alphalink.com.au
Web site: www.ozhypnosis.com.au
Publications:
Australian Journal of Clinical and Experimental Hypnosis (AJCEH)
P.O. Box 592, Heidelberg Vic. 3084
Australia
Phone: +61 3 9496 4621
Fax: +61 3 9496 4564
E-mail: bevans@alphalink.com.au
Web site: www.ozhypnosis.com.au/journal.html

British Association of Medical Hypnosis (BAMH)

E-mail: secretary@bamh.org.uk
Web site: http://www.hypnoforum.com/bamh/

British Society of Clinical Hypnosis (BSCH)

Organising Secretary
125 Queensgate
Bridlington
East Yorkshire Y0167JQ
Phone: 01262 403103
E-mail: sec@bsch.org.uk
Website: http://www.bsch.org.uk/

British Society of Experimental and Clinical Hypnosis (BSECH)

Hollybank House, Lees Road
Mossley, Ashton-u-Lyne
OL5 OPL
UK
Phone/Fax: 01457 839363
E-mail: honsec@bsech.com
Web site: http://www.bsech.com
Publications:
Contemporary Hypnosis
Editor: John Gruzelier
Blackhorse Road
Letchworth
Herts SG6 1HN
Phone: 01462 672555
Fax: 01462 480947

British Society of Medical and Dental Hypnosis (BSMDH)

28 Dale Park Gardens
Cookridge, Leeds
LS16 7PT
UK
Phone/Fax: 07000 560309
E-mail: nat.office@bsmdh.org
Web site: http://www.bsmdh.org

Centro Ericksoniano de Mexico (CEM)

E-mail: erickmex@hipnosis.com.mx
Web site: www.hipnosis.com.mx

Centro Italiano Ipnosi Clinico-Sperimentale (CIICS)

E-mail: ciics@seleneweb.com

Centro Studi de Ipnosi Clinica e Psiocoterapia "H. Bernheim" (CSICHB)

Italy
E-mail: dirsan@villarosa.it

Danish Society of Clinical Hypnosis

Web site: www.hypnoterapi.com

Dansk Selskab for Klinisk Hypnose (DSKH)

Rosenborggade 12
1130 Copenhagen K
Denmark
E-mail: hypnosis@get2net.dk

Deutsche Gesellschaft für ärztliche Hypnose und Autogenes Training E.V. (DGAHAT)

Sekretariat
Postfach 1365
41463 Neuss
Germany
Web site: www.dgaehat.de

Deutsche Gesellschaft für zahnärztliche Hypnose (DGZH)

Esslinger Straße 40
70182 Stuttgart
Germany
E-mail: mail@dgzh.de
Web site: www.dgzh.de

Dutch Society of Hypnosis (Nvvh—Nederlandse vereniging voor hypnose)

Nvvh, Herenstraat 1-B
3512KA Utrecht
The Netherlands
E-mail: secretariaat@nvvh.com or info@nvvh.com
Web site: http://www.nvvh.com

Publication:
International Journal of Clinical and Experimental Hypnosis
Official journal of the society (see above for details)

European Society of Hypnosis (ESH)

DGZH E.V.
Esslinger Str. 40
70182 Stuttgart
Germany
E-mail: mail@esh-hypnosis.org
Web site: www.esh-hypnosis.org
Publications:
European Journal of Clinical Hypnosis (EJCH)
British Association of Medical Hypnosis
15 Connaught Square
London W2 2HG
United Kingdom
Phone: +44 0171- 706 7775
Fax: +44 0171- 262 1237
E-mail: editor@ejch.com
Web site: www.ejch.com

Flemish Society of Hypnosis (VHYP—Vlaams Wetenschappelijke Hypnose Vereniging)

Correspondentie-adres
Honingstraat 5 2220 Heist-op-den-Berg
Phone/Fax: 015 245183
E-mail: vhyp@village.uunet.be
Web site: http://www.vhyp.be
Universitair Centrum Sint-Jozef.
Leuvensesteenweg 517
3070 Kortenberg

German Society of Hypnosis (DGH)

Druffelsweg 3
48653 Coesfeld
Germany
E-mail: DGH-Geschaeftsstelle@t-online.de
Publications:

Experimentelle und Klinische Hypnose

Hypnosis Society of New Zealand (NZSH)

Wellington
New Zealand
Phone: 04 385 6998
E-mail: cmc89@telstra.net.nz
Web site: http://www.opotiki.com/hypnosisnz/

Hungarian Association of Hypnosis (HAH)

E-mail: mhesecretary@hotmail.com or GGACS@IZABELL.ELTE.HU

Indian Society of Clinical and Experimental Hypnosis (ISCEH)

E-mail: mrs_shovajana@im.eth.net

Israel Society of Hypnosis (IsSH)

E-mail: ewa@netvision.net.il
Web site: www.hypno.co.il or www.hypno.org.il

Japan Institute of Hypnosis (JIH)

E-mail: endo-s@nms.ac.jp

Japan Society of Hypnosis (JSH)

E-mail: jsh@human.tsukuba.ac.jp

MEG, Milton H. Erickson Gesellschaft für Klinische Hypnose E.V.

Waisenhausstraβe 55
80637 Munich
Germany
E-mail: monika-kohl@t-online.de
Web site: http://www.milton-erickson-gesellschaft.de or www.MEG-hypnose.de
Publications:
Hypnose und Kognition

Mexican Society of Hypnosis (MSH)

E-mail: ericksmh@iwm.com.mx

Norwegian Society for Clinical and Experimentel Hypnosis (NFKEH—Norsk Forening for Klinisk og Ekspeimentell Hypnose)

E-mail: guro@smerteklinikken.com
Web site: www.hypnoseforeningen.no

Österreichische Gesellschaft für Autogenes Training und Allgemeine Psychotherapie (OGATAP)

OGATAP Secretariat
Kaiserstr. 14/13
1070 Vienna
Austria
E-mail: office@oegatap.at

Sociedade Brasileira de Hipnose

Rua Jacirendi, 60
CEP 030066-000 Tatuapé
Sao Paulo
Brazil
E-mail: joelpriori@starmedia.com
Web site: www.sbhipnose.com.br

Società Italiana di Ipnosi (SII)

E-mail: ipnosii@tin.it
Web site: http://www.hypnosis.it

Societe Quebecoise d'Hypnose inc (SQH)

Bureau 485
1575 Boul. Henri-Bourassa ouest
Montréal, Québec H3M 3A9
Canada
E-mail: cpgb@qc.aira.com

South African Society of Clinical Hypnosis (SASCH)

E-mail: sasch@cis.co.za

Swedish Society of Clinical and Experimental Hypnosis (SSCEH)

SFKH's kansli, Flat 3, S-931 85 Skellefteå
E-mail: ssceh@telia.com
Web site: http://www.hypnos-se.org
Publication:
Hypnos

Swiss Medical Society of Hypnosis (SMSH)

E-mail: smsh@smile.ch
Web site: www.smsh.ch

Swiss Society for Clinical Hypnosis (SHypS)

E-mail: peter.hain@bluewin.ch
Web site: www.hypnos.ch

Tieteellinen Hypnoosi–Vetenskaplig Hypnose (TH-VH)

Kylätie 8 M 6
16300 Orimattila
Finland
E-mail: timo.heinonen@pp2.inet.fi
Web site: www.hypnoosi.net

Vlaamse Wetenschappelijke Hypnose Vereniging

517 3070 Kortenberg
Belgium
E-mail: vhyp@village.uunet.be
Web site: www.vhyp.be

References

Aaronson, B. (1968). Hypnosis, time rate perception and personality, *Journal of Schizophrenia, 2,* 11–41.

Achterberg, J., Simonton, O., & Simonton, S. (1976). *Stress, Psychological Factors and Cancer.* Fort Worth, TX: New Medicine Press.

Alexander, F. (1939). Psychological aspects of medicine. *Psychosomatic Medicine, 1,* 7–18.

Alexander, R. (1997). Comparison of eye movement desensitization and reprocessing and hypnosis. Unpublished doctoral dissertation, Washington State University.

Ambrose, G. (1963). Hypnotherapy for children. In J. M. Schneck (Ed.), *Hypnosis in Modern Medicine.* Springfield, IL: Charles C. Thomas.

Ament, P. (1955). Time distortion with hypnodontics. *Journal of American Society of Psychosomatic Medicine and Dentistry, 2,* 11–12.

Anbar, R. (2001). Automatic word processing: A new forum for hypnotic expression. *American Journal of Clinical Hypnosis, 44,* 27–36.

Anderson, K., Barabasz, A., Barabasz, M., & Warner, D. (2000). The effects of Barabasz' INAP alert hypnosis on QEEG in children with ADHD. *Child Study Journal, 30*(1), 51–62.

Appel, P. (1992). The use of hypnosis in physical medicine and rehabilitation. *Psychiatric Medicine, 10,* 133–148.

Aston-Jones, G., Rajkowski, R., & Cohen, J. (1999). Role of locus coeruleus in attention and behavioral flexibility. *Biological Psychiatry, 46,* 1309–1320.

August, R. V. (1961). *Hypnosis in Obstetrics.* New York: McGraw-Hill.

Azin, N., & Nunn, R. (1978). *Habit Control in a Day.* New York: Simon & Schuster.

Baer, L. (1980). Effect of a time slowing suggestion on performance accuracy on a perceptual motor task. *Perceptual and Motor Skills, 51,* 167–176.

Baker, E. (1990). Hypnoanalysis for structural pathology: Impairments of self-representation and capacity for object involvement. In M. L. Fass & D. Brown (Eds.), *Creative Mastery in Hypnosis and Hypnoanalysis: A Festschrift for Erika Fromm* (pp. 279–286). Hillsdale, NJ: Erlbaum.

Bailey, C. (1991). *The New Fit or Fat.* New York: Houghton-Mifflin.

Banerjee, S., Srivastav, A., & Palan, B. (1993). Hypnosis and self-hypnosis in the management of nocturnal enuresis: A comparative study with Imipramine therapy. *American Journal of Clinical Hypnosis, 36,* 113–119.

Barabasz, A. (1973). Group desensitization of test anxiety in elementary school. *Journal of Psychology, 83,* 295–301.

Barabasz, A. (1977). *New Techniques in Behavior Therapy and Hypnosis.* South Orange, NJ: Power Publishers.

Barabasz, A. (1979). Isolation, EEG alpha and hypnotizability in Antarctica. In G. Burrows (Eds.), *Hypnosis 1979* (pp. 3–18). Amsterdam: Elsevier/North Holland Biomedica Press.

451

Barabasz, A. (1980a). EEG alpha, skin conductance and hypnotizability in Antarctica. *International Journal of Clinical and Experimental Hypnosis, 28*, 63–74.

Barabasz, A. (1980b). Effects of hypnosis and perceptual deprivation on vigilance in a simulated radar target detection task. *Perceptual and Motor Skills, 50*, 19–24.

Barabasz, A. (1980c). Enhancement of hypnotic susceptibility following perceptual deprivation: Pain tolerance, electrodermal and EEG correlates. In M. Pajntar, E. Roskar, & M. Lavric (Eds.), *Hypnosis in Psychotherapy and Psychosomatic Medicine* (pp. 13–18). Ljubljana, Yugoslavia: University Press (Univerzitetna Tiskarna).

Barabasz, A. (1982). Restricted environmental stimulation and the enhancement of hypnotizability: Pain, EEG alpha, skin conductance and temperature responses. *International Journal of Clinical and Experimental Hypnosis, 30*(2), 147–166.

Barabasz, A. (1984a). Antarctic isolation and imaginative involvement: Preliminary findings. *International Journal of Clinical and Experimental Hypnosis, 32*, 296–300.

Barabasz, A. (1984b, April 7). *Hypnosis in the treatment of HPV.* Paper presented at Massachusetts General Hospital, Boston.

Barabasz, A. (1985, March). Enchantment of military pilot reliability by hypnosis and psychophysiological monitoring: In-flight and simulator data. *Aviation, Space, and Environment Medicine, 56*, 248–250.

Barabasz, A. (1990a). Effects of isolation on states of consciousness. In A. Harrison, Y. Clearwater, & C. McKay (Eds.), *The Human Experience in Antarctica: Applications to Life in Space* (pp. 201–208). New York: Springer-Verlag.

Barabasz, A. (1990b). Eingeschränke stimulation durch die Umwelt ruft spontane Hypnose fur die Schmerzkontrolle beim cold pressor test hervor *Experimentelle und Klinische Hypnose,* 4(Heft 2), 95–105. (Nominated for the Donald Hebb award for the best research paper 1990-1992, International REST Investigators Society)

Barabasz, A. (1990c). Flotation restricted environmental stimulation elicits spontaneous hypnosis. In R. Van Dyck, A. J. Spinhoven, W. Vander Does, Y. R. Van Rood, & W. Demoor (Eds.), *Hypnosis: Current Theory, Research and Practice.* Amsterdam: Free University Press. (Based on an invited address to the European Congress of Hypnosis and Psychosomatic Medicine, Oxford University, Oxford, England)

Barabasz, A. (1993). Neo-dissociation accounts for pain relief and hypnotic susceptibility findings: Flotation REST elicits hypnosis. In A. Barabasz & M. Barabasz (Eds.), *Clinical and Experimental Restricted Environmental Stimulation: New Developments and Perspectives* (pp. 41–52). New York: Springer-Verlag.

Barabasz, A. (1994). Schnell neuronale Aktivierung. Reduzierte Stimulation und psychophysiologische Aufziechnungen bei der Behandlung eines phobischen Piloten. *Experimentelle und Klinische Hypnose, 10*, 167–176.

Barabasz, A. (1995). Enhancement of military reliability by hypnosis and psychophysiological monitoring: In-flight and simulator data. *Aviation, Space, and Environmental Medicine, 66*, 248–250.

Barabasz, A. (2000). EEG markers of alert hypnosis: The induction makes a difference. *Sleep and Hypnosis, 2*(4), 164–169.

Barabasz, A. (2001a, March). *Arrests and Convictions from Hypnotically Constructed Memory: Corroboration and Confabulation.* Paper presented at the annual meeting of the American Society of Clinical Hypnosis, Reno, Nevada.

Barabasz, A. (2001b, November 7-11). *Presidential Address: The State of Hypnosis.* Paper presented at the 52nd annual scientific meeting of the Society for Clinical and Experimental Hypnosis, San Antonio, Texas.

Barabasz, A. (2003a, August 7-10). Presidential Address: Hypnosis for real-induction can make the difference. Paper presented at 111th annual convention of the American Psychological Association, Toronto, Canada.

Barabasz, A. (2003b, September 10-16). The reality of trance. Keynote address presented at the annual conference of the Australian Society of Hypnosis, Gold Coast Australia.

Barabasz, A. (2004). Theories of hypnosis: Issues, convergence and research breakthroughs. *Hypnose-konzept Fragen und Durchbruche in der Forchung, Hypnose* (Hykog), 21, 1–2.

Barabasz, A. (in press). A verbal non-verbal dissociation induction for resistant subjects. *International Journal of Clinical and Experimental Hypnosis.*

Barabasz, A. (in press). Effects of tailored, symptom neutralizing hypnosis on irritable bowel syndrome. *International Journal of Clinical and Experimental Hypnosis.*

Barabasz, A., Baer, L., Sheehan, D., & Barabasz, M. (1986). A three year clinical follow-up of hypnosis and restricted environmental stimulation therapy for smoking. *International Journal of Clinical and Experimental Hypnosis, 34,* 169–181.

Barabasz, A., & Barabasz, M. (1981). Effects of rational-emotive therapy on psychophysiological and reported measures of test anxiety arousal. *Journal of Clinical Psychology, 37*(3), 511–514.

Barabasz, A., & Barabasz, M. (1989). Effects of restricted environmental stimulation: Enhancement of hypnotizability for experimental and chronic pain control. *International Journal of Clinical and Experimental Hypnosis, 37*(3), 217–231.

Barabasz, A., & Barabasz, M. (1992). Research design considerations. In E. Fromm & M. Nash (Eds.), *Contemporary Hypnosis Research* (pp. 173–200). New York: Guilford.

Barabasz, A., & Barabasz, M. (1994a, October). EEG responses to a reading comprehension task during active alert hypnosis and waking states. Paper presented at the 45th annual scientific meeting of the Society for Clinical and Experimental Hypnosis, San Francisco, California.

Barabasz, A., & Barabasz, M. (1994b, August 12–16). Effects of focused attention on EEG topography during a reading task. Symposium: Behavioral Medicine, Psychophysiology and Hypnosis, presented at the 102nd annual convention of the American Psychological Association (APA Division 30), Los Angeles, California.

Barabasz, A., & Barabasz, M. (1995). Attention deficit hyperactivity disorder: Neurological basis and treatment alternatives. *Journal of Neurotherapy, 1,* 1–10.

Barabasz, A., & Barabasz, M. (1996). Neurotherapy and alert hypnosis in the treatment of attention deficit hyperactivity disorder. In S. Lynn, I. Kirsch, & J. Rhue (Eds.), *Clinical Hypnosis Casebook* (pp. 271–292). Washington, D.C.: American Psychological Association.

Barabasz, A., & Barabasz, M. (2000). Treating AD/HD with hypnosis and neurotherapy. *Child Study Journal, 30*(1), 25–32.

Barabasz, A., & Barabasz, M. (2002, August 22–25). Hypnotic realities: Trance and suggestion. Invited address presented at the 110th annual convention of the American Psychological Association, Chicago.

Barabasz, A., Barabasz, M., & Bauman, J. (1993). Restricted environmental stimulation technique improves human performance: Rifle marksmanship. *Perceptual and Motor Skills, 76,* 867–873.

Barabasz, A., Barabasz, M., Higley, L., & Christensen, C. (in press). Hypnosis in the treatment of genital human papillomavirus in females. *International Journal of Clinical and Experimental Hypnosis.*

Barabasz, A., Barabasz, M., Jensen, S., Calvin, S., Trevison, M., & Warner, D. (1999). Cortical event related potentials show the structure of hypnotic suggestions is crucial. *International Journal of Clinical and Experimental Hypnosis, 47*(1), 5–22.

Barabasz, A., Barabasz, M., Lin-Roark, I., Roark, J., Sanchez, O., & Christensen, C. (2003, November 12–16). Age regression produced focal point dependence: Experience makes a difference. Presented at 54th annual scientific program of the Society for Clinical and Experimental Hypnosis, Chicago.

Barabasz, A. & Christensen, C. (in press). Age regression: Tailored vs. scripted inductions. *American Journal of Clinical Hypnosis.*

Barabasz, A., Christensen, C., & Barabasz, M. (2004, July 30). Clinician experience and hypnotic depth: Effects on age regression phenomena. Paper presented at the 112th annual convention of the American Psychological Association, Honolulu, Hawaii.

Barabasz, A., Crawford, H., & Barabasz, M. (1993, October). EEG topographic map differences in attention deficit disordered and normal children: Moderating effects from focused active alert instructions during reading, math, and listening tasks. Paper presented at the 33rd annual meeting of the Society for Psychophysiological Research, Rottach-Egern, Germany.

Barabasz, A., & Lonsdale, C. (1983). Effects of hypnosis on P300 olfactory evoked potential amplitudes. *Journal of Abnormal Psychology, 92,* 520–525.

Barabasz, A., & Lonsdale, C. (1985). EEG evoked potentials, hypnotic and transient olfactory stimulation in high and low susceptibility subjects. In *Modern Trends in Hypnosis* (pp. 138–139). New York: Plenum.

Barabasz, A., & McGeorge, C. (1978). Biofeedback, meditated biofeedback and hypnosis in peripheral vasodilation training. *American Journal of Clinical Hypnosis, 21,* 23–37.

Barabasz, A., & Wright, G. (1975). Treatment of collagen vascular disease by hypnotic imagery. *Hypnosis Quarterly, 19,* 15–18.

Barabasz, M. (1987). Trichotillomania: A new treatment. *International Journal of Clinical and Experimental Hypnosis, 35*(3), 146–154.

Barabasz, M. (1996). Hypnosis, hypnotizability and eating disorders. Presented at the 47th annual workshops and scientific program of the Society for Clinical and Experimental Hypnosis, Tampa.

Barabasz, M., & Barabasz, A. (1996). Attention-deficit disorder: Diagnosis, etiology and treatment [Special issue]. *Child Study Journal, 26*(1), 1–37.

Barabasz, M., Barabasz, A., Darakjy-Jaeger, J., & Warner, D. (2001, November 7-11). Dry flotation restricted environment stimulation (REST) enhances hypnotizability: Pain, EEG and skin conductance. Presented at the 52nd annual scientific program of the Society for Clinical and Experimental Hypnosis, San Antonio, Texas.

Barabasz, M., Barabasz, A., & Mullin, C. (1983). Effects of brief Antarctic isolation on absorption and hypnotic susceptibility: Preliminary results and recommendations. *International Journal of Clinical and Experimental Hypnosis, 31,* 235–238.

Barabasz, M., & Spiegel, D. (1989). Hypnotizability and weight loss in obese subjects. *International Journal of Eating Disorders, 8,* 335–341.

Barber, J. (1977). Rapid induction analgesia: A clinical report. *American Journal of Clinical Hypnosis, 19,* 138–147.

Barber, J. (1996). Hypnotic analgesia: Clinical considerations. In J. Barber (Ed.), *Hypnosis and Suggestion in the Treatment of Pain* (pp. 85–118). New York: W. W. Norton.

Barber, J., & Mayer, D. (1977). Evaluation of the efficacy and neural mechanism of a hypnotic analgesia procedure in experimental and clinical dental pain. *Pain, 4,* 41–48.

Barber, T. (1966). The effects of hypnosis and suggestion on strength and endurance: A critical review of research studies. *British Journal of Social and Clinical Psychology, 5,* 42–50.

Barber, T. (1969). *Hypnosis: A Scientific Approach.* New York: Van Nostrand Reinhold.

Barber, T. (1970). *LSD, Marijuana, Yoga, and Hypnosis.* Chicago: Aldine.

Barber, T., & Calverley, D. (1964). Toward a theory of "hypnotic" behavior: Enhancement of strength and endurance. *Canadian Journal of Psychology, 28,* 156–157.

Barber, T., & Glass, L. (1962). Significant factors in hypnotic behavior. *Journal of Abnormal and Social Psychology, 64,* 222–228.

Barnier, A., & McConkey, K. (2003). Hypnosis, human nature, and complexity: Integrating neuroscience approaches into hypnosis research. *International Journal of Clinical and Experimental Hypnosis, 51*(3), 282–308.

Barrett, D. (1990). Deep trance subjects: A schema of two distinct subgroups. In R. G. Kunzendorf (Ed.), *Mental Iimagery* (pp. 101–112). New York: Plenum.

Bauman, F. (1970). Hypnosis and the adolescent drug abuser. *American Journal of Clinical Hypnosis, 13*(1), 17–21.

Beahrs, J. (1986). *Limits of Scientific Psychiatry: Role of Uncertainty in Mental Health.* New York: Brunner.

Belsky, J., & Khanna, P. (1994). The effects of self-hypnosis for children with cystic fibrosis: A pilot study. *American Journal of Clinical Hypnosis, 36,* 282–292.

Bennett, H. (1993). Preparing for surgery and medical procedures. In D. Goleman & J. Gurin (Eds.), *Mind-Body Medicine* (pp. 401–427). Yonkers, NY: Consumer Reports Books.

Bernhiem, H. (1964). *Hypnosis and Suggestion in Psychotherapy.* New York: University Books. (Original work published 1886 under the title *Suggestive Therapeutics*)

Blanck, G., & Blanck, R. (1974). *Ego Psychology: Theory and Practice.* New York: Columbia University Press.

Bonello, F., Doberneck, R., & Papermaster, A. (1960). Hypnosis in surgery: The post-gastrectomy dumping syndrome. *American Journal of Clinical Hypnosis, 2,* 215–219.

Bowers, K. (1976). *Hypnosis for the Seriously Curious.* Monterey, CA: Brooks/Cole.

Bowers, K. (1992). Imagination and dissociation in hypnotic responding. *International Journal of Clinical and Experimental Hypnosis, 40,* 253–275.

Bowers, K., & Van der Meulen, S. (1972, Fall). A comparison of psychological and chemical techniques in the control of pain. Paper presented at the Society for Clinical and Experimental Hypnosis.

Brady, J. P., Luborsky, C., & Cron, D. (1974). Blood pressure reduction in patients with essential hypertension through metronome-conditioned relaxation: A preliminary report. *Behavior Therapy, 5,* 203–209.

Braid, J. (1843). *The Power of the Mind over the Body.* London: Churchill

Braid, J. (1960). *Braid on Hypnotism: The Beginnings of Modern Hypnosis* (Rev. ed. by A. E. Waite). New York: Julian Press.

Braid, J. (1970). The physiology of fascination and the critics criticized. In M. M. Tinterow (Ed.), *Foundations of Hypnosis: From Mesmer to Freud* (pp. 365–389). Springfield, IL: Charles C. Thomas.

Bramwell, J. (1956). *Hypnotism: Its History, Practice and Theory.* New York: Institute for Research in Hypnosis and Julian Press. (Original work published in 1903 by Grant Richards, England)

Brann, L., & Guzvica, S. (1987). Comparison of hypnosis with conventional relaxation for antenatal and intrapartum use. *Journal of the Royal College of General Practitioners, 37,* 437–440.

Breuer, J., & Freud, S. (1957). *Studies on Hysteria.* New York: Basic Books.

Brown, D., & Fromm, E. (1987). *Hypnosis and Behavioral Medicine.* Hillside, NJ: Erlbaum.

Bucknell, R. (1993). Reinterpreting the jhanas. *Journal of International Association of Buddhist Studies, 16*(2), 375–409.

Burgess, T. (1952). Hypnosis in dentistry. In L. LeCron (Ed.), *Experimental Hypnosis* (pp. 322–351). New York: Macmillan.

Burrows, G., & Dennerstein, L. (Eds.). (1980). *Handbook of Hypnosis and Psychosomatic Medicine.* Amsterdam: Elsevier/North Holland Biomedical Press.

Calvin, S. (2000, October 25-29). ERP markers of Barabasz's instant alert hypnosis: Inductions and instructions make a difference. Paper presented at the 51st annual scientific meeting of the Society for Clinical and Experimental Hypnosis, Seattle, Washington.

Campbell, P. (2004). Can anecdotes add to an understanding of hypnosis? *International Journal of Clinical and Experimental Hypnosis, 52,* 218–231.

Cardena. E. (in press). The phenomenology of quiescent and physically active deep hypnosis. *International Journal of Clinical and Experimental Hypnosis.*

Chang, J. (1977). *The Tao of Lore.* New York: Penguin.

Charcot, J. (1888). Essai d'une distinction nosographique des divers états compris sous le nom d' hypnotisme. In A. Binet & C. Fere (Eds.), *Animal Magnetism* (pp. 154–163). New York: D. Appleton. (Original work published *Comptes Rendus de l' Academic des Sciences,* 1882)

Charcot, J. (1889). *Lectures on Diseases of the Nervous System.* London: New Sydenham Society.

Chaves, J. (1986). Hypnosis in the management of phantom limb pain. In E. Dowd & J. Healy (Eds.), *Case Studies in Hypnotherapy* (pp. 198–209). New York: Guilford.

Chaves, J. (1989). Hypnotic control of clinical pain. In N. P. Spanos & J. F. Chaves (Eds.), *Hypnosis: The Cognitive-Behavioral Perspective.* Buffalo, NY: Prometheus Books.

Chaves, J. (1994). Recent advances in the application of hypnosis to pain management. *American Journal of Clinical Hypnosis, 37,* 117–129.

Chaves, J., & Dworkin, S. (1997). Hypnotic control of pain: Historical perspectives and future prospects. *International Journal of Clinical and Experimental Hypnosis, 45,* 356–376.

Cheek, D. (1962). Ideomotor questioning for investigation of subconscious "pain" and target organ vulnerability. *American Journal of Clinical Hypnosis, 5,* 30–41.

Cheek, D. (1964). Further evidence of persistence of hearing under chemo-anesthesia: A detailed case report. *American Journal of Clinical Hypnosis, 7,* 55–59.

Cheek, D. B., & LeCron, L. M. (1968). *Clinical Hypnotherapy.* New York: Grune & Stratton.

Chia, M. (1983). *Awaken Healing Energy through the Tao.* Santa Fe, NM: Aurora.

Christensen, C. (2004). Preferences for descriptors of hypnosis. Presented at the International Congress of Hypnosis, Singapore, October 17–23.

Clarke, J. (1996). Teaching hypnosis in U.S. and Canadian dental schools. Presented at the Annual Meeting of the American Society of Clinical Hypnosis, 39(2).

Clarke, J. (1997). *The role of Hypnosis in Treating Bruxism* (Hypnosis International Monographs, 3: Hypnosis in Dentistry). Munich, Germany: Per-Olof Wikstrom.

Clarke, J., & Persichetti, S. (1988). Hypnosis and concurrent denture construction for a patient with a hyper-sensitive gag reflex. *American Journal of Clinical Hypnosis, 30*(4), 485–488.

Clarke, J., & Reynolds, P. (1991). Suggestive hypnotherapy for nocturnal bruxism: A pilot study. *American Journal of Clinical Hypnosis, 33*(4), 248–253.

Coe, W. (1992). Hypnosis: Wherefore art thou? *International Journal of Clinical and Experimental Hypnosis, 4,* 219–237.

Cohn, P. (1991). An exploratory study on peak performance in golf. *Sport Psychologist, 54,* 1–14.

Coleman, J. C., Butcher, J. N., & Carson, R. C. (1980). *Abnormal psychology and modern life* (6th ed.). New York: Scott, Foresman.

Colgan, S., Faragher, E., & Whorwell, P. (1988). Controlled trial of hypnotherapy in relapse prevention of duodenal ulceration. *Lancet, 11,* 1299–1300.

Collison, D. R. (1975). Which asthmatic patients should be treated by hypnotherapy? *Medical Journal of Australia, 1,* 776–781.

Collison, D. R. (1978). Hypnotherapy in asthmatic patients and the importance of trance depth. In F. H. Frankel & H. S. Zamansky (Eds.), *Hypnosis at its bicentennial.* New York: Plenum Press.

Conn, J. (1959). Cultural and clinical aspects of suggestion. *International Journal of Clinical and Experimental Hypnosis, 7,* 175–185.

Cooke, C. E., & Van Vogt, A. E. (1956). *The Hypnotism Handbook.* Alhambra, CA: Borden. (Reprinted in American Society of Clinical Hypnosis: *A Syllabus on Hypnosis and a Handbook of Therapeutic Suggestions.* 1983, pp. 44–45.).

Cooper, K. (1970). *The New Aerobics.* New York: M. Evans.

Cooper, L., & Erickson, M. (1959). *Time Distortion in Hypnosis.* Baltimore: Williams & Wilkins.

Cooper, L., & London, P. (1971). The development of hypnotic susceptibility: A longitudinal (convergence) study. *Child Development, 42,* 487–503.

Copeland, D. (1986). The application of object relations theory to the hypnotherapy of developmental arrests: The borderline patient. *International Journal of Clinical and Experimental Hypnosis, 34,* 157–168.

Cornelius, A. (2002a). Intervention techniques in sport psychology. In J. M. Silva & D. E. Stevens (Eds.), *Psychological Foundations of Sport* (pp. 197–223). Boston: Allyn & Bacon.

Cornelius, A. (2002b). Psychological interventions for the injured athlete. In J. M. Silva & D. E. Stevens (Eds.), *Psychological Foundations of Sport* (pp. 224–243). Boston: Allyn & Bacon.

Cotecha, B., & Shneerson, J. (2003). Cheapened options of snoring and sleep apnoea. *Journal of the Royal Society of Medicine, 96,* 343–344.

Coue, E. (1923). *How to Practice Suggestion and Autosuggestion.* New York: American Library Service.

Cox, J. L., Murray, D., & Chapman, G. (1993). A controlled study of the onset, duration and prevalence of postnatal major depressive disorder. *British Journal of Psychiatry, 163,* 27–31.

Cox, R. (2002). *Sport Psychology: Concepts and Applications* (5th ed.). New York, W. C. Brown/McGraw-Hill.

Craft, T. (2003). The use of direct suggestion in the successful treatment of a case of snoring. *Contemporary Hypnosis, 20*(2), 98–101.

Crasilneck, H. (1995). The use of the Crasilneck bombardment technique in problems of intractable organic pain. *American Journal of Clinical Hypnosis, 37,* 255–266.

Crasilneck, H., & Fogelman, M. (1957). The effects of hypnosis on blood coagulation. *International Journal of Clinical and Experimental Hypnosis, 5,* 132–137.

Crasilneck, H., & Hall, J. (1985). *Clinical Hypnosis: Principals and Applications.* Orlando, FL: Grune and Stratton.

Crawford, H. (1990). Cognitive and psychophysiological correlates of hypnotic responsiveness and hypnosis. In M. L. Mass & D. Brown (Eds.), *Creative Mastery in Hypnosis and Hypnoanalysis: A Festschrift for Erika Fromm* (pp. 47–54). Hillsdale, NJ: Erlbaum.

Crawford, H. (1994). Brain dynamics and hypnosis: Attentional and disattentional processes. *International Journal of Clinical and Experimental Hypnosis, 42,* 204–232.

Crawford, H. (2001). Neuropsychophysiology of hypnosis: Towards understanding of how hypnotic interventions work. In G. D. Burrows, R. O. Stanley, & P. B. Bloom, (Eds.), *International handbook of clinical hypnosis* (pp. 61–84). New York: Wiley.

Crawford, H., Gur, R., Skolnick, B., Gur, R., & Benson, D. (1993). Effects of hypnosis on regional cerebral blood flow during ischemic pain with and without suggested hypnotic analgesia. *International Journal of Psychophysiology, 15,* 181–195.

Crawford, H., Knebel, T., Kaplan, L., Vendemia, J., Xie, M., Jamison, S., & Pribram, K. (1998). Hypnotic analgesia: 1. Somatosensory event-related potential changes to noxious stimuli and 2. Transfer learning to reduce chronic low back pain. *International Journal of Clinical and Experimental Hypnosis, 46*, 92–132.

Crawford, H., McClain-Furmanski, D., Castagnoli, N., & Castagnoli, K. (2002). Enhancement of auditory sensory gating and stimulus-bound gamma band (40 Hz) oscillations in heavy tobacco smokers. *Neuroscience Letters, 317*, 151–155.

Csikszentmihalyi, M. (1990). *Flow: The Psychology of Optimal Experience.* New York: Harper and Row.

Dane, J. (1996). Hypnosis for pain and neuromuscular rehabilitation with multiple sclerosis: Case summary, literature review, and analysis of outcomes. *International Journal of Clinical and Experimental Hypnosis, 44*, 208–231.

David, D., & Brown, R. J. (2002). Suggestibility and negative priming: Two replication studies. *International Journal of Clinical and Experimental Hypnosis, 50*(30), 215–228.

Davidson, J. (1962). Assessment of the value of hypnosis in pregnancy and labor. *British Medical Journal, 2*, 951–953.

Davis, L., & Husband, R. (1931). A study of hypnotic susceptibility in relation to personality traits. *Journal of Abnormal and Social Psychology, 26*, 175–182.

Deabler, H., Fidel, D., & Dillenkoffer, M. (1973). The use of relaxation and hypnosis in lowering high blood pressure. *American Journal of Clinical Hypnosis, 16*, 73–83.

Derlega, V. J., & Janda, L. H. (1978). *Personal Adjustment: The Psychology of Everyday Life.* Morristown, NJ: General Learning Press.

De Pascalis, V., Magurano, M., & Bellusci, A. (1999). Pain perception, somatosensory event-related potentials and skin conductance responses to painful stimuli in high, mid, and low hypnotizable subjects: Effects of differential pain reduction strategies. *Pain, 83*, 499–508.

De Pascalis, V., Magurano, M., Bellusci, A., & Chen, A. (2001). Somatosensory event-related potential and autonomic activity to varying pain reduction cognitive strategies in hypnosis. *Clinical Neurophysiology, 112*, 1475–1485.

Dick-Read, G. (1968). *Childbirth without Fear.* New York: Heineman.

Dikle, W., & Olness, K. (1980). Self-hypnosis, biofeedback, and voluntary peripheral temperature control in children. *Pediatrics, 66*, 335–340.

Dinges, D., Whitehouse, W., Orne, E., Bloom, P., Karlin, M., Bauer, N., Gillen, K., Shapiro, B., Ohene, F., Dampier, C., & Orne, M. (1997). Self hypnosis training as an adjunctive treatment in the management of pain associated with sickle cell disease, *International Journal of Clinical and Experimental Hypnosis, 45*, 417–432.

Dixon, M., & Laurence, J. (1992). Two hundred years of hypnosis research: Questions resolved? Questions unanswered! In E. Fromm & M. Nash (Eds.), *Contemporary Hypnosis Research* (pp. 34–66). New York: Guilford.

Doberneck, R., Griffen, W., Papermaster, A., Bonello, F., & Wangensteen, O. (1959). Hypnosis as an adjunct to surgical therapy. *Surgery, 46*, 299–304.

Dorcus, R., & Goodwin, P. (1955). The treatment of patients with the dumping syndrome by hypnosis. *Journal of Clinical and Experimental Hypnosis, 3*, 200–202.

du Maurier, G. (1941). *Trilby.* New York: E. P. Dutton.

Dunbar, F. (1947). *Mind and Body: Psychosomatic Medicine.* New York: Random House.

Eastwood, J., Gaskovski, P., & Bowers, K. (1998). The folly of effort: Ironic effects in the mental control of pain. *International Journal of Clinical and Experimental Hypnosis, 46*, 77–91.

Edel, J. W. (1959). Nosebleed controlled by hypnosis. *American Journal of Clinical Hypnosis, 2*, 89–91.

Edwards, S., & van der Spuy, H. (1985). Hypnotherapy as a treatment for enuresis. *Journal of Child Clinical Psychology, Psychiatry and Allied Health Disciplines, 26*, 161–170.

Eichman, W., & Umstead, J. (1971). Profile of mood states. In *Eighth Mental Measurements Yearbook*, Lincoln, Nebraska, Buros Institute of Mental Measurement. (pp. 1015–1019).

Elkins, G., & Hasanrajab, M. (2004). Clinical hypnosis for smoking cessation: Preliminary results of a three session intervention. *International Journal of Clinical and Experimental Hypnosis, 52*(1), 73–81.

Elliotson, J. (1843). *Numerous Cases of Surgical Operations without Pain in the Mesmeric State.* Philadelphia: Lea & Blanchard.

Ellis, A., & Russell, G. (1977). *Handbook of Rational-Emotive Therapy.* New York: Springer.

Emmerson, G. (2003). *Ego State Therapy*. Williston, VT: Crown.

Erickson, M. (1938a). A study of clinical and experimental findings on hypnotic deafness: I. Clinical experimentation and findings. *Journal of Genetic Psychology, 19,* 127–150.

Erickson, M. (1938b). A study of clinical and experimental findings on hypnotic deafness: II. Experimental findings with a conditioned response technique. *Journal of Genetic Psychology, 19,* 151–167.

Erickson, M. (1952). Deep hypnosis and its induction. In L. M. LeCron (Ed.), *Experimental Hypnosis* (pp. 70–112). New York: Macmillan.

Erickson, M. (1958). Naturalistic techniques of hypnosis. *American Journal of Clinical Hypnosis, 1,* 3–8.

Erickson, M. (1965). Hypnosis and examination panics. *American Journal of Clinical Hypnosis, 7,* 356–357. (See also *American Journal of Clinical Hypnosis* (1973) 15, p. 106).

Erickson, M. (1967). An introduction to the study and application of hypnosis for pain control. In J. Lassner (Ed.), *Hypnosis and Psychosomatic Medicine: Proceedings of the International Congress of Hypnosis and Psychosomatic Medicine.* New York: Springer-Verlag.

Erickson, M. (1973). Hypnosis and examination panics. *American Journal of Clinical Hypnosis, 7,* 356–357.

Erickson, M. H., Hershman, S., & Secter, I. I. (1961). *The Practical Application of Medical and Dental Hypnosis.* New York: Julian Press.

Erickson, M., Rossi, E., & Rossi, S. (1976). *Hypnotic Realities: The Induction of Clinical Hypnosis and Forms of Indirect Suggestion.* New York: Irvington.

Esdaile, J. (1957). *Hypnosis in Medicine and Surgery.* New York: Institute for Research in Hypnosis and Julian Press. (Original copyright Mesmerism in India, 1850)

Evans, F. (1979). Hypnosis and sleep: Techniques for exploring cognitive activity during sleep. In E. Fromm & R. E. Shor (Eds.), *Hypnosis: Developments in Research and New Perspectives* (2nd ed., pp. 139–183). New York: Aldine.

Evans, F. (1989). Hypnosis and chronic pain: Two contrasting case studies. *Clinical Journal of Pain, 5,* 169–176.

Ewin, D. M. (1974). Condyloma acuminatum: Successful treatment of four cases by hypnosis. *American Journal of Clinical Hypnosis, 17,* 73–78.

Ewin, D. (1983). Emergency room hypnosis for the burned patient. *American Journal of Clinical Hypnosis, 26,* 5–8.

Ewin, D. (1986a). The effect of hypnosis and mental set on major surgery and burns. *Psychiatric Annals, 16,* 115–118.

Ewin, D. (1986b). Emergency room hypnosis for the burned patient. *American Journal of Clinical Hypnosis, 29,* 7–21.

Ewin, D. (1990). Hypnotic technique for recall of sounds heard under general anaesthesia. In B. Benno, W. Fitch, & K. Millar (Eds.), *Memory and Awareness in Anaesthesia.* Amsterdam: Swets & Zeitlinger.

Ewin, D. (1992). Rapid eye-roll induction. In D. C. Hammond (Ed.), *Hypnotic Induction and Suggestion* (p. 49). Bloomingdale, IL: American Society of Clinical Hypnosis.

Ewin, D. (2003, November 12-16). *Using Ideomotor Signals in Hypnoanalysis.* Presented at the 54th annual workshops and scientific program of the Society of Experimental and Clinical Hypnosis, Chicago.

Ewin, D. (2004). Single visit hypnotic cure of stentorian snoring: A brief communication. *International Journal of Clinical and Experimental Hypnosis, 4,* (in press).

Faria, J. C. (1819). *De la Cause du Sommeil Lucide: ou Etude de la Nature de l'Homme* [Of the Cause of Lucid Sleep: Or the Study of the Nature of Man]. Paris: Mme. Horiac.

Federn, P. (1952). *Ego psychology and the psychoses.* New York: Basic Books.

Ferenczi, S. (1926). *Further Contributions to the Theory and Technique of Psychoanalysis.* London: Hogarth.

Feussner, G. (1998). Diversion, trafficking, and abuse of methylpheidate. National Institutes of Health Concensus Development. Conference on Diagnosis and Treatment of ADHD, Bethesda, Maryland, March.

Finer, B. (1982). Treatment in an interdisciplinary pain clinic. In J. Barber & C. Adrian (Eds.), *Psychological Approaches to the Management of Pain* (pp. 186–204). New York: Brunner.

Finer, B. & Nylen, B. (1961). Cardiac arrest in the treatment of burns, and report on hypnosis as a substitute for anesthesia. *Plastic Reconstructive Surgery, 27,* 49–55.

Finkelstein, S. (2003). Rapid hypnotic inductions and therapeutic suggestions in the dental setting. *International Journal of Clinical and Experimental Hypnosis, 51*(1), 77–85.

Frankl, F. (1976). *Hypnosis: Trance as a Coping Mechanism.* New York: Plenum.

Frankl, F., & Orne, M. (1976). Hypnotizability and phobic behavior. *Archives of General Psychiatry, 33,* 1259–1261.

Frankl, V. (1963). *Man's Search for Meaning.* New York: Simon & Schuster.

Franklin, B., de Bory, G., Lavoisier, A., Bailly, J., Majault, Sallin, D'Arcet, J., Guillotin, J., & Leroy, J. (1784). *Rapport des Commissaires Charges par le Roy de l'Examen du Magnetisme Animal* Paris: Bibliothèque Royale.

Fredericks, L. (2001). *The Use of Hypnosis in Anesthesiology.* Springfield, IL: Charles C. Thomas.

Freeman, R., Barabasz, A., Barabasz, M., & Warner, D. (2000). Hypnosis and distraction differ in their effects on cold pressor pain. *American Journal of Clinical Hypnosis, 43*(2), 137–148.

French, T., & Alexander, F. (1941). *Psychogenic Factors in Bronchial Asthma. Psychosomatic Medicine* [Monograph 4]. Washington, DC: National Research Council.

Freud, A. (1946). *The Ego and Mechanisms of Defense.* New York: International Universities Press.

Freud, S. (1910). Five lectures on psychoanalysis. In The *Standard Edition of the Complete Psychological Works of Sigmund Freud* (Vol. 11, pp. 9–55). London: Hogarth.

Freud, S. (1922). *The Infantile Genital Organization of the LIbido: A Supplement to the Theory of Sexuality; Collected Papers* (Vol. II, pp. 244–248. London: Hogarth.

Freud, S. (1935). *A General Introduction to Psychoanalysis.* New York: Liveright.

Freud, S. (1938). *A General Introduction to Psychoanalysis.* New York: Pocket.

Freud, S. (1953). *A General Introduction to Psychoanalysis.* New York: Liverright.

Freud, S. (1900-1953). *Collected Papers* (Vols. I-V). London: Hogarth and Institute of Psycho-Analysis.

Frischholz, E., Tryon, W., Vellios, A., Fisher, S., Maruffi, B., & Spiegel, H. (1980). The relationship between the Hypnotic Induction Profile and the Stanford Hypnotic Susceptibility Scale, Form C: A replication. *American Journal of Clinical Hypnosis, 22,* 185–196.

Fromm, E. (1965). Awareness versus consciousness. *Psychological Reports, 16,* 711–712.

Fromm, E. (1972). Activity and passivity of the ego in hypnosis. *International Journal of Clinical and Experimental Hypnosis, 20,* 238–251.

Fromm, E. (1976). Altered states of consciousness and ego psychology. *Social Service Review, 50,* 557–569.

Fromm, E. (1977). An ego psychological theory of altered states of consciousness. *International Journal of Clinical and Experimental Hypnosis, 25,* 372–387.

Fromm, E. (1979). The nature of hypnosis and other altered states of consciousness: An ego-psychological theory. In E. Fromm & R. E. Shor (Eds.), *Hypnosis: Developments in Research and New Perspectives* (2nd ed., pp. 1098–1131). New York: Aldine.

Fromm, E. (1981). How to write a clinical paper: A brief communication. *International Journal of Clinical and Experimental Hypnosis, 29,* 5–9.

Fromm, E. (1988). Self-hypnosis and the creative imagination. In I. Shafer (Ed.), *The Incarnate Imagination: Essays in Theology, the Arts and Social Sciences in Honor of Andrew Greeley; A Festschrift* (pp. 15–24). Bowling Green, OH: Popular Press.

Fromm, E. (1992). An ego-psychological theory of hypnosis. In E. Fromm & M. Nash (Eds.), *Contemporary Hypnosis Research* (pp. 131–148). New York: Guilford.

Fromm, E., Brown, D. P., Hurt, S. W., Oberlander, J. Z., Boxer, A. M., & Pfeifer, G. (1981). The phenomena and characteristics of self-hypnosis. *International Journal of Clinical and Experimental Hypnosis, 29,* 189–246.

Fromm, E., & Kahn, S. (1990). *Self-Hypnosis: The Chicago Paradigm.* New York: Guilford.

Fromm, E., & Nash, M. (1997). *Psychoanalysis and Hypnoanalysis.* Madison, CT: International Universities.

Fromm, E., Oberlander, M., & Gruenewald, D. (1970). Perceptual and cognitive processes in different states of consciousness: The waking state and hypnosis. *Journal of Projective Techniques and Personality Assessment, 34,* 375–387.

Gaddes, W., & Edgell, D. (1994). *Learning Disabilities and Brain Function.* New York: Springer-Verlag.

Gainer, M. J. (1992). Hypnotherapy for reflex sympathetic dystrophy. *American Journal of Clinical Hypnosis, 34,* 227–232.

Galovski, T. E., & Blanchard, E. B. (1998). The treatment of irritable bowel syndrome with hypnotherapy. *Applied Psychophysiological Biofeedback, 23,* 219–232.

Gardner, G. G. (1976). Childhood, death, and human dignity: Hypnotherapy for David. *International Journal of Clinical and Experimental Hypnosis, 24,* 122–139.

Gardner, G., & Olness, K. (1981). *Hypnosis and Hypnotherapy with Children.* New York: Grune and Stratton.

Garver, R. (1977). The enhancement of human performance with hypnosis through neuromotor facilitation and control of arousal level. *American Journal of Clinical Hypnosis, 19*(3), 177–181.

Gatchel, R. J., & Epker, J. (1999). Psychosocial predictors of chronic pain and response to treatment. In R. J. Gatchel & D. C. Turk (Eds.), *Psychosocial factors in pain: Clinical perspectives* (pp. 412–434). New York: Guilford.

Gauld, A. (1988). Reflections on mesmeric analgesia. *British Journal of Experimental and Clinical Hypnosis, 5,* 177–124.

Gilboa, D., Borenstein, A., Seidman, D., & Tsur, H. (1990). Burn patients' use of autohypnosis: Making a painful experience bearable. *Burns, 16,* 441–444.

Gill, M., & Brenman, M. (1959). *Hypnosis and Related States.* New York: International Universities Press.

Giovino, G., Henningfield, J., Tomar, S., Escobedo, L., & Slade, J. (1995). Epidemiology of tobacco use and dependence. *Epidemiological Review, 17,* 48–65.

Gliedman, L., Nash, H., Imber, S., Stone, A. Frank, J. (1958). Reduction of symptoms by pharmacologically inert substances and by short term psychotherapy. *Archives of Neurology and Psychiatry, 79,* 345–351.

Goldberg, F. (1996). Psychoanalytic practice and managed care: Comparison of Division 39 and other psychologist survey results. *Psychologist-Psychoanalyst, 16*(3), 1–5.

Gonsalkorale, W. M., Houghton, L. A., & Whorwell, P. J. (2002). Hypnotherapy in irritable bowel syndrome: A large-scale audit of clinical service with examination of factors influencing responsiveness. *American Journal Gastroenterology, 97,* 954–961.

Gonsalkorale, W., Miller, V., Afzol, A., & Whorwell, P. (2003). Long term benefits of hypnotherapy for irritable bowel syndrome. *GUT, 52*(11), 1623–1629.

Goodman, A. (2004). Private-practice notes. San Diego, CA.

Gordin, R. (1995). Hypnosis in sport. In K. P. Henschen & W. F. Straub (Eds.), *Sport Psychology: An Analysis of Athlete Behavior* (pp. 193–201). Longmeadow, MA: Movement Publications.

Gorton, B. E. (1959). Physiologic aspects of hypnosis. In J. M. Schneck (Ed.), *Hypnosis in modern medicine* (pp. 246–280). Springfield, IL: Charles C. Thomas.

Gravitz, M. (2004). The historical role of hypnosis in the theoretical origins of transference. *International Journal of Clinical and Experimental Hypnosis, 52*(2), 91–201.

Gravitz, M., & Gravitz, R. (1977). The collected writing of Milton H. Erickson: The complete bibliography, 1929–1977. *American Journal of Clinical Hypnosis, 20,* 84–94.

Green, J. (2004). Presidential address, Annual Convention of the American Psychological Association, Honolulu, July 28–August 1.

Green, J., Barabasz, A. Barrett, D., & Montgomery. (in press). Forging ahead: The 2003 APA definition of hypnosis. *International Journal of Clinical and Experimental Hypnosis.*

Green, J., & Lynn, S. (2000). Hypnosis and suggestion-based approaches to smoking cessation: An examination of the evidence. *International Journal of Clinical and Experimental Hypnosis, 48*(2), 191–220.

Grinker, R., & Spiegel, H. (1945). *War Neuroses.* Philadelphia: Blakiston.

Gruenewald, D. (1965). Hypnotherapy in a case of nailbiting. *International Journal of Clinical and Experimental Hypnosis.*

Gruzelier, J., Allison, J., & Conway, A. (1988). A psychophysiological differentiation between hypnotic behavior and simulation. *International Journal of Psychophysiology, 6,* 331–338.

Guillotin, J., & LeRoy, J. (1784). *Rapport des Commissaires Chargés par le Roy de l'Examen du Magnetisme Animal.* Paris: Bibliothèque Royale.

Haanen, H. C., Hoenderdos, H. T., van Romunde, L. K., Hop, W. C., Mallee, C., Terwiel, J. P., & Hekster, G. B. (1991). Controlled trial of hypnotherapy in the treatment of refractory fibromyalgia. *Journal of Rheumatology, 18,* 72–75.

Haley, J. (1967). *Advanced Techniques of Hypnosis and Therapy: Selected Papers of Milton H. Erickson, M.D.* New York: Grune and Stratton.

Haley, J. (1973). *Uncommon Therapy, the Psychiatric Techniques of Milton H. Erickson M.D.* New York: W. W. Norton.

Hall, H., Minnes, L., Tosi, M., & Olness, K. (1992). Voluntary modulation of neutrophil adhesiveness using a cyberphysiological strategy. *International Journal of Neuroscience, 63,* 287–297.

Hall, W. (1967). Gastric function during hypnosis and hypnotically induced gastro-intestinal symptoms. *Journal of Psychosomatic Research, 11,* 263–266.

Hammond, D. (1990). *Handbook of Hypnotic Suggestions and Metaphors.* New York: W. W. Norton.

Hanin, Y. (1978). A study of anxiety in sports. In W. F. Straub (Ed.), *Sport Psychology: An Analysis of Athlete Behavior* (pp. 236–249). Ithaca, NY: Movement.

Hanin, Y. (1999). *Emotions in Sport.* Champaign, IL: Human Kinetics.

Harding, H. (1967). Hypnosis in the treatment of migraine. In J. Lassner (Ed.), *Hypnosis and Psychosomatic Medicine* (pp. 131–134). New York: Springer-Verlag.

Hargadon, R., Bowers, K. S., & Woody, E. Z. (1995). Does counterpain imagery mediate hypnotic analgesia? *Journal of Abnormal Psychology, 104,* 508–516.

Harmon, T., Hynan, M., & Tyre, T. (1990). Improved obstetric outcomes using hypnotic analgesia and skill mastery combined with childbirth education. *Journal of Consulting and Clinical Psychology, 58*(5), 525–530.

Hartland, J. (1966). *Medical and Dental Hypnosis.* Baltimore: Williams & Wilkins.

Hartland, J. (1971). Further observations of the use of "ego-strengthening" techniques. *American Journal of Clinical Hypnosis, 14,* 1–8.

Hartmann, H. (1958). *Ego Psychology and the Problem of Adaptation* (D. Rapaport, Trans.) New York: International Universities Press. (Original work published 1939)

Harvey, R., Hinton, R., Gunary, R., & Barry, R. (1989). Individual and group hypnotherapy in the treatment of refractory irritable bowel syndrome. *Lancet,* 1:8635, 424–425.

Hatfield, E. C. (1961). The validity of the LeCron method of evaluating hypnotic depth. *International Journal of Clinical and Experimental Hypnosis, 9,* 215–221.

Hatfield, F. (2000). *Fitness: The Complete Guide.* Santa Barbara, California: International Sports Science Association.

Hebert, R. (Ed.). (1998). *Minding the Body: The Science of Hypnosis.* Washington, DC: Center for the Advancement of Health.

Helzer, J., Robins, L., & L. McEvoy. (1987). PTSD in the general population. *New England Journal of Medicine, 317,* 1630–1634.

Heron, W. (1953). *Clinical Applications of Suggestion and Hypnosis* (2nd ed.). Springfield, IL: Charles C. Thomas.

Hesse, H. (1951). *Siddartha* (Hilda Rosner, Trans.). Toronto, Canada; New York: Bantam Books.

Hilgard, E. (1965). *Hypnotic Susceptibility.* New York: Harcourt, Brace, and World.

Hilgard, E. (1969). Pain as a puzzle for psychology and physiology. *American Psychologist, 24,* 103–113.

Hilgard, E. (1973). The domain of hypnosis: With some comments on alternate paradigms. *American Psychologist, 28,* 972–982.

Hilgard, E. (1977). *Divided Consciousness: Multiple Controls in Human Thought and Action.* New York: John Wiley.

Hilgard, E. (1979). A Saga of Hypnosis: Two Decades of the Stanford Laboratory of Hypnosis Research 1957–1979. Unpublished manuscript, Stanford University.

Hilgard, E. (1992). Dissociation and theories of hypnosis. In E. Fromm & N. Nash (Eds.), *Contemporary Hypnosis Research* (pp. 69–101). New York: Guilford.

Hilgard, E., & Hilgard, J. (1975). *Hypnosis in the Relief of Pain.* Las Altos, CA: William Kaufman.

Hilgard, E., & Hilgard, J. (1983). *Hypnosis in the Relief of Pain* (2nd ed.). Los Altos, CA: William Kaufman.

Hilgard, E., & Hilgard, J. (1994). *Hypnosis in the Relief of Pain* (Rev. ed.). New York: Brunner/ Mazel.

Hilgard, E., & Loftus, E. (1979). Effective interrogation of the eye witness. *International Journal of Clinical and Experimental Hypnosis, 27,* 342–357.

Hilgard, E., Morgan, A., & MacDonald, H. (1975). Pain and dissociation in the cold pressor test: A study of hypnotic analgesia with "hidden reports" through automatic key pressing and automatic talking. *Journal of Abnormal Psychology, 87,* 17–31.

Hilgard, E., & Tart, C. (1966). Responsiveness to suggestions following waking and imagination instructions and following induction of hypnosis. *Journal of Abnormal Psychology, 71*(3), 196–208.

Hilgard, J. (1974). Imaginative involvement: Some characteristics of the highly hypnotizable and non-hypnotizable. *International Journal of Clinical and Experimental Hypnosis, 22,* 138–156.

Hilgard, J. (1979). Imaginative and sensory-effective involvements in everyday life and in hypnosis. In E. Fromm & R. E. Shor (Eds.), *Hypnosis: Developments in Research and New Perspectives* (2nd ed., pp. 483–517). New York: Aldine.

Hilgard, J., & LeBaron, S. (1984). *Hypnotherapy of Pain in Children with Cancer.* Los Altos, CA: William Kaufman.

Hofbauer, R., Rainville, P., Duncan, G., & Bushnell, M. (1998). Cognitive modulation of pain sensation alters activity in human cerebral cortex. *Abstracts—Society for Neuroscience, 24.*

Holroyd, J. (1980). Hypnosis treatment for smoking: An evaluative review. *International Journal of Clinical and Experimental Hypnosis, 28,* 341–357.

Holroyd, J. (1991). The uncertain relationship between hypnotizability and smoking treatment outcome. *International Journal of Clinical and Experimental Hypnosis, 39,* 93–102.

Holroyd, J. (1996). Hypnosis treatment of clinical pain: Understanding why hypnosis is useful. *International Journal of Clinical and Experimental Hypnosis, 44,* 33–51.

Holroyd, J. (2003). The science of meditation and the state of hypnosis. *American Journal of Clinical Hypnosis, 46,* 109–128.

Holt, R. (1963). *Manual for the scoring of primary process manifestations in Rorschach responses* (9th ed.). New York: Research Center for Mental Health, New York University. (Mimeograph)

Horan, J. (1950). Management of neurodermatitis by hypnotic suggestion. *British Journal of Medical Hypnosis, 2,* 43.

Horevitz, R. (1992). Hypnosis in the treatment of multiple personality disorders. In S. Lynn, J. Rhue, & I. Kirsch (Eds.), *Handbook of Clinical Hypnosis* (pp. 176–195). Washington, DC: American Psychological Association.

Houghton, L., Heyman, D., & Whorwell, P. (1996). Symtomatology, quality of life and economic features of irritable bowel syndrome: The effect of hypnotherapy. *Alimentary Pharmacological Therapy, 10,* 91–95.

Hull, C. (1933). *Hypnosis and Suggestibility.* New York: Appleton.

Ikali, M., & Steinhaus, A. (1961). Some factors modifying the expression of human strength. *Journal of Applied Psychology, 16,* 157–163.

Ikemi, Y., & Nakagawa, S. A. (1962). A psychosomatic study of contagious dermatitis. *Kyushu Journal of Medical Science, 13,* 335–352.

Iserson, K. (1999). Hypnosis for pediatric fracture reduction. *Journal of Emergency Medicine, 17,* 53–56.

Jack, M. (1999). The use of hypnosis for a patient with chronic pain. *Contemporary Hypnosis, 16,* 231–237.

Jacknow, D., Tschann, J., Link, M., & Boyce, W. (1994). Hypnosis in the prevention of chemotherapy-related nausea and vomiting in children: A prospective study. *Developmental and Behavioral Pediatrics, 25,* 258–264.

Jacobs, S., & Gotthelf, C. (1986). Effects of hypnosis on physical and athletic performance. In F. A. De Piano & H. C. Salzberg (Eds.), *Clinical applications of hypnosis* (pp. 98–117). Norwood, NJ: Ablex.

Jacobs, S., & Salzberg, H. (1987). The effects of posthypnotic performance enhancing instructions on cognitive-behavior performance. *International Journal of Clinical and Experimental Hypnosis, 35,* 41–50.

Jacobson, A., Hackett, T., Surmon, O., & Silverberg, A. (1973). Raynaud phenomenon: Treatment with hypnotic and operant technique. *Journal of American Medical Association, 225,* 739–740.

Jacobson, E. (1938). *Progressive Relaxation.* Chicago: University of Chicago Press.

James, W. (1890). *Principles of Psychology.* New York: Holt.

James, W. (1935). *The Variety of Religious Experience.* New York: Longman.

Janet, P. (1889). *L' Automatisme Psychologique.* Paris: Felix Alcan.

Janet, P. (1925). *Psychological Healing: A historical and Clinical Study* (E. Paul & C. Paul, Trans.). New York: Macmillan. (Original work published 1919)

Janis, I. (1958). *Psychological Stress.* New York: Wiley.

Jasiukaitis, P., Nouriani, B., & Spiegel, D. (1996). Left hemisphere superiority for event-related potential effects of hypnotic obstruction. *Neuropsychological, 34,* 661–668.

Jencks, B. (1978). Utilizing the phases of breathing rhythm in hypnosis. In F.H. Frankel & H. S. Zamansky (Eds.), *Hypnosis at Its Bicentennial* (pp. 169–182). New York: Plenum.

Jenkins, M., & Pritchard, M. (1993). Hypnosis: Practical applications and theoretical considerations in normal labor. *British Journal of Obstetrics and Gynecology, 100,* 221–228.

Jensen, M. (1996). Enhancing motivation to change in pain treatment. In R. J. Gatchel & D. C. Turk (Eds.), *Psychological Approaches to Pain Management: A Practitioner's Handbook* (pp. 78–111). New York: Guilford.

Jensen, M., & Barber, J. (2000). Hypnotic analgesia of spinal cord injury pain. *Australian Journal of Clinical and Experimental Hypnosis, 28,* 150–168.

Jensen, S., Barabasz, A., Barabasz, M., & Warner, D. (2001). EEG P300 event related markers of hypnosis. *American Journal of Clinical Hypnosis, 44*(2), 127–139.

Johnson, L. (1981). Current research in self-hypnotic phenomenology: The Chicago paradigm. *International Journal of Clinical and Experimental Hypnosis, 29,* 247–258.

Johnson, L., Johnson, D., Olson, M., & Newman, J. (1981). The uses of hypnotherapy with learning-disabled children. *Journal of Clinical Psychology, 37,* 291–299.

Johnson, W. (1961a). Body movement awareness in the non-hypnotic and hypnotic states. *Research Quarterly, 32,* 263–264.

Johnson, W. (1961b). Hypnosis and muscular performance. *Journal of Sports Medicine and Physical Fitness, 1,* 71–79.

Jones, G., & Hardy, L. (1990.) Stress in sports: Experiences of some elite performers. In G. Jones & L. Hardy (Eds.), *Stress and Performance in Sports* (pp. 247–277). Chichester, UK: Wiley.

Kahn, S., & Fromm, E. (1992). Self-hypnosis, personality and the experiential method. In E. Fromm & M. Nash (Eds.), *Contemporary Hypnosis Research* (pp. 390–404). New York: Guilford.

Kahn, S., & Fromm, E. (2001). *Changes in the Therapist.* Mahwah, NJ: Erlbaum.

Kasanin, J. (1944). *Language and thought in Schizophrenia.* Berkeley: University of California Press.

Katchan, F., & Belozerski, G. (1940). Obstetrical analgesia by hypnosis. *Tsent. nauch-issled acouch–guinek, Lenigrad Institute, 6,* 19–89.

Katz, E. R., Kellerman, J., & Ellenberg, L. (1987). Hypnosis in the reduction of acute pain and distress in children with cancer. *Journal of Pediatric Psychology, 12,* 379–394.

Kelsey, D., & Barrow, J. D. (1958). Maintenance of posture by hypnotic suggestion in patient undergoing plastic surgery. *British Medical Journal,* 756–757.

Kendall, G., Hrycaiko, D., Martin, G., & Kendall, T. (1990). The effects of an imagery rehearsal, relaxation, and self-talk package on basketball game performance. *Journal of Sport and Exercise Psychology, 12,* 157–166.

Khema, A. (1997). *Who is My Self? A Guide to Buddhist Meditation.* Boston: Wisdom Publications. (Based on Sutta 9: the States of Consciousness Sutta, in M. Walshe, Trans., 1987, *The Long Discourses of the Buddha.* Boston: Wisdom)

Kiecolt-Glaser, J., Glaser, R., Williger, D., Stout, J., Messick, G., Sheppard, S., Ricker, D., Romisher, S., Briner, W., Bonnell, G., & Donnerberg, R. (1985). Psychosocial entrancement of immunocompetence in a geriatric population. *Health Psychology, 4,* 25–41.

Kihlstrom, J. (1987). The cognitive unconscious. *Science, 237,* 1445–1452.

Kihlstrom, J. (1992). Hypnosis: A sesquicentennial essay. *International Journal of Clinical and Experimental Hypnosis, 50,* 301–314.

Kihlstrom, J. (1997). Convergence in understanding hypnosis? Perhaps, but perhaps not quite so fast. *International Journal of Clinical and Experimental Hypnosis, 45,* 324–332.

Kihlstrom, J. (2003). The fox, the hedgehog and hypnosis. *International Journal of Clinical and Experimental Hypnosis, 51*(2), 166–189.

Kihlstrom, J., & Evans, F. (1979). *Functional disorders of memory.* Hillsdale, NJ: Erlbaum.

Killeen, P., & Nash, M. (2003). The four causes of hypnosis. *International Journal of Clinical and Experimental Hypnosis, 51*(3), 195–231.

Kinnunen, T., Zamansky, H. S., & Nordstrom, B. L. (2001). Is the hypnotized subject complying? *International Journal of Clinical and Experimental Hypnosis, 49*(2), 83–94.

Kirsch, I. (1990). *Changing Expectations: A Key to Effective Psychotherapy.* Pacific Grove, CA: Brooks/Cole.

Kirsch, I. (1993). Professional opinions about hypnosis: Results of the APA Division 30 survey. *Bulletin of Division 30 Psychological Hypnosis, APA, 2,* 4–5.

Kirsch, I. (1996) Hypnotic enhancement of cognitive-behavioral weight loss treatments: Another meta-reanalysis. *Journal of Consulting and Clinical Psychology,* 64, 517–519.

Kirsch, I. (2002) Yes, there is a placebo effect, but is there a powerful antidepressant drug effect? *Prevention & Treatment,* http://journals.apa.org/prevention/volume 5/pre0050022i.html.

Kirsch, I. (2003). *The Debate Goes On.* Invited address presented at the annual convention of the American Psychological Association, Toronto, Ontario, August 8–12.

Kirsch, I., & Council, J. (1989). Response expectancy as a determinant of hypnotic behavior. In N. P. Spanos & J. F. Chaves (Eds.), *Hypnosis: A Cognitive-Behavioral Perspective* (pp. 360–379). Buffalo, NY: Prometheus Books.

Kirsch, I., & Lynn, S. (1995). The altered state of hypnosis. *American Psychologist, 50*(10), 846–858.

Kirsch, I., & Lynn, S. (1999, November). The socio-cognitive theory of hypnosis. Paper presented at the 50th annual scientific program of the Society for Clinical and Experimental Hypnosis, New Orleans.

Kirsch, I., Montgomery, G., & Sapirstein, G. (1995). Special feature: Hypnosis as an adjunct to cognitive-behavioral psychotherapy; A meta-analysis. *Journal of Consulting and Clinical Psychology, 63*(2), 214–220.

Klein, K., & Spiegel, D. (1989). Modulation of gastric acid secretion by hypnosis. *Gastroenterology, 96,* 1383–1387.

Kline, M. (1950). Situational cardiovascular symptomatology and hypnosis. *British Journal of Medical Hypnotism, 1,* 33–36.

Kline, M. (1953). Delimited hypnotherapy: The acceptance of resistance in the treatment of a long standing neurodermatitis with a sensory-imagery technique. *Journal of Clinical and Experimental Hypnosis, 1*(4), 18–22.

Kline, M. (1954). Psoriasis and hypnotherapy: A case report. *International Journal of Clinical and Experimental Hypnosis, 2,* 318–322.

Kline, M. (1958). *Freud and Hypnosis.* New York: Julian Press.

Kline, M. (1966). Hypnotic amnesia in psychotherapy. *International Journal of Clinical and Experimental Hypnosis, 14,* 112–120.

Kline, M., Guze, H., Haggarty, T. (1954). An experimental study of the nature of hypnotic deafness, *Journal of Clinical and Experimental Hypnosis, 2,* 145–156.

Kluft, R. (1987). An update on multiple personality disorder. *Hospital and Community Psychiatry, 38,* 363–373.

Kluft, R. (2003). Antaeus and androgyny: Negotiating paradigm exhaustion and pursuing professional growth in clinical practice; Comment. *American Journal of Clinical Hypnosis, 45*(4), 323–331.

Koch, T., Lang, E., Hatsiopoulou, O., Anderson, B., Berbaum, K., & Spiegel, D. (2003). Adverse short-term effects of attention control treatment on hypnotizability: A challenge in designing controlled hypnosis trials. *International Journal of Clinical and Experimental Hypnosis, 52*(4), 357–368.

Koe, G., & Oldridge, O. (1988). The effect of hypnotically induced on reading performance. *International Journal of Clinical and Experimental Hypnosis, 34*(4), 275–283.

Kogan, M., Biswas, A., & Spiegel, D. (1997). Effect of medical and psychotherapeutic treatment on the survival of women with metastatic breast carcinoma. *Cancer, 80,* 225–230.

Kohen, D., (1986). Applications of relaxation/mental imagery (self-hypnosis) in pediatric emergency. *International Journal of Clinical and Experimental Hypnosis, 34*(4), 283–294.

Kohen, D., & Olness, K. (1993). Hypnotherapy with children. In J. W. Rhue, S. J. Lynn, & I. Kirsch (Eds.), *Handbook of Clinical Hypnosis* (pp. 357–381). Washington, DC: American Psychological Association.

Kosslyn, S., Thompson, W., Constantini-Ferrando, M., Alpert, N., & Spiegel, D. (2000). Hypnotic visual illusion alters color processing in the brain. *American Journal of Psychiatry, 157,* 1279–1284.

Kramer, E., & Tucker, G. (1967). Hypnotically suggested deafness and delayed auditory feed-back. *International Journal of Clinical and Experimental Hypnosis, 15,* 37–43.

Kripper, S. (1966). The use of hypnosis with elementary and secondary school children in a summer reading clinic. *American Journal of Clinical Hypnosis, 8,* 261–266.

Krippner, S., & Rubin, D. (1973). *Galaxies of Life.* New York: Gordon & Breach.

Kroger, W. (1963). *Clinical and Experimental Hypnosis.* Philadelphia: Lippincott.

Kroger, W. (1977). *Clinical and Experimental Hypnosis* (2nd ed.). Philadelphia: Lippincott.

Kroger, W., & Fezler, W. (1976). *Hypnosis and Behavior Modification: Imagery Conditioning.* Philadelphia: Lippincott.

Kroger, W. S., & Freed, S. C. (1951). *Psychosomatic Gynecology.* Philadelphia: Saunders.

Kropotov, J., Crawford, H., & Polyakov, Y. (1997). Somatosensory event-related potential changes to painful stimuli during hypnotic analgesia: Anterior cingulated cortex and anterior temporal cortex intracranial recordings. *International Journal of Psychophysiology, 27*(1), 1–8.

Kubie, L. S., & Margolin, D. (1944). The process of hypnotism and the nature of the hypnotic state. *American Journal of Psychiatry, 100,* 611–622.

Kuttner, L. (1987). *No Fears, No Tears: Children with Cancer Coping with Pain* [film]. Canadian Cancer Society, British Columbia/Yukon Division: Vancouver, British Columbia.

Kuttner, L., Bowman, M., & Teasdale, M. (1988). Psychological treatment of distress, pain, and anxiety for young children with cancer. *Journal of Developmental and Behavioral Pediatrics, 9,* 374–381.

LaClave, L., & Blix, S. (1989). Hypnosis in the management of symptoms in a young girl with malignant astrocytoma: A challenge to the therapist. *International Journal of Clinical and Experimental Hypnosis, 37*(1), 6–14.

Lait, V. S. (1972). A case of recurrent compulsive vomiting. *American Journal of Clinical Hypnosis, 14,* 196–198.

Lamaze, F. (1958). *Painless childbirth.* London: Burke.

Lang, E., Benotsch, E., Fick, L., Lutgendorf, S., Berbaum, M., Berbaum, K., Logan, H., & Spiegel, D. (2000). Adjunctive non-pharmacological analgesia for invasive medical procedures: A randomised trial. *Lancet, 355,* 1486–1490.

Lang, E., & Berbaum, K. (1997). Educating interventional radiology personnel in nonpharmacologic analgesia: Effect on patients' pain perception. *Academic Radiology, 4*(11), 753–757.

Lang, E., Joyce, J., Spiegel, D., Hamilton, D., & Lee, K. (1996). Self-hypnotic relaxation during interventional radiological procedures: Effects on pain perception and intravenous drug use. *International Journal of Clinical and Experimental Hypnosis, 44,* 106–119.

Lang, E., & Rosen, M. (2002). Cost analysis of adjunct hypnosis with sedation during outpatient interventional radiologic procedures. *Radiology, 222*(2), 375–382.

Lavoie, G. (1990). Clinical hypnosis: A psychodynamic approach. In M. L. Fass & D. P. Brown (Eds.), *Creative Mastery in Hypnosis and Hypnoanalysis: A Festschrift for Erika Fromm* (pp. 77–105). Hillsdale, NJ: Erlbaum.

Lea, P., Ware, P., & Monroe, R. (1960). The hypnotic control of intractable pain. *American Journal of Clinical Hypnosis, 3,* 3–8.

LeCron, L. (1953). A method of measuring the depth of hypnosis. *Journal of Clinical and Experimental Hypnosis, 1,* 4–7.

LeCron, L. (1968). *Experimental Hypnosis.* New York: Citadel.

Lembo, T., Naliboff, B., Martin, K., Munakata, J., Parker, R., Gracely, R., & Mayer, E. (2000). Irritable bowel syndrome patients show altered sensitivity to exogenous opioids. *Pain, 87,* 137–147.

Levin, L., & Harrison, R. (1976). Hypnosis and age regression in the service of the ego. *International Journal of Clinical and Experimental Hypnosis, 24,* 400–418.

Levinson, B. (1965). State of awareness during general anesthesia. *British Journal of Anesthesiology, 37,* 544–546.

Levitan, A. (1990). Setting sun metaphor. In D. C. Hammond (Ed.), *Handbook of Hypnotic Suggestions and Metaphors.* New York: W. W. Norton.

Liebeault, A. (1866). *Du Sommeil et des Etats Analogues Consideres surtout au Point de Vue de l'Action Moral sur le Physique.* Paris: Masson.

Liggett, D. (2000a). Enhancing imagery through hypnosis: A performance aid for athletes. *American Journal of Clinical Hypnosis, 43*(2), 149–157.

Liggett, D. (2000b). *Sport Hypnosis.* Champaign, IL: Human Kinetics.

Liggett, D., & Hamada, S. (1993). Enhancing the visualization of gymnasts. *American Journal of Clinical Hypnosis, 35*(3), 190–197.

Liossi, C., & Hatira, P. (1999). Clinical hypnosis versus cognitive behavioral training for pain management with pediatric cancer patients undergoing bone marrow aspirations. *International Journal of Clinical and Experimental Hypnosis, 47,* 104–116.

Liossi, C., & Hatira, P. (2003). Clinical hypnosis in the alleviation of procedure-related pain in pediatric oncology patients. *International Journal of Clinical and Experimental Hypnosis, 51*(1), 4–28.

London, P. (1963). *Children's Hypnotic Susceptibility Scale.* Palo Alto, CA: Consulting Psychologists Press.

Low, C. (1999). Attention deficit hyperactivity disorder: Dissociation and adaptation (a theoretical presentation and case study). *American Journal of Clinical Hypnosis, 41*(3), 253–261.

Lubar, J. (1991). Discourse on the development of EEG diagnostics and biofeedback for attention-deficit/hyperactivity disorders. *Biofeedback and Self-Regulation, 16,* 201–225.

Ludwig, A., Lyle, M., & Miller, M. (1964). Group hypnotherapy techniques with drug addicts. *International Journal of Clinical and Experimental Hypnosis, 12,* 53–66.

Lynn, S.J. (2003, November). Hypnosis and Buddhism in practice: Acceptance based approaches in psychotherapy. Paper presented at the 54th annual workshops and scientific program of the Society for Clinical and Experimental Hypnosis, Chicago.

Lynn, S. J., Kirsch, I., Barabasz, A., Cardena, E., & Patterson, D. (2000). Hypnosis as an empirically supported clinical intervention: The state of the evidence and a look to the future. *International Journal of Clinical and Experimental Hypnosis, 48*(2), 239–259.

Lynn, S. J., Rhue, J. W., & Weekes, J. R. (1990). Hypnotic involuntariness: A social cognitive analysis. *Psychological Review, 97,* 169–184.

Magaw, A. (1906). A review of over 14 thousand surgical anaesthesias. *Surgery, Gynecology and Obstetrics, 3,* 795–797.

Malzack, R. (1974, October). Acupuncture and pain mechanisms. Paper presented at the 26th Annual Meeting of the Society for Clinical and Experimental Hypnosis, Montreal.

Malzack, R. (1993). Labor pain as a model for acute pain. *Pain, 53,* 117–120.

Malzack, R., & Wall, P. (1965). Pain mechanism: A new theory. *Science, 150,* 971–979.

Mann, C., Lubar, J., Zimmerman, W., Miller, C., & Muenchen, R. (1992). Quantitative analysis of EEG in boys with attention deficit hyperactivity disorder: Controlled study with clinical implications. *Pediatric Neurology, 8,* 30–36.

Marchesi, C. (1949). The hypnotic treatment of bronchial asthma. *British Journal of Medical Hypnotism, 1,* 14–19.

Marcus, H. W. (1963). Hypnosis in dentistry. In J. M. Schneck (Ed.), *Hypnosis in Modern Medicine* (3rd ed., pp. 229–279). Springfield, IL: Charles C. Thomas.

Marmer, M. (1959). *Hypnosis in Anesthesiology.* Springfield, IL: Charles C. Thomas.

Maslach, C., Marshall, G., & Zimbardo, P. (1972). Hypnotic control of peripheral skin temperature: A case report. *Psychophysiology, 9,* 600–605.

Mason, A. (1952). A case of congenital icthyosiform erythroderma of Brocq treated hypnosis. *British Medical Journal, 2,* 422–423.

Mauer, M., Burnett, K., Ouellette, E., Ironson, G., & Dandes, H. (1999). Medical hypnosis and orthopedic hand surgery: Pain perception, postoperative recovery, and therapeutic comfort. *International Journal of Clinical and Experimental Hypnosis, 47,* 144–161.

McAleney, P., Barabasz, A., & Barabasz, M. (1990). Effects of floatation restricted environmental stimulation on intercollegiate tennis performance. *Perceptual Motor Skills, 71,* 1023–1028.

McCarney, S. (1989). *Attention Deficit Disorders Evaluation Scale.* Columbia, MO: Hawthorne Educational Services.

McCarthy, P. (2001). Hypnosis in obstetrics and gynecology. In L. E. Fredericks (Ed.), *The Use of Hypnosis in Surgery and Anesthesiology* (pp. 163–211). Springfield, IL: Charles C. Thomas.

McConkey, K., Szeps, A., & Barnier, A. J. (2001). Indexing the experience of sex change in hypnosis and imagination. *International Journal of Clinical and Experimental Hypnosis, 49,* 131–140.

McConkey, K., Wende, V., & Barnier, A. J. (1999). Measuring change in the subjective experience of hypnosis. *International Journal of Clinical and Experimental Hypnosis, 47,* 23–39.

McGlashan, T. H., Evans, F. J., & Orne, M. T. (1969). The nature of hypnotic analgesia and placebo response to experimental pain. *Psychosomatic Medicine, 31,* 227–246.

McNair, D., Lorr, M., & Droppleman, L. (1971). *Profile of Mood States: Manual.* San Diego, CA: Educational and Industrial Testing Service.

Meares, A. (1961). *A System of Medical Hypnosis*. Philadelphia: Saunders.

Meares, A. (1982-1983). A form of intensive meditation associated with the regression of cancer. *American Journal of Clinical Hypnosis, 25,* 114–121.

Meddis, S. (1994, May 12). Nation's drug (scene) again degenerating. *USA Today,* p. 3A.

Meldman, M. (1960). Personality decomposition after hypnotic symptom suppression. *Journal of American Medical Association, 173,* 359–361.

Mertz, H., Fullerton, S., Naliboff, B., & Mayer, E. (1998). Symptoms and visceral perception in severe functional and organic dyspepsia. *Gut, 42,* 814–822.

Mesmer, F. (1781). *Précis Historique des Faits Relatifs au Magnetisme Animal jusques en Avril 1781.* London: n.p.

Miller, M., Barabasz, A., & Barabasz, M. (1991). Effects of active alert and relaxation hypnotic inductions on cold pressor pain. *American Psychological Association, 100,* 223–226.

Milling, L., & Costanino, C. (2000). Clinical hypnosis with children: First steps toward empirical support. *International Journal of Clinical and Experimental Hypnosis, 48*(2), 113–137.

Milling, L., Kirsch, I., & Burgess, C. A. (1999). Brief modification of suggestibility and hypnotic analgesia: Too good to be true? *International Journal of Clinical and Experimental Hypnosis, 47,* 91–103.

Montgomery, G., DuHamel, K., & Redd, W. (2000). A meta-analysis of hypnotically induced analgesia: How effective is hypnosis? *International Journal of Clinical and Experimental Hypnosis, 48,* 138–153.

Morgan, A., & Hilgard, J. (1978–1979). The Stanford Hypnotic Clinical Scale for Adults. *American Journal of Clinical Hypnosis, 21,* 134–147.

Morgan, A. & Hilgard, J. (1978–1979). The Stanford Hypnotic Clinical Scale for Children. *American Journal of Clinical Hypnosis,* 21, 148–169.

Morgan, W. (1972). Hypnosis and muscular performance. In W. P. Morgan (Ed.), *Ergogenic Aids and Muscular Performance* (pp. 193–233). New York: Academic Press.

Morgan, W. (1980). Hypnosis and sports medicine. In G. D. Burrows, D. R. Collison, & L. Dennerstein (Eds.), *Handbook of Hypnosis and Psychosomatic Medicine* (pp. 359–375). Amsterdam: Elsevier/North Holland Biomedical Press.

Morgan, W. (1985). Psychogenic factors and exercise metabolism. *Medicine and Science in Sports and Exercise, 17,* 309–316.

Morgan, W. (1993). Hypnosis and sport psychology. In J. Rhue, S. J. Lynn, & I. Kirsch (Eds.), *Handbook of Clinical Hypnosis* (pp. 649–670). Washington, DC: American Psychological Association.

Morgan, W. (1996). Hypnosis in sport and exercise psychology. In J. L. Van Raalte & B. W. Brewer (Eds.), *Exploring Sport and Exercise Psychology* (pp. 107–130). Washington, DC: American Psychological Association.

Morgan, W., & Brown, D. (1983). Hypnosis. In W. H. Williams (Ed.), *Ergogenic Aids in Sport* (pp. 223–252). Champaign, IL: Human Kinetics.

Moss, A. (1952). Hypnodontics: Hypnosis in dentistry. Brooklyn, NY: Dental Items of Interest.

Naliboff, B., Munakata, J., Chang, L., & Mayer, E. (1998). Toward a biobehavioral model of visceral hypersensitivity in irritable bowel syndrome. *Journal of Psychosomatic Research,* 45, 6, 485–492.

Nanamoli, B., & Bodhi, B. (Trans.). (1995). Sutta 30 [The shorter discourse on the simile of the Heartwood], Sutta 77 [The greater discourse to Sakuludayin], Sutta 118 [Mindfulness of breathing]. In *The Middle Length Discourse of the Buddha: A New Translation of the Majjhima Nikaya.* Boston: Wisdom Publications.

Naruse, G. (1965). The hypnotic treatment of stage fright in champion athletes. *International Journal of Clinical and Experimental Hypnosis, 13,* 63–70.

Nash, M. (1992). Hypnosis, psychopathology, and psychological regression. In E. Fromm & M. Nash (Eds.), *Contemporary Hypnosis Research* (pp. 149–172). New York: Guilford.

Nash, M. (2000). The status of hypnosis as an empirically validated clinical intervention: A preamble to the special issue. *International Journal of Clinical and Experimental Hypnosis, 48*(2), 107–112.

Nash, M. (2001, July). The truth in the hype of hypnosis. *Scientific American,* 47–55.

Nash, M., Miton, A., & Baldridge, J. (1988). Twenty years of scientific hypnosis in dentistry, medicine, and psychology. *International Journal of Clinical and Experimental Hypnosis, 36,* 198–205.

National Institutes of Health. (1996). Technology assessment panel on integration of behavioral and relaxation approaches into the treatment of chronic pain and insomnia. *Journal of the American Medical Association, 276,* 313–318.

Nelson, M., & Denny, E. (1960). *The Nelson-Denny Reading Test: Vocabulary Comprehension Rate.* Ontario, Canada: Houghton-Mifflin.

Newman, M. (1971). Hypnotic handling of the chronic bleeder in extraction: A case report. *American Journal of Clinical Hypnosis, 14,* 126–127.

Newman, M. (1974). Hypnosis and hemophiliacs. *Journal of American Dental Association, 88,* 273.

Newton, B. (1982-1983). The use of hypnosis in the treatment of cancer patients. *American Journal of Clinical Hypnosis, 25,* 104–113.

Nideffer, R. (1981). *The Ethics and Practice of Applied Sport Psychology.* Ithaca, NY: Movement.

Nishith, P., Barabasz, A., Barabasz, M., & Warner, D. (1999). Brief hypnosis substitutes for alprazolam use in college students: Transient experiences and quantitative EEG responses. *American Journal of Clinical Hypnosis, 41*(3), 262–268.

Norris, A., & Huston, P. (1956). Raynaud's disease studied by hypnosis. *Diseases of the Nervous System, 17,* 163–165.

Olness, K., Culbert, T., & Uden, D. (1989). Self-regulation of salivary immunoglobulin A by children. *Pediatrics, 83,* 66–71.

Olness, K., & Kohen, D. (1996). *Hypnosis and Hypnotherapy with Children* (3rd ed.). New York: Guilford.

Orlick, T. (1980). *In the Pursuit of Excellence.* Ottawa: Coaching Association of Canada.

Orne, M. (1959). The nature of hypnosis: Artifact and essence. *Journal of Abnormal and Social Psychology, 58,* 277–299.

Orne, M. (1966). Hypnosis, motivation, and compliance. *American Journal of Psychiatry, 122,* 721–726.

Orne, M. (1974). Pain suppression by hypnosis and related phenomena. In J. J. Bonica (Ed.), *Advances in Neurology* (Vol. 4, pp. 563–572). New York: Raven Press.

Orne, M. (1979). On the simulating subject as a quasi-control group in hypnosis research: What, why, and how. In E. Fromm & R. E. Shor (Eds.), *Hypnosis: Developments in Research and New Perspectives* (2nd ed., pp. 519–566). New York: Aldine.

Orne, M., & McConkey, K. (1981). Toward convergent inquiry into self-hypnosis. *International Journal of Clinical and Experimental Hypnosis, 29,* 313–323.

Oster, M. (1994). Psychological preparation for labor and delivery using hypnosis. *American Journal of Clinical Hypnosis, 37*(1), 12–21.

Oster, M., & Sauer, C. (2001). Hypnosis for childbirth preparation. In L. M. Hornyak & J. Green (Eds.), *Healing from Within: Hypnosis in Women's Health Care.* Washington, DC: APA Books.

Page, R., & Handley, G. (1993). The use of hypnosis in cocaine addiction. *American Journal of Clinical Hypnosis, 36*(2), 120–123.

Palsson, O. (1998 & 2004). *Standardized Hypnosis Treatment Protocol for Irritable Bowel Syndrome.* Chapel Hill, North Carolina, self published.

Palsson, O., Tuner, M., & Johnson, D. (2002). Hypnosis treatment for severe irritable bowel syndrome: Investigation of mechanisms and effects on symptoms. *Digestive Disorders Science, 47,* 2605–2614.

Pates, J., Cummings, A., & Maynard, I. (2002). The effects of hypnosis on flow states and three-point shooting performance in basketball players. *Sport Psychologist, 16,* 34–47.

Pates, J., & Maynard, I. (2000). Effects of hypnosis on flow states and golf performance. *Perceptual and Motor Skills, 91*(3), 1057–1075.

Pates, J., Maynard, I., & Westbury, A. (2001). An investigation into the effects of hypnosis on basketball performance. *Journal of Applied Sport Psychology, 13,* 84–102.

Pates, J., Oliver, R., & Maynard, I. (2001). The effects of hypnosis on flow states and golf-putting performance. *Journal of Applied Sport Psychology, 13,* 341–354.

Patterson, D. (2001). Is hypnotic pain control effortless or effortful? *Hypnos, 28,* 132–134.

Patterson, D., Adcock, R., & Bombardier, C. (1997). Factors predicting hypnotic analgesia in clinical burn pain. *International Journal of Clinical and Experimental Hypnosis, 45,* 377–395.

Patterson, D., & Jensen, M. (2003). Hypnosis and clinical pain. *Psychological Bulletin, 129*(4), 495–521.

Patterson, D., & Ptacek, J. (1997). Baseline pain as a moderator of hypnotic analgesia for burn injury treatment. *Journal of Consulting and Clinical Psychology, 65,* 60–67.

Patterson, D., Questad, K., & Boltwood, M. (1987). Hypnotherapy as a treatment for pain in patients with burns: Research and clinical considerations. *Journal of Burn Care and Rehabilitation, 8,* 263–268.

Pearson, R. (1961). Response to suggestions given under general anesthesia. *American Journal of Clinical Hypnosis,* 4, 106–114.

Perry, C. (1992). Theorizing about hypnosis in either/or terms. *International Journal of Clinical and Experimental Hypnosis, 40*(4), 238–252.

Perry, C. (2004). Can anecdotes add to an understanding of hypnosis? *International Journal of Clinical and Experimental Hypnosis,* 3, 218–236.

Perry, C., & Laurence, J. R. (1980). Hypnotic depth and hypnotic susceptibility: A replicated finding. *International Journal of Clinical and Experimental Hypnosis, 28,* 272–280.

Perry, C., Nadon, R., & Button, J. (1992). The measurement of hypnotic ability. In E. Fromm & M. Nash (Eds.), *Contemporary Hypnosis Research* (pp. 459–490). New York: Guilford.

Piccione, C., Hilgard, E. & Zimbardo, P. (1989). On the degree of stability of measured hypnotizability over a 25-year period. *Journal of Personality and Social Psychology,* 56, 289–206.

Pratt, G., & Korn, E. (1986). Using hypnosis to enhance athletic performance. In B. Zilbergeld, M. G. Edelstein, & D. L. Araoz (Eds.), *Hypnosis: Questions and Answers* (pp. 204–231). New York: W. W. Norton.

Pressman, M. (1979). Psychological techniques for the advancement of sport potential. In P. Klavora & J. Daniel (Eds.), *Coach, Athlete and the Sport Psychologist* (pp. 133–143). Toronto, Canada: University of Toronto.

Prince, M. (1906). *Dissociation of Personality.* New York: Longman-Green.

Prussack, H. (2002, March). Patient with Torticollis. Video presented at the annual conference of the American Society for Clinical Hypnosis, Reno, Nevada.

Pulos, L. (1979). Athletes and self-hypnosis. In P. Klavora & J. V. Daniel (Eds.), *Coach, Athlete and the Sport Psychologist* (pp. 144–154). Toronto, Canada: University of Toronto.

Raginsky, B. (1963). Temporary cardiac arrest under hypnosis. In M. Kline (Ed.), *Clinical Correlations of Experimental Hypnosis* (pp. 434–455). Springfield, IL: Charles C. Thomas

Rainville, P., Carrier, B., Hofbauer, R., Bushnell, M., & Duncan, G. (1999). Dissociation of sensory and affective dimensions of pain using hypnotic modulation. *Pain, 82,* 159–171.

Rainville, P., Duncan, G., Price, D., Carrier, B., & Bushnell, M. (1997). Pain affect encoded in human anterior cingulate but somatosensory cortex. *Science, 277,* 968–971.

Rainville, P., Hofbauer, R., Paus, T., Duncan, G., Bushnell, M., & Price, D. (1999). Cerebral mechanisms of hypnotic induction and suggestion. *Journal of Cognitive Neuroscience, 11,* 110–125.

Rainville, P., & Price, D. (2003). Hypnosis phenomenology and neurobiology of consciousness. *International Journal of Clinical and Experimental Hypnosis, 51*(2), 105–129.

Rank, O. (1952). *The Trauma of Birth.* New York: Brunner.

Rather, N., Barabasz, M., & Barabasz, A. (1993, August 20-24). Effects of study skills training on the academic self-efficacy and performance of provisional college student. Paper presented at the 101st annual convention of the American Psychological Association, Toronto, Canada.

Rausch, V. (1980). Cholecystectomy with self-hypnosis. *American Journal of Clinical Hypnosis, 22,* 124–129.

Ray, W., & De Pascalis, V. (2003). Temporal aspects of hypnotic processes. *International Journal of Clinical and Experimental Hypnosis, 51*(2), 147–165.

Ray, W., & Tucker, D. (2003). Evolutionary approaches to understanding the hypnotic experience. *International Journal of Clinical and Experimental Hypnosis, 51*(3), 256–281.

Reich, W. (1945). *Character Analysis: Principles and Techniques for Psychoanalysts in Practice and in Training 2nd ed.,* Oxford, U.K., Orgone Institute Press.

Resnick, H., Kilpatrick, D., Dansky, B., Saunders, B., & Best, C. (1993). Prevalence of civilian trauma and PTSD in a representative national sample of women. *Journal of Consulting and Clinical Psychology, 61,* 984–991.

Reyher, J. (1964). Brain mechanisms, intrapsychic processes and behavior: A theory of hypnosis and psychopathology. *American Journal of Clinical Hypnosis,* 7, 107–119.

Reynolds, J. (1997). Post-traumatic stress disorder after childbirth: The phenomenon of traumatic birth. *Canadian Medical Journal, 156,* 831–835.

Rhue, J., & Lynn, S. (1989). Fantasy proneness, absorption, and hypnosis: A re-examination. *International Journal of Clinical and Experimental Hypnosis, 37,* 100–106.

Rhue, J., Lynn, S., Bukh, K., & Henry, S. (1991). Fantasy Proneness, Hypnotizability and Creativity. Unpublished manuscript, Ohio University.

Rhue, J., Lynn, S., & Kirsch, I. (1993). *Handbook of Clinical Hypnosis*. Washington, DC: American Psychological Association.

Rice, F. G. (1961). The hypnotic induction of labor: Six cases. *American Journal of Clinical Hypnosis, 4*, 119–122.

Rodolfa, E., Kraft, W., & Reilley, R. (1990). Etiology and treatment of dental anxiety and phobia. *American Journal of Clinical Hypnosis, 33*(1), 22–28.

Rosenberg, S. (1982–1983). Hypnosis in cancer care: Imagery to enhance the control of physiological and psychological "side-effects" of cancer therapy. *American Journal of Clinical Hypnosis, 25*, 122–127.

Russell, L. (2002). Hypnotic Intervention for Genital Human Papillomavirus Infections in Female Patients. Unpublished doctoral dissertation, Washington State University.

Russell, R. (1980). The effects of hypnosis and mastery imagery on task performance. *Dissertation Abstracts International, 41*, 2368.

Russell, L., & Barabasz, A. (2001, November 7–11). Papilloma virus (vaginal warts): Hypnotizability versus expectation. Presented at the 52nd annual scientific meeting of the Society for Clinical and Experimental Hypnosis, San Antonio, Texas.

Ruzyla-Smith, P., Barabasz, A., Barabasz, M., & Warner, D. W. (1995). Effects of hypnosis on the immune response: B-cells, T-cells, helper and suppressor cells. *American Journal of Clinical Hypnosis, 38*, 71–79.

Ryde, D. (1964). A personal study of some uses of hypnosis in sports and sports injuries. *Journal of Sports Medicine and Physical Fitness, 4*, 241–246.

Sacerdote, P. (1972). Theory and practice of pain control in malignancy and other protracted or recurring painful illnesses. *International Journal of Clinical and Experimental Hypnosis, 20*, 1–14.

Sacerdote, P. (1981). Teaching self-hypnosis to adults. *International Journal of Clinical and Experimental Hypnosis, 29*, 282–299.

Sanders S. (1977). Mutual group hypnosis and smoking. *American Journal of Clinical Hypnosis, 20*, 131–135.

Sarbin, T. (1950). Contributions to roll-taking theory: I. Hypnotic behavior. *Psychological Review, 57*, 255–270.

Sarbin, T. (2002, August). Suggestibility and Hypnosis. Invited address presented at the 110th Annual Convention of the American Psychological Association, Chicago.

Sarbin, T. (2004). Unresolved Issues in Hypnosis. Presented at the 112th Annual Convention of the American Psychological Association, Honolulu, July 28–August 1.

Sarbin, T., & Coe, W. (1972). *Hypnosis: A Social Psychological Analysis of Influence Communication*. New York: Holt, Rinehart and Winston.

Schaper, A. M., Rooney, B. L., Kay, N. R., & Silva, P. D. (1994). Use of the Edinburgh Postnatal Major Depressive Disorder Scale to identify postpartum major depressive disorder in a clinical setting. *Journal of Reproductive Medicine, 39*(8), 620–624.

Scheibe, K., Gray, F., & Keim, J. (1968). Hypnotically induced deafness and delayed auditory feedback: A comparison of real and simulating subjects. *International Journal of Clinical and Experimental Hypnosis, 16*, 158–164.

Schreiber, E. (1991). Using hypnosis to improve performance of college basketball players. *Perceptual and Motor Skills, 72*, 536–538.

Schreiber, F. (1974). *Sybil*. New York: Warner.

Schultz-Stubner, S. (1996). Hypnosis: A side effect-free alternative to medical sedation in regional anesthesia. *Anaesthetist, 45*(10), 956–969.

Schwarzkopf, N. (with Petre, P.). (1992). *The Autobiography: It Doesn't Take a Hero*. New York: Bantam.

Scott, M. (1960). *Hypnosis in Skin and Allergic Diseases*. Springfield, IL: Charles C. Thomas.

Secter, I. I. (1960). Some notes on controlling the exaggerated gag reflex. *American Journal of Clinical Hypnosis, 2*, 149–153.

Secter, I. I. (1961). Tongue thrust and nail biting simultaneously treated during hypnosis. *American Journal of Clinical Hypnosis, 6*, 51–53.

Secter, I. I. (1973). Swallowing difficulties. In *A Syllabus on Hypnosis and a Handbook of Therapeutic Suggestions* (p. 116). Des Plaines, IL: American Society of Clinical Hypnosis.

Shapiro, A., & Moris, L. (1978). Placebo effect in medical and psychological therapies. In A Bergin & S. Garfield (Eds.), *Handbook of Psychotherapy and Behavior Change: An Empirical Analysis*. New York: John Wiley.

Shear, J., & Jevning, R. (1999). Pure consciousness: Scientific exploration of meditation techniques. *Journal of Consciousness Studies, Special Issue: The View from Within: First-Person Approaches to the Study of Consciousness*, 6(2-3), pp. 189–209. Abstract retrieved from http://www.imprint.co.uk/jcs_6_2-3.html.

Sheehan, P. (1977). Incongruity in trance behavior: A defining property of hypnosis? In W. E. Edmonston, Jr. (Ed.), *Conceptual and Investigative Approaches to Hypnosis and Hypnotic Phenomena* (Vol. 296). New York: New York Academy of Sciences.

Sherman, S. (1971). Very Deep Hypnosis: An Experiential and Electroencephalographic Investigation. Unpublished doctoral dissertation, Stanford University.

Shephard, B. (2001). *A War of Nerves: Soldiers and Psychiatrists in the Twentieth Century*. Cambridge, MA: Harvard University Press.

Shor, R. (1969). Hypnosis and the concept of the generalized reality-orientation. In C. E. Tart (Ed.), *Altered States of Consciousness: A Book of Readings* (pp. 233–250). New York: Wiley. (Original work published 1959)

Shor, R. (1978). *Inventory of Self-Hypnosis, Form A*. Palo Alto, CA: Consulting Psychologists Press.

Shor, R. (1979). A phenomenological method for the measurement of variables important to an understanding of the nature of hypnosis. In E. Fromm & R. E. Shor (Eds.), *Hypnosis: Developments in Research and New Perspectives* (2nd ed., pp. 105–135). New York: Aldine.

Shor, R., & Orne, E. (1962). *The Harvard Group Scale of Hypnotic Susceptibility, Form A*. Palo Alto, CA: Consulting Psychologists Press.

Simmel, E. (1944). War neuroses. In S. Lorand (Ed.), *Psychoanalysis Today* (pp. 227–248). New York: International Universities Press.

Simon, E., & Lewis, D. (2000). Medical hypnosis for temporomandibular disorders: Treatment efficacy and medical utilization outcome. *Oral Surgery, Oral Medicine, Oral Pathology and Oral Radiology*, 90(1), 54–63.

Sinclair-Geben, A., & Chalmers, D. (1959). Treatment of warts by hypnosis. *Lancet*, II. 480–482.

Smith, G., McKenzie, J., Marmer, D., & Steele, R. (1985). Psychologic modulation of the human immune response to varicella zoster. *Archives of Internal Medicine*, 145, 2110–2112.

Smith, J., Barabasz, A., & Barabasz, M. (1996). A comparison of hypnosis and distraction in severely ill children undergoing painful medical procedures. *Journal of Counseling Psychology*, 43(2), 187–195.

Smith, P., Barabasz, A., Barabasz, M., & Warner, D. (1995). The effects of hypnosis on the immune response: B cells, T cells, helper and suppressor cells. *American Journal of Clinical Hypnosis*, 38(2), 71–79.

Smith, S., & Balaban, A. (1983). A multidimensional approach to pain relief: Case report of a patient with systemic lupus erythematosus. *International Journal of Clinical and Experimental Hypnosis*, 31, 72–81.

Spanos, N. (1982). A social psychological approach to hypnotic behavior. In G. Weary & H. L. Mirels (Eds.), *Integrations of Clinical and Social Psychology* (pp. 231–271). New York: Oxford University Press.

Spanos, N. (1986). Hypnotic behavior: A social psychological interpretation of amnesia, analgesia and trance logic. *Behavioral and Brain Sciences*, 9, 449–467.

Spanos, N., & Barber, T. (1974). Toward a convergence in hypnosis research. *American Psychologist*, 29, 500–511.

Spanos, N., & Chaves, J. (1989). The cognitive-behavioral alternative in hypnosis research. In N. P. Spanos & J. F. Chaves (Eds.), *Hypnosis: The Cognitive-Behavioral Perspective* (pp. 9–16). Buffalo, NY: Prometheus Books.

Spanos, N., & Coe, W. (1992). A socio-psychological approach to hypnosis. In E. Fromm & M. Nash (Eds.), *Contemporary Hypnosis Research* (pp. 102–129). New York: Guilford.

Spanos, N., Gwynn, M., Dellamalva, C., & Bertrand, L. (1988). Social psychological factors in the genesis of posthypnotic source amnesia. *Journal of Abnormal Psychology*, 88, 527–546.

Spanos, N., Perlini, A., & Robertson, L. (1989). Hypnosis, suggestion, and placebo in the reduction of experimental pain. *Journal of Abnormal Psychology*, 98, 285–293.

Spanos, N., Radtke, H., Hodgins, D., Stam, H., & Bertrand, L. (1983). The Carleton University Responsiveness to Suggestion Scale: Normative data and psychometric properties. *Psychological Reports, 53*, 523–535.

Spanos, N., Salas, J., Menary, E., & Brett, P. (1986). Comparison of overt and subjective responses to the Carleton University Responsiveness to Suggestion Scale and the Stanford Hypnotic Susceptibility Scale under conditions of group administration. *Psychological Reports, 58*, 847–856.

Spiegel, D. (1991a). Neurophysiological correlates of hypnosis and dissociation. *Journal of Neuropsychiatry and Clinical Neuroscience, 3*, 440–445.

Spiegel, D. (1991b). Uses of hypnosis in managing medical symptoms. *Psychiatric Medicine, 9*(4) 521–533.

Spiegel, D. (1997). Imagery and hypnosis in the treatment of cancer patients. *Oncology* 1179–1195.

Spiegel, D. (2003). Negative and positive visual hypnotic hallucinations: Attending inside and out. *International Journal of Clinical and Experimental Hypnosis, 51*(2), 130–146.

Spiegel, D., & Barabasz, A. (1987). Psychophysiology of hypnotic hallucinations. In R. G. Kunzendorf & A. A. Sheikh (Eds.), *Psychophysiology of mental imagery: Theory, research, and application* (pp. 133–145). New York: Baywood.

Spiegel, D., & Barabasz, A. (1988). Effects of hypnotic hallucination on P300 evoked potential amplitudes: A reconciling conflicting findings. *American Journal of Clinical Hypnosis, 31*, 11–17.

Spiegel, D., & Barabasz, A. (1990). In R. G. Kunzendorf & A. A. Sheikth (Eds.), *Psychophysiology of Hypnotic Hallucinations, Psychophysiology of Mental Imagery: Theory, Research, and Application* (pp. 133–146). Boston: Baywood.

Spiegel, D., Bierre, P., & Rootenberg, J. (1989). Hypnotic alteration of somatosensory perception. *American Journal of Psychiatry, 146*, 749–754.

Spiegel, D., & Bloom, J. (1983). Group therapy and hypnosis reduce metastatic breast carcinoma pain. *Psychosomatic Medicine*, 333–339.

Spiegel, D., Bloom, J., Kraemer, H., & Gottheil, E. (1989). Effect of psychosocial treatment on survival of patients with metastatic breast cancer. *Lancet, 2*, 888–891.

Spiegel, D., Cutcomb, S., Ren, C., & Pribram, K. (1985). Hypnotic hallucinations alter evoked potentials. *Journal of Abnormal Psychology, 94*, 249–255.

Spiegel, H. (1970). A single-treatment method to stop smoking using ancillary self-hypnosis. *International Journal of Clinical and Experimental Hypnosis.*

Spiegel, H. (1998). Defining hypnosis: Controlled imagination. In R. Hebert (Ed.), *Minding the Body: The Science of Hypnosis*. Washington, DC: Center for Advancement of Health.

Spiegel, H., & Bridger, A. (1970). *Manual for Hypnotic Induction Profile: Eye-roll Levitation Method*. New York: Soni Medica.

Spiegel, H., & Spiegel, D. (1978-1987). *Trance and Treatment: Clinical Uses of Hypnosis*. New York: Basic Books; Washington, DC: American Psychiatric Press.

Spiegel, H., & Spiegel, D. (2004). *Trance and Treatment: Clinical Uses of Hypnosis* (2nd ed.). Arlington, VA: American Psychiatric Publishing.

Spinhoven, P. (1988). Similarities and dissimilarities in hypnotic and nonhypnotic procedures for headache control: A review. *American Journal of Clinical Hypnosis, 30*, 183–194.

Spinhoven, P., Linssen, A. C., Van Dyck, R., & Zitman, F. G. (1992). Autogenic training and self-hypnosis in the control of tension headache. *General Hospital Psychiatry, 14*, 408–415.

Stanton, H. (1993). Using hypnotherapy to overcome examination anxiety. *American Journal of Clinical Hypnosis, 35*(3), 198–204.

Stanton, H. (1994). Self-hypnosis: One path to reduce test anxiety. *Contemporary Hypnosis, 11*, 14–18.

Sterman, B. (2000). EEG markers for attention deficit disorder: Pharmacological and neurofeedback applications. *Child Study Journal, 30*, 1–24.

Stolzenberg, J. (1955). Clinical applications of hypnosis in producing hypno-anesthesia control of hemorrhage and salivation during surgery: A case report. *Journal Clinical and Experimental Hypnosis, 3*, 24–27.

Strasberg, I. (1960). Control of gagging by light hypnosis. *American Journal of Clinical Hypnosis, 2*, 148–149.

Stunkard, A. (1972). Foreword. In R. B. Stuart & B. Davis (Eds.), *Slim Chance in a Fat World: Behavioral Control of Obesity*. Champagne, IL: Research Press.

Suinn, R. (1980). *Psychology in Sports: Methods and Applications*. Minneapolis, MN: Burgess.

Sutcher, H. (1997). Hypnosis as adjunctive therapy for multiple sclerosis: A progress report. *American Journal of Clinical Hypnosis, 39*, 283–290.

Sutcliffe, J. (1961). "Credulous" and "skeptical" views of hypnotic phenomena: Experiments on aesthesia, hallucination, and delusion. *Journal of Abnormal and Social Psychology, 62*, 189–200.

Sutcliffe, J. (1965). "Credulous" and "skeptical" views of hypnotic phenomena: A review of certain evidence and methodology. In R. E. Shor & M. T. Orne (Eds.), *The Nature of Hypnosis: Selected Basic Readings* (pp. 124–152). New York: Holt.

Szechtman, H., Woody, E., Bowers, K., & Nahmias, C. (1998). Where the imaginal appears real: A positron emission tomography study of auditory hallucinations. *Proceedings of the National Academy of Sciences of the United States of America, 95*, 1956–1960.

Tart, C. (1963). Hypnotic depth and basal skin resistance. *International Journal of Clinical and Experimental Hypnosis, 11*, 81–92.

Tart, C. (1969). *Altered States of Consciousness*. New York: Wiley.

Tart, C. (1972). Measuring the depth of an altered state of consciousness, with particular reference to self report scales of hypnotic depth. In E. Fromm & R. Shor (Eds.), *Hypnosis: Research Developments and Perspectives* (pp. 445–447). Chicago: Aldine.

Tasini, M., & Hackett, T. (1977). Hypnosis in the treatment of a child with warts. *American Journal of Clinical Hypnosis, 15*, 12–14.

Taylor, J., & Gerson, A. (1992). *A conceptual model of the effects of imagery administration on cognitive/affective and behavioral change*. Unpublished manuscript.

Taylor, J., Horevitz, R., & Balague, G. (1993). The use of hypnosis in applied sport psychology. *Sport Psychologist, 7*, 58–78.

Tellegen, A. (1981). Practicing the two disciplines for relaxation and enlightenment: Comment on "Role of the feedback signal in electromyograph biofeedback: The relevance of attention" by Qualls and Sheehan. *Journal of Experimental Psychology: General, 110*, 217–226.

Tellegen, A., & Atkinson, G. (1974). Openness to absorbing and self-altering experiences ("absorption"), a trait related to hypnotic susceptibility. *Journal of Abnormal Psychology, 33*, 142–148.

Troffer, F. (1965). *Hypnotic age regression and cognitive function*. Unpublished doctoral dissertation, Stanford University.

Trustman, R. B., Dubovsky, S., & Titley, R. (1977). Auditory perception during general anesthesia—Myth or fact? *International Journal of Clinical and Experimental Hypnosis, 25*, 88–105.

Ulett, A., Akpinar, S., Itil, T., & Fakuda, T. (1971). The neurophysiological basis of hypnosis-objective techniques. *Folia Psychiatrica Et Neurilogica Japonica, 25*(3), 203–211.

Unestahl, L. (1979). Hypnotic preparation of athletes. In G. D. Burrows, D. R. Collison, & L. Dennerstein (Eds.), *Hypnosis 1979* (pp. 47–61). Amsterdam: Elsevier/North Holland Biomedical Press.

Unestahl, L. (1981). *New paths of sport learning excellence* [Monograph]. Orebro, Sweden: Orebro University, Department of Sport Psychology.

Unestahl, L. (1983). *Inner mental training: A systematic self-instructional program for self-hypnosis*. Orebro, Sweden: Veje.

Unestahl, L. (1986). The ideal performance. In L.-E. Unestahl (Ed.), *Sport psychology in theory and practice* (pp. 21–38). Orebro, Sweden: Veje.

U.S. Department of Health and Human Services. (1990). *The health benefits of smoking cessation: A report of the surgeon general* (DHHS Publication No. CDC 90–8416). Washington, DC: U.S. Government Printing Office.

Van Pelt, S. J. (1949). Hypnotherapy in medical practice. *British Journal of Medical Hypnotism, 1*, 8–13.

Venkatesh, S., Raju, T. R., Shivani, Y., Tompkins, G., & Meti, B. L. (1997). A study of structure of phenomenology of consciousness in meditative and nonmeditative states. *Indian Journal of Physiology and Pharmacology, 41*, 149–153.

Vermetten, E. (2004). *Brain imagery and recall of traumatic events*. Manuscript in preparation.

Vogt, O. (1896). Zur Kenntnis des Wesens und der psychologischen Bedeutung des Hypnotismus *Zeitschrift fur Hypnotismus, 4*, 122–129.

Wagaman, J., Barabasz, A., & Barabasz, M. (1991). Flotation rest and imagery in the improvement of collegiate basketball performance. *Perceptual and Motor Skills, 72*, 119–122.

Wagstaff, G. (1981). *Hypnosis, Compliance and Belief*. New York: St. Martin's.

Wain, H. (1980). Pain control through the use of hypnosis. *American Journal of Clinical Hypnosis, 23*, 41–46.

Wald, A., & Kline, M. (1955). A university program in dental hypnosis. *Journal of Clinical and Experimental Hypnosis, 3*, 183–187.

Wall, V., & Womack, W. (1989). Hypnotic versus active cognitive strategies for alleviation of procedural distress in pediatric oncology patients. *American Journal of Clinical Hypnosis, 31*(3), 181–189.

Wallace, B. (1999). The Buddhist tradition of samatha: Methods for refining and examining consciousness. *Journal of Consciousness Studies, 6*, 175–187.

Wark, D. (1996). Teaching college students better learning skills using self-hypnosis. *American Journal of Clinical Hypnosis 38*(4), 277–287.

Warner, D., Barabasz, A., & Barabasz, M. (2000). The efficacy of Barabasz' alert hypnosis and neurotherapy on attentiveness, impulsivity, and hyperactivity in children with ADHD. *Child Study Journal, 30*(1), 43–49.

Watkins, H. (1976). Hypnosis and smoking: A five-session approach. *International Journal of Clinical and Experimental Hypnosis, 24*, 381–390.

Watkins, J. (1949). *Hypnotherapy of War Neuroses*. New York: Ronald.

Watkins, J. (1954). Trance and transference. *Journal of Clinical and Experimental Hypnosis, 2*, 284–290.

Watkins, J. (1963). Transference aspects of the hypnotic relationship. In M. V. Kline (Ed.), *Clinical Correlations of Experimental Hypnosis* (pp. 5–24). Springfield, IL: Charles C. Thomas.

Watkins, J. (1966). Symposium on posthypnotic amnesia: Discussion. *International Journal of Clinical and Experimental Hypnosis, 14*, 139–149.

Watkins, J. (1967). *Hypnosis and Consciousness from the View Point of Existentialism*. Springfield, IL: Charles C. Thomas.

Watkins, J. (1971). The affect bridge: A hypnoanalytic technique. *International Journal of Clinical and Experimental Hypnosis, 19*, 21–27.

Watkins, J. (1978). *The Therapeutic Self*. New York: Human Sciences Press.

Watkins, J. (1987). *Hypnotherapeutic Techniques*. New York: Irvington.

Watkins, J. (1992). *Hypnotherapeutic Techniques*. New York: Irvington.

Watkins, J. (1992a). *Hypnoanalytic Techniques: Clinical Hypnosis* (Vol. 2). New York: Irvington.

Watkins, J. (1992b). Psychoanalyse, hypnoanalyse, ego-state therapie: Auf der Suche nach einer effektiven Therapy. *Hypnose und Kognition, Bend, 9*, 85–97. (Translated from the English by Monica Amler)

Watkins, J. (2001). *Adventures in Human Understanding: Stories for Exploring the Self*. Wales, UK: Crown House.

Watkins, J., & Johnson, R. (1982). *We, the Divided Self*. New York: Irvington.

Watkins, J., & Watkins, H. (1979-1980). Ego states and hidden observers. *Journal of Altered States of Consciousness, 5*, 3–18.

Watkins, J., & Watkins, H. (1981). Ego state therapy. In R. J. Corsini (Ed.), *Handbook of Innovative Psychotherapies* (pp. 252–270). New York: Wiley.

Watkins, J., & Watkins, H. (1982). Ego-state therapy. In L. E. Abt & I. N. Stuart (Eds.), *The New Therapies: A Source Book* (pp. 95–121). New York: Van Nostrand Reinhold.

Watkins, J., & Watkins, H. (1990). Dissociation and displacement: Where goes the "ouch"? *American Journal of Clinical Hypnosis, 33*(1), 1–10.

Watkins, J., & Watkins, H. (1997). *Ego states: Theory and Therapy*. New York: W. W. Norton.

Watts, A. (1957). *A Way of Zen*. New York: Pantheon.

Weinberg, R., & Gould, D. (1995). *Foundations of Sport and Exercise Psychology*. Champaign, IL: Human Kinetics.

Weinberg, R., & Gould, D. (2003). *Foundations of Sport and Exercise Psychology* (3rd ed.). Champaign, IL: Human Kinetics.

Weinberg, R., Seabourne, T., & Jackson, A. (1981). Effects of visuo-motor behavioral rehearsal, relaxation, and imagery on karate performance. *Journal of Sport Psychology, 3*, 228–238

Weitzenhoffer, A. (1953). *Hypnotism: An Objective Study of Suggestibility*. New York: Wiley.

Weitzenhoffer, A., & Hilgard, E. (1959). *Stanford Hypnotic Susceptibility Scale: Forms A and B*. Palo Alto, CA: Consulting Psychologists Press.

Weitzenhoffer, A., & Hilgard, E. (1962). *Stanford Hypnotic Susceptibility Scale: Form C.* Palo Alto, CA: Consulting Psychologists Press.

Whorwell, P., Prior, A., & Colgan, S. (1987). Hypnotherapy in severe irritable bowel syndrome: Further experience. *Gut, 28,* 2(8414), 423–425.

Whorwell, P., Prior, A., & Faragher, E. (1984). Controlled trial of hyponotherapy in the treatment of severe refractory irritable bowel syndrome. *Lancet,* 1232–1234.

Wilson, G. (1978). *The Secrets of Sexual Fantasy.* London: Dent.

Williams, G. (1968). Hypnosis in perspective. In L. M. LeCron (Ed.), *Experimental Hypnosis* (pp. 4–21). New York: Citadel.

Williams, J., & Harris, D. (1998). Relaxation and energizing techniques for regulation of arousal. In J. M. Williams (Ed.), *Applied Sport Psychology: Personal Growth to Peak Performance* (3rd ed.). Mountain View, CA: Mayfield.

Williamson, J., McColl, R., Mathews, D., Mitchell, J., Raven, P., & Morgan, W. (2002). Brain activation by central command during actual and imagined handgrip under hypnosis. *Journal of Applied Physiology, 92,* 1317–1324.

Wilson, G. (1978). *The Secrets of Sexual Fantasy.* London: Dent.

Wilson, K. (2000). Performance hypnosis: A key to the zone. Retrieved December from http://AmericasDoctor.com/library_main.cf.

Wolf, M. (1978). Social validity: The case for subjective measurement or how applied behavioral analysis is finding its heart. *Journal of Applied Behavioral Analysis, 11,* 203–214.

Wolfe, L. S. (1961). Hypnosis in anesthesiology. In L. M. LeCron (Ed.), *Techniques of Hypnotherapy* (pp. 188–212). New York: Julian Press.

Wolfe, L. S., & Millet, J. B. (1960). Control of post-operative pain by suggestion under general anesthesia. *American Journal of Clinical Hypnosis, 3,* 109–112.

Wolpe, J., & Lazarus, A. (1966). *Behavior Therapy Techniques.* Oxford, UK: Pergamon.

Woody, E., & McConkey, K. (2003). What we don't know about the brain and hypnosis, but need to: A view from the Buckhorn Inn. *International Journal of Clinical and Experimental Hypnosis, 51*(3), 282–308.

Wookey, E. E. (1938). Uses and limitations of hypnosis in dental treatment. *British Dental Journal,* 65.

Wright, E. (1966). Symposium on posthypnotic amnesia: Discussion. *International Journal of Clinical and Experimental Hypnosis, 14,* 135–138.

Yapko, M. D. (1992). *Hypnosis and the Treatment of Depressions: Strategies for Change.* New York: Brunner.

Yapko, M. D. (1997). *Breaking the Patterns of Depression.* New York: Doubleday.

Zachariae, R., & Bjerring, P. (1993). Increase and decrease of delayed cutaneous reactions obtained by hypnotic suggestions during sensitization. *Allergy,* 48(1),1–6.

Zamansky, H. S., Scharf, B., & Brightbill, R. (1964). The effect of expectancy for hypnosis on pre-hypnotic performance. *Journal of Personality, 32,* 236–248.

Zarren, J., & Eimer, B. (2001). *Brief Cognitive Hypnosis: Facilitating the Change of Dysfunctional Behavior.* New York: Springer.

Zeig, J. K. (1982). *Ericksonian Approaches to Hypnosis and Psychotherapy.* New York: Brunner/Mazel.

Zeltzer, L., Dolgin, M., LeBaron, S., & LeBaron, C. (1991). A randomized, controlled study of behavioral intervention for chemotherapy distress in children with cancer. *Pediatrics, 88,* 34–42.

Zeltzer, L., Fanurik, D., & LeBaron, S. (1989). The cold pressor paradigm in children: Feasibility of an intervention model: II. *Pain, 37,* 305–313.

Zeltzer, L., & LeBaron, S. (1982). Hypnosis and the nonhypnotic techniques for reduction of pain and anxiety during painful procedures in children and adolescents with cancer. *Journal of Pediatrics, 101,* 1032–1035.

Zeltzer, L., & LeBaron, S. (1984). *The Stanford Hypnotic Clinical Scale for Children–Revised.* Unpublished manuscript.

Zeltzer, L., LeBaron, S., & Zeltzer, P. (1984). The effectiveness of behavioral intervention for reduction of nausea and vomiting in children and adolescents receiving chemotherapy. *Journal of Clinical Oncology, 2,* 683–690.

Zimbardo, P., Marshall, G., & Maslachg, V. (1971). Liberating behavior from time-bound control: Expanding the present through hypnosis. *Journal of Applied Social Psychology, 1,* 305–323.

Index

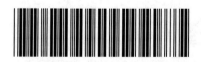